An Early Start for Your Child with Autism

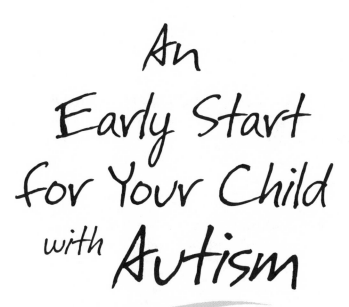

An
Early Start
for Your Child
with Autism

Using **Everyday Activities**
to Help Kids Connect,
Communicate,
and Learn

Sally J. Rogers, PhD
Geraldine Dawson, PhD
Laurie A. Vismara, PhD

THE GUILFORD PRESS
New York   London

*To all parents of children and adults with autism, for their courage,
their hope, their generosity, and their perseverance*
—S. J. R.

*To my loving husband, Joseph, and my wonderful children,
Chris and Maggie, who have supported my work with patience,
understanding, and a shared commitment to improving the lives
of people with autism*
—G. D.

*To my father, for his commitment to improving the lives
of individuals with autism, and to all the courageous individuals
and their families who are overcoming the challenges of autism*
—L. A. V.

© 2012 The Guilford Press
A Division of Guilford Publications, Inc.
370 Seventh Avenue, Suite 1200, New York, NY 10001
www.guilford.com

The information in this volume is not intended as a substitute for consultation with
healthcare professionals. Each individual's health concerns should be evaluated by a
qualified professional.

Printed in the United States of America

This book is printed on acid-free paper.

Last digit is print number: 9   8   7

Library of Congress Cataloging-in-Publication Data

Rogers, Sally J.
   An early start for your child with autism : using everyday activities to help kids connect,
   communicate, and learn / Sally J. Rogers, Geraldine Dawson, and Laurie A. Vismara.
       p. cm.
   Includes bibliographical references and index.
   ISBN 978-1-60918-470-4 (pbk. : alk. paper)
   ISBN 978-1-4625-0389-6 (hardcover : alk. paper)
   1. Autism in children—Treatment—Popular works. 2. Children with disabilities—Means
of communication. I. Dawson, Geraldine. II. Vismara, Laurie A. III. Title.
RJ506.A9R642 2012
618.92′85882—dc23
                                                            2012015186

Contents

Authors' Note

To protect the identities of the families with whom we have worked, all the stories about families and the examples in this book are composites of real people created to reflect common challenges and successes that we have witnessed many times. The comments from parents scattered throughout the book have been reprinted in their own words with their permission, but their names have been omitted to protect their privacy. We are grateful for their candor and support.

A word about our use of pronouns in this book may also be helpful. In most of the text, we alternate between "he" and "she" to refer to your child with autism. However, in items for your personal use (such as forms, boxes, Activity Checklists, and tables), as well as in the Part II Chapter Summaries and in Chapter 14, we use "he or she."

Acknowledgments

We want to begin by expressing our deep appreciation for the support we have received from Rochelle Serwator, Chris Benton, and Kitty Moore at The Guilford Press, for motivating and encouraging us, believing in the value of this book, and helping us produce a better one than we would have thought possible. We also want to share our individual acknowledgments.

From Sally:

My preparation for writing this book began with the very first parents and toddlers with whom I worked in Ann Arbor, Michigan. My experiences with children like Laura Ann and Peter, as well as their parents, taught me so much about the first few years of a family's life when a child has developmental disabilities. I appreciate what I learned from them about supporting their relationships, their interactional styles, and their child-raising and family values as they provided interventions for their children. I am extremely grateful to the families in Denver with whom my colleagues and I worked. They are the families from whom I learned not only about early autism and its effects on families, but also about the resilience, hope, and determination of parents to seek out what is best for their children—who persist, across years and decades, to improve the quality of their children's day-to-day lives and prepare themselves and their children for the future. I appreciate all that I learned from my Denver colleagues in the Developmental Psychobiology Research Group about parent–child relationships and measurement approaches, and I appreciate their challenges to me (especially those of Bob Emde and Gordon Farley) to move from clinical services to well-controlled studies of early intervention.

I particularly appreciate what I have learned in the collaborations with my two coauthors, who are also friends and colleagues. Geri's work allowed for tremendous growth in the definition and rigor of the intervention approach, and she has been a tireless, enthusiastic, and optimistic partner in our shared work with the Early Start Denver Model (ESDM). Laurie and I together worked out much of the methodology for the ESDM parent training package, which she first studied and published in her postdoctoral research program. The three of us share both belief and experience in the power of parent-delivered interventions embedded in daily routines to teach young children with autism language, play, and social engagement, and these beliefs and experiences were linchpins for developing our research programs in parent interventions and for writing this book.

I also want to thank my two daughters, Sara and Amy, for giving me my only direct experience in parenting toddlers, and for embracing my autism work throughout their lives. My assistant, Diane Larzelere, provided talented and speedy help for manuscript development, and constant cheerful encouragement.

From Geri:

I want to begin by thanking the many parents and children with whom I have had the privilege of working over the past 25 years. They are my true heroes and best teachers. Nothing is as rewarding as sharing the excitement of a new ability being achieved. It has been my delight to watch parents interacting with their young children with autism, drawing them into closer interactions, and helping them learn to communicate and play. It was my privilege to provide suggestions and advice from the perspective of a seasoned clinician and developmental psychologist and then to witness the unfolding of each child's skills over time. Throughout the process of therapy, the persistence, humor, insight, and unconditional love that family members show have been my inspiration.

Early on, my perspectives on autism were shaped by Eric Schopler, Michael Rutter, and Marian Sigman. At a time when other professionals were blaming parents for autism, Eric, a pioneer, showed us that parents are our most important partners, ideally positioned to help their child with autism. Michael's insights about the interface between the social and thinking brain ring truer today than ever and are consistent with the ESDM. Marian's landmark studies described the development of autism in exquisite detail, providing a roadmap for creating developmentally informed treatments.

I gratefully acknowledge my graduate students and colleagues at the University of Washington for their openness to new ideas and willingness to pursue them, and for their humor and passion for improving the lives of children with autism and their families. I especially want to acknowledge the hard work of the UW team in completing the randomized clinical trial of the ESDM, which helped lay the foundation for the work discussed in this book.

Finally, I wish to thank my husband, Joe, and my children, Chris and Maggie, whose constant love and support made this book and my life's work possible.

From Laurie:

I did not intentionally set out to become an autism researcher or clinician. Rather, autism chose me—my half-brother was diagnosed at a very young age. At the time,

I did not fully comprehend what it meant for him to have autism or the minute-by-minute challenges that he and so many other individuals with autism would come to face. What I did come to grasp was the amount of pain my father and stepmother experienced in coping with his diagnosis, coupled with the unconditional love and desire to protect and help him in whatever way humanly possible. Their commitment and dedication to creating an enriched and dignified life for my brother has been my daily inspiration for helping other parents do the same for their children with autism. This book represents the unselfish willingness of parents to share the trials and triumphs through which they have helped their children with autism learn, as well as to help others understand what living with autism is like.

I would also like to acknowledge the incredible mentoring of Drs. Robert and Lynn Koegel and Sally Rogers. The Koegels taught me the value of embracing parents as equal, collaborative partners in helping their children overcome daily challenges. It was because of the Koegels' teaching that my own brother found his voice, and for this accomplishment I will always be indebted to them. When I came to work with Sally, she expanded my thinking and approach to interacting with families. She helped me listen better to families' needs, understanding their emotions and struggles with the everyday demands that their children face. I admire her and Geri Dawson's lifelong dedication to finding answers, through science, to improve the quality of life for individuals with disabilities and their families. I am honored to be a part of this book with them and hope to follow their example of using science to better individuals' lives. Lastly, thank you to my parents and friends for their unending love and tolerance for my work schedule. They have always understood my passion and at times compulsion to pursue a career in research and academics, and I am grateful for their encouragement and patience.

Introduction

If you are a parent of a child recently diagnosed with autism, you are not alone. A 2009 study by the U.S. Centers for Disease Control and Prevention in Atlanta, Georgia, found that autism spectrum disorders (ASD) affect 1 in 110 children in the United States, meaning that hundreds of thousands of parents have learned that their child has an ASD. This year, more children will be diagnosed with ASD than with cystic fibrosis, AIDS, and cancer combined. Children from all economic and racial backgrounds are affected equally. You are not alone in the chaos of feelings, questions, and concerns that you have now. Please be assured, however, that, equipped with solid knowledge and skills, parents of a child newly diagnosed with ASD can put the pieces in place to have satisfying and happy lives. Children with ASD can lead meaningful, productive, and fulfilling lives. This book will help you take action right now that will put you and your child on the road to that kind of life.

The goal of this book is to provide parents[1] like you, and the other people who love and care for your child, with tools and strategies to help your child move onto a positive developmental path as soon as possible. No matter how difficult life may seem right now, there are things you can do starting tomorrow that will, over time, make a tremendous difference in your child's future. You can teach your child to interact with you and others, communicate, enjoy social exchanges, and play. You can be hopeful that your child can learn, engage, and relate to others.

We know that many parents are left to fend for themselves for quite a while after their child has received a diagnosis of ASD. Either trained therapists are not available in their area, or there are long waiting lists to get into intervention programs. We know you are eager to begin helping your child. So to ease your frustration and worry while you wait for intervention to start, or to enhance the

---

[1]Although we generally use the term "parents," this book is designed more broadly for all types of caregivers, including extended family members, legal guardians, and others who provide care for a young child with ASD.

intervention your child may be receiving now, in this book we offer information, tools, and strategies that you can use immediately, on your own. The strategies described here are designed to be used during your everyday interactions with your child—playing, changing, dressing, bathing, meals, outings, book time, and even household chores. They can transform your day-to-day experiences with your child into enriched learning opportunities, and they can also give your child's treatment a boost as you continue to use them once intervention begins.

With these strategies in hand, we are confident that you will help your child learn, communicate, and play. You will likely see changes in your child day by day, week by week. As you begin to use these strategies, you will see how effectively you can help your child with ASD and how responsive your child can be to new learning opportunities. We hope that some of your feelings of fear and frustration will be replaced with a sense of hope, determination, and confidence in yourself as a parent, in your family, and in your child.

This book is based on our extensive and ongoing work with families like yours, using the Early Start Denver Model to help children become active, curious, and engaged learners in the world. The strategies you'll learn come from formal scientific studies that show children's accelerated development when the Early Start Denver Model is delivered combined with parents' use of these skills. Although children with ASD benefit from and need intensive early intervention services from trained professionals, we believe that parents and other family caregivers can make an enormous difference in their child's learning.

We three authors of this book have all worked for many years directly as clinicians teaching families how to promote engagement, learning, and communication during the daily routines that naturally occur with children. We have found that parents are as effective as therapists in teaching core skills affected by autism. They can use these strategies to make every interaction with their child count toward learning. Parents also have the opportunity to teach skills or behaviors at home that children may not learn elsewhere or may not have much opportunity to practice in other settings.

The Early Start Denver Model supports parents' relationships with their children. It helps parents develop learning opportunities via simple games, communicative interactions during caregiving, and fun exchanges during other daily routines. No special background or prior knowledge is required. The strategies described here are designed to help parent–child interactions become more fun, more emotionally rich, and more meaningful, while at the same time providing children with more learning opportunities. We hope that parents from many different walks of life and many different backgrounds will find the strategies helpful for developing richer learning experiences for their children from the everyday activities involving playing with toys, bathing, eating meals, grocery shopping, or other activities in their daily lives.

We also understand that each child with ASD is unique, with a personal set of special gifts and challenges. As someone once said, "If you have met one child with autism, you have met one child with autism." Like each typically developing child, each child with ASD has a unique personality, set of likes and dislikes, talents, and challenges. But all young children with ASD, by definition, have trouble relating and communicating with others and playing with toys in a typical way.

From decades of research on early development and intervention in children with ASD, we have learned a great deal about the kinds of difficulties that young children with ASD have. It can be hard for them to pay attention to the people around them—including others' language and activities. It is often hard for them to share their feelings—happiness, anger, sadness, frustration—with other people by sending emotional messages to others through their facial expressions, gestures, and sounds or words. They experience a full range of emotions but may not share them in a way that is easy to understand. They may not be very interested in playing with other children and may not respond very well to other children's efforts to play with them. They often do not use many gestures to communicate and don't seem to understand the gestures of others. They are less likely to imitate others readily, so it can be hard to teach them by showing them how to do something and expecting them to copy it. Many children with ASD enjoy toys, but they often play with them in unusual ways, and their play can be very repetitive. Developing speech, and responding to others' speech, can be very difficult for many children with ASD, even for those who learn how to repeat other people's words. It is also not unusual for children with ASD to have some "challenging behaviors." These challenging behaviors are often seen in other young children as well, but young children with ASD do not respond to the typical ways parents try to teach children how to behave. They may throw tantrums, hit or bite others, destroy objects, and sometimes hurt themselves (this is called *self-injurious behavior*).

This book will teach you strategies for helping your child in each of these areas. Many studies, including studies we authors have conducted ourselves, have shown that early intervention can be tremendously helpful for children with ASD, resulting in significant gains in learning, communicating, and social skills. Some children even lose their diagnosis of ASD as a result of early intervention; others may still have challenges but are able to participate well in regular classrooms, develop friendships, and communicate well with others. Still others may

> ### *Areas in Which Most Children with ASD Have Difficulties*
>
> - Paying attention to other people
> - Using social smiles
> - Taking turns and engaging in social play
> - Using gestures and language
> - Imitating others
> - Coordinating attention (eye gaze) with others
> - Playing in typical ways with toys

continue to have significant challenges requiring ongoing special services, but early intervention will help them progress.

Most of the research on early intervention has focused on studies in which the treatment is delivered by trained therapists. The research on *parent-delivered* early intervention is still at an early stage. However, studies show that parents and other caregivers can learn to use many treatment strategies as well as trained therapists, and that when parents use these strategies, the quality of their interactions with their children improves and the children become more socially engaged and learn to communicate better with others. We have helped many parents learn to use these strategies at home with their young children, and they have told us again and again how helpful these approaches are for teaching their children to learn, interact with others, communicate, and play in more typical ways. In our work with many children over the years, we have discovered that *every single child with ASD can learn* to communicate, improve social interactions with others, and increase play skills. We are confident that these techniques will help you feel more effective as a parent, a playmate, and a first teacher for your child. And as you use the techniques and see your child learn from them, you will experience a sense of parental pride and pleasure that comes from seeing your child achieve and knowing that you are part of your child's successes.

This book is designed for parents of young children with symptoms of ASD who are in the infant through preschool years/kindergarten. You can use it whether you only suspect your child has ASD or your child has already been diagnosed. It will provide you with step-by-step instructions and examples through which you can use your typical everyday activities to help your child become more engaged, communicative, and interactive with you and with your family.

How to Use This Book

Each chapter of this book is designed to address questions, concerns, and challenges that most parents of young children with ASD experience. Among the issues that we address are feelings and concerns related to leading your life as a parent of a child with ASD, including knowing what you need to do at this early stage. Getting the best professional help will be uppermost in your mind, so this topic is covered in Chapter 1. Because parenting a child with ASD can be stressful, it will be essential that you begin this journey by considering how you will make sure to take care of yourself and the rest of the family, and avoid setting aside those needs to focus solely on the child with ASD. Doing so would mean that you would be less effective and more likely to become worn out in the process. These issues are addressed in Chapter 2. Then, to lay the groundwork for the intervention strategies described in the remaining chapters, Chapter 3 offers a fundamental understanding of what is known about ASD. This provides a context for the treatment approach offered in this book. Each of the remaining chapters describes the intervention strategies in detail, with each chapter building on the previous ones. So it will make sense for most people to read the chapters in order. However, Chapters 9 and 13 are not as dependent on earlier chapters as are the others. You may find it helpful to read them earlier in the process and refer to them as you move along in the book. We recognize that some parents will find some chapters more helpful than others, however, depending on their child's unique challenges.

> *"It's extremely overwhelming to get the diagnosis of autism, then to find out all of the therapies that are available and how many hours they entail. You want to act immediately, you want to make up for lost time, you want to try everything to get your baby back. You hear numbers such as '40-hour-a-week program,' and you start to panic. Breathe. You can do this. The beauty of the strategies in this book, which are based on the Early Start Denver Model, is that it gives you the tools to interact and teach your child in a naturalistic environment without making therapy a significant strain and burden on your family. The goal is to give your child as many opportunities as a neurotypical child, and this workbook outlines the steps for your family to carry that out in a comfortable and natural way."*

As you begin to practice the intervention strategies and incorporate them into your everyday interactions with your child, please keep in mind that the goal of this book is not to transform you from a parent into a therapist! Nor will you spend many hours with your child "providing therapy." Rather, these strategies are meant to be used during the typical routines that are part of your daily experience, such as during bath time, at the park, or while you are putting your child to bed. They should not take more time than your typical activities with your child would. The strategies build on the loving, caring relationship you already have with your child, and they use that foundation to help your child overcome some of the difficulties that are part of ASD. So let's get started.

Part I

Getting Started

1

Setting Up Your Child's Early Intervention Program

Carmen and Roberto received a diagnosis of autism for their 3-year-old, Teresa, last week. They spent a whole day at a clinic where Teresa saw person after person who asked her to play with toys, draw, swing on a swing, and do all kinds of other things. Carmen and Roberto were surprised at how much Teresa did for the doctors. These people really seemed to understand Teresa and know just what to do to encourage her to play. Teresa enjoyed herself and did some things for the doctors that her parents had never seen. They were proud of her and glad that it had gone so well.

The doctors were kind and friendly to Carmen and Roberto. They spent a lot of time with them, asking them all sorts of questions. At the end, the parents met with the psychologist on the team, Dr. Avila, who spoke both Spanish and English. She said that Teresa had some talents and abilities—she was already beginning to read! But she was also having problems learning to communicate and play. Dr. Avila said that Teresa had autism. This was the reason for her lack of speech, her odd finger movements, her big tantrums, and other problems, too. The doctor was so sure about this. That helped Carmen and Roberto. Their daughter wasn't stubborn or spoiled. She had autism, a biological condition. The diagnosis explained everything about her. And she was smart.

Dr. Avila reassured Carmen and Roberto that they had not caused Teresa's autism, nor could they have prevented it. However, they could help Teresa a great deal by finding her a good treatment program. The doctor also said that autism was something that did not go away by itself. That was hard to hear, but also, in a way, a kind of relief. Carmen and Roberto now had a name for what was wrong—a diagnosis, a way to explain Teresa.

Dr. Avila gave them phone numbers and names of people to call, as well as handouts to read (even some in Spanish for the grandmas), a list of books and websites, a fact sheet about autism, and names of parent groups. Carmen and Roberto went home in a sea of worry, grief, and questions. For a few days they were just numb and couldn't talk about it or even think clearly about anything. They went through the next few days like robots—going through the motions of everything they had to do at work and at home, but feeling numb and sad.

On the weekend, though, over breakfast, Carmen started to talk to Roberto about it all. So many different feelings were going through her at once. She was desperately worried about Teresa, about her future, about what to do, about how to help her do well. She wanted to start finding treatments as the doctor had advised, but she didn't know where to begin. Roberto listened closely to Carmen as she expressed her feelings. Carmen had words for the thoughts and feelings that he was having, too. They were a close couple. He reached out and squeezed her hand. "We'll get through this," he said. "We'll pray, and we'll work with her, and we'll get through this." Carmen squeezed his hand back, wiped away a few tears, and felt grateful for her husband—he listened, he joined, he was there with her. She was not alone. "But what should we do now?" she asked. "Who should we call first?" There was so much information on the sheet the doctor had given them; she had no idea where to start.

The news about autism probably opened up a huge new set of feelings and thoughts for you, as it did for Carmen and Roberto, including those involved in finding and beginning treatment for your child. On the one hand, you may feel a sense of urgency to get started. On the other hand, you may find yourself somewhat overwhelmed and even a little reluctant to start the process. The amount of new information and new terminology can be daunting. The numerous phone calls and appointments can make the process seem never-ending. Perhaps you even feel that if you can put off seeking help for a little longer, things will get better on their own. All of these feelings have been shared by countless parents and other family members who have stood in your shoes. We hope to make the process a little easier for you by providing straightforward information and techniques that can set you on the right path.

Starting in Chapter 4, we describe concrete ways to help your child increase his social and emotional interactions, communication, and play during your typical daily routines, so that you can increase your child's learning opportunities throughout the day. These parent-delivered strategies can be used together with other interventions for your child, which may involve a number of different people. In this first chapter, we offer information and tips for finding and pulling together the essential ingredients of a successful early intervention program for your child.

Getting Started: Knowledge Is Power

At first, the new terms, the difficulty in finding good treatment, and the uncertainty that lies ahead make many parents feel like getting into bed and hiding under the covers. Fortunately, this feeling is soon overshadowed by the determination to find out what is best for their child and to find the best intervention available. But getting these answers can be difficult. There is so much out there—so many different opinions and so much disagreement among people.

A recent survey of thousands of parents found that a large majority of parents (81%!) turn to the Internet to gain an understanding of and help for ASD.[1] The Internet allows parents across the globe to access an enormous amount of information, much of which is valuable. However, the information found on the web can also be misleading and unreliable. As you read and listen to others, keep these questions in mind:

- Who is the author? Does the author have the background and expertise needed to provide reliable, authoritative information?
- Has the information been tested thoroughly by research? Has it been published in scientific journals?
- What is the date of the information? Is it current?
- Is the website trying to sell you something? Products, assessments, treatments?
- Does the website claim to have a miraculous "cure" for ASD?
- Does the site seem biased? Does it discuss different points of view or only one?

Be skeptical! If you don't feel comfortable with your answers to any of these questions, question the truth of the information you are reading on the Internet.

To make it easier to sort through the information and options presented on the web, one group—Autism Speaks, the world's largest autism science and advocacy organization—brought parents and professionals together to create a set of tools to help parents walk through those first overwhelming days after diagnosis.

> **Helpful Tip**
>
> The National Cancer Institute offers these tips for evaluating health-related information on the Internet:
>
> - A website should make it easy for people to learn who is responsible for the site and its information.
> - If the person in charge of the website did not write the materials, the original source should be clearly identified.
> - Health-related websites should give information about the medical credentials of the people who prepare or review the material on the site.

[1]Law, P. *Interactive Autism Network Survey*. Presented at the conference on Ethics of Communicating Scientific Findings of Autism Risk, Drexel University, Philadelphia, PA, October 6, 2009.

As a parent of a young child with ASD, you will find a lot of useful information on the Autism Speaks website,[2] under "Family Services." If you still have questions about whether your child has ASD or what the specific symptoms of ASD look like, you can check out the ASD Video Glossary at *www.autismspeaks. org/what-autism/video-glossary.* The glossary contains more than a hundred video clips of children's behavior, illustrating the sometimes subtle differences between typical and atypical behavior. The ASD Video Glossary can help you learn more about your child's symptoms of ASD.

A second important tool for you is the "100 Day Kit." You can download the kit for free at *www.autismspeaks.org/family-services/tool-kits/100-day-kit.* This kit, which is available in Spanish, gives information on ASD diagnosis and causes, your child's educational rights, different therapies and treatments, and 10 things your child wishes you knew, as well as safety tips, useful forms, and a glossary. The kit will provide you with a detailed plan for what to do in the next 100 days. Knowledge is power, and the 100 Day Kit will help you feel better prepared for the start of your journey down the new road that has opened up in front of you as a parent of a child with ASD.

The strategies that you will learn starting in Chapter 4 will help you work with your child at home right now, while you are waiting for intervention to begin. They will continue to be helpful once your child is enrolled in an intervention program. That is, they will ensure that your child is learning not only while with teachers and therapists, but also throughout the day-to-day moments with you. You are, after all, your child's most valuable teacher—just as parents of children without an ASD diagnosis are—because you know your child best and you're the person with whom your child spends the most time. Those daily activities with you are the most important and most frequent learning opportunities your child has, and you are there and ready to make the most of them.

Helpful Tip

The 100 Day Kit from Autism Speaks provides these things:

- General diagnostic and medical information
- Help with family issues
- Guidance for finding services
- Descriptions of different types of treatments
- An action plan for getting started
- A glossary and resources

---

[2]If you have trouble accessing this information on a computer, you can call 888-AUTISM2 (888-288-4762) and speak with an Autism Response Team Coordinator. The 100 Day Kit will be sent to your home for free.

Finding the Best Intervention Program

In 2001, the National Research Council,3 an organization that advises the U.S. Congress on policy, made a set of recommendations about **best practices** for early intervention with young children with ASD. These straightforward recommendations can serve as a basic guide and yardstick by which to assess the effectiveness of an intervention program you're considering. The criteria are as follows:

- ✓ Intervention should begin as soon as possible.
- ✓ The intervention program should be individualized for each child, taking into account each child's unique characteristics, strengths, and challenges.
- ✓ The intervention program should be designed and overseen by a trained, professional, interdisciplinary team.
- ✓ A curriculum that focuses on the specific areas of challenges in ASD should be used.
- ✓ The program should provide for ongoing data collection on the progress the child is making in each skill area, and adjustments to the program should be made when progress is not evident.
- ✓ The child should be actively engaged in the intervention activities and should receive at least 25 hours of structured intervention each week.
- ✓ Parents should be closely involved in the intervention, as well as in setting goals and priorities, and should be taught how to implement the intervention strategies at home.

We would add another criterion to this list: The intervention provided for your child should be based on **evidence-based practices (EBPs)**. You may run into this phrase often as you read about autism interventions. It means that the intervention has been tested in scientific studies and published in scientific journals, and that the results showed those intervention practices to be more helpful for young children with ASD than no intervention. With all the claims and all the hype about autism treatment these days, you will want to be sure that your child is receiving interventions that have been tested and found to be effective.

How will you know? You can ask the providers if their intervention is based on EBPs, and if you want, you can ask them to share with you the research articles that demonstrated its success. You can find trustworthy information about EBPs on the National Standards Project website (*www.nationalautismcenter.org/*

---

[3]Committee on Educational Interventions for Children with Autism, National Research Council. *Educating children with autism.* Washington, DC: National Academy Press, 2001.

affiliates) and on the website for the National Professional Development Center on ASD (*http://autismpdc.fpg.unc.edu*).

Receiving appropriate early intervention based on best practices is not just a goal. It is a legal right of your child's, thanks to a law called the ***Individuals with Disabilities Education Improvement Act (IDEA)***, which was enacted in 1975 and revised in 2004. This law guarantees the rights of all children, including those with ASD, to a free and appropriate education that meets their unique and individual needs. This means your child with ASD is eligible for free education that addresses her specific needs (even as a toddler).

How do you find an early intervention provider? The professional who provided you with the diagnosis may also have provided you with a name and phone number to call to begin the process of starting early intervention services. If this did not happen, your child's doctor may well know the agency and phone number to call. Another route is to call your school district's special education department, say your child has just received a diagnosis of ASD, and ask whom you should speak to. You can also find information on how to find and access early intervention services

> ### ✍ Helpful Tip
> You can locate early intervention services in your community by calling your school district's special education department. Even if your child is much younger than school age, your school district can help you. Your child's doctor is another source of information about services. There is also information on the Autism Speaks website (*www. autismspeaks.org/family-services/ resource-guide*) and on the Autism Society of America's website (*www. autism-society.org*).

in your state on the Autism Speaks website (*www.autismspeaks.org/family-services/ resource-guide*) and the Autism Society's website (*www.autism-society.org*).

A good early intervention program can be provided in different ways:

- **If your child is under age 3,** you will work with the early intervention provider to develop an ***individualized family service plan (IFSP)***. This is a document that you and others will write together. It will describe your child's specific intervention needs and goals, and the types of services your child and family will receive to reach those goals.
- **If your child is 3 years old or older,** he will receive an evaluation, and you and the preschool services agency staff members will develop an ***individualized education program (IEP)*** for your child, usually under the direction of your local school district. Your child's intervention will move from "early intervention" to "preschool" services at age 3, even if you started out with an IFSP.

Choosing a Birth-to-3 Program or Preschool Program

Because the needs of each child with ASD are unique, there are many ways to construct an early intervention program that can help your child, and many types of intervention models to draw from. Some children receive all of their services at a specialized clinic- or school-based program, whereas others receive most of their interventions from people who work with the children at home. It is common for young children with autism to receive their intervention from a combination of school-, clinic-, and/or home-based intervention programs. In some places, services are delivered by people working for the public agency. In other places, the public agency contracts with private groups to serve children.

As we have said above, high-quality programs use EBPs. Most EBPs have come from the field of ***applied behavior analysis (ABA)***. What is ABA? ABA is the use of teaching practices that come from the scientific study of learning to teach or change behavior. The principles of ABA can be used to teach new skills, shape existing behaviors into new ones, and reduce the frequency of problem behaviors. Later in this book (Chapter 9), we describe the principles of ABA in more detail. For now, the important thing is to look for early intervention programs that use EBPs in their approach. As noted earlier, you can ask any early intervention provider directly whether the program uses EBPs in its teaching approach. If the answer is no, look for additional options.

Providers of early intervention programs and services may include early educators, speech–language therapists, behavior analysts, occupational therapists, or other professionals, along with educational or therapy assistants. Although the amount of intervention for preschoolers recommended by the National Research Council (see the checklist on page 13) is 25 hours per week, we don't know what the best number of hours is for children under 3, and public services in many places may provide only a few hours per week of intervention. You can use the intervention strategies described later in this book, and those you learn from your intervention team, at home to increase the number of hours of high-quality learning experiences your child receives. This will also help your child learn to bring (***generalize***) the skills learned in other settings into daily life at home and in your family activities.

If you have a choice of intervention programs, try to visit and observe different programs in action, meet with the director and teachers, and talk with other parents of children participating in the program. As you observe the program and talk with the teachers and parents, imagine your child in this program. Is the intervention approach based on EBPs? Does it seem right for your child? Is this the kind of approach you think will work best for your child? Programs differ in their degree of structure and routine, how they work with parents, how they teach language, how quiet or noisy they are, whether they are delivered at home or in a group, and so on. How do these qualities match your child's individual personality, learning style, and abilities? How do they match your preferences, values, and expectations for how others should interact with your child? The National Research Council recommendations mentioned earlier can be broken down into more specific criteria that you can use to evaluate an early intervention program.[4] You may not be able to determine whether all of the criteria in the checklists in the box on pages 18–19 are being met without delving into a lot of detail with the providers, but you can get a fairly good idea of whether many of them are being met by observing the program closely and asking questions as they arise.

Use of Additional Therapists

Public agency intervention programs will have speech–language therapists, occupational therapists, psychologists, and physical therapists on staff. If you go through your public agency for services, your child is likely to receive an evaluation by a speech–language therapist, and perhaps an occupational therapist as well. Their information is typically used to build the goals and service plans that appear on your child's IFSP or IEP. Sometimes these therapists work directly with children separately from other children; sometimes they work with a small group of children, or children and parents; and sometimes they consult with those who are providing the ongoing intervention, rather than working directly with children. Some families also use these types of therapists privately, using their children's medical insurance to cover the costs, if possible. If your child is not making enough progress in developing spoken language, discuss this with your team members and ask them whether additional therapy from a speech–language therapist might be helpful. You can ask them for referral sources, and your child's physician should also be able to refer you to a speech–language pathologist whose services are covered by your child's health care insurance. Their treatment may focus on general communication, including use of gesture and developing word use, articulation and speech development, and even social interaction and play.

If your child's motor coordination or responses to sensory stimuli are very concerning to you, you can follow the same process just described to find an occupational therapist. Discuss this with your team and your child's physician; ask whether additional occupational therapy or physical therapy may be helpful to your child; ask for a referral to a professional whose services are covered by your child's health care insurance; and seek additional treatment. A list of therapists who have experience working with young children with autism in your area is also provided in the "Resource Guide" section of the Autism Speaks website.

---

[4]Adapted from Librera, W. L., et al. *Autism program quality indicators: A self-review and quality improvement guide for programs serving young students with autism spectrum disorders.* Trenton: New Jersey Department of Education, 2004. Available at *www.eric.ed.gov.*

Therapists in the Home Setting

When an intervention is delivered at home, typically a professional person acts as a ***program manager*** or supervisor of the program. The program manager has expertise in early intervention and supervises a team of ***therapists***, who may be paraprofessionals who should receive training and ongoing close supervision by the program manager. These paraprofessionals (sometimes also referred to as ***tutors***, ***aides***, ***interventionists***, or ***home therapists***) come to the home regularly to work with the child. In some areas, these services are paid for by the public early intervention service agency. In other areas, health insurance will pay for these early intervention services. Sometimes parents pay out of pocket. Reforming insurance coverage practices to cover such services is an important goal for advocacy organizations. If you have home-based therapy, it is important to ensure that the program manager is professionally trained and credentialed, will see your child frequently, will observe and supervise the others working with your child frequently, and is using EBPs. Use the checklist in the box on page 21 to determine whether a home-delivered intervention you are considering will be effective for your child.

The Role of Your Child's Physician in Early Intervention

Only recently has the impact of your child's medical health on her ability to learn and benefit from early intervention been fully recognized. We have learned that ASD not only affects the brain and behavior, but can also affect the whole body. Thus your child's physician will play an ongoing role in your child's treatment. Common medical issues that children with ASD may experience include sleep disturbances, such as difficulty falling asleep and frequent awakening; eating difficulties, such as finicky eating and food aversions; gastrointestinal problems, such as constipation and diarrhea; and seizures. Less common medical problems include rare inborn problems with metabolism. A physician should screen for these metabolic conditions as part of the diagnostic workup.

> ### 🖐️ *Helpful Tip*
>
> If your diagnosis came from a medical center team, your child probably had a medical workup as part of the process, including a blood draw, urinalysis, and other tests. If your diagnosis came from an independent professional, you may not have had a complete medical workup for your child's autism yet. If you have not, ask your child's doctor to carry out a full medical workup for autism. It is quite important, because in some cases there is a known medical reason that is contributing to autism, and it may affect your child's treatment.

Not all physicians are familiar

Criteria for Measuring the Quality of an Early Intervention Program

1. Does the program engage the children sufficiently?

- ✓ Are all children involved in the classroom activities? Or are some children wandering or isolated?
- ✓ Does the program give your child at least 25 hours a week of structured intervention when added to other interventions the child is receiving?
- ✓ Is each teacher or other adult staff member in charge of only two to three students?
- ✓ Is the program offered year-round?
- ✓ Are the educational activities planned systematically and appropriate for the developmental age of the children?
- ✓ Does the program track daily progress so that the methods can be assessed for effectiveness?

2. Are staff members well qualified?

- ✓ Do they know how to develop an IEP to meet the unique needs of a child with ASD?
- ✓ Do they know how to use a comprehensive curriculum specifically for ASD?
- ✓ Can they adapt the learning environment and use instructional methods known to help children with ASD learn?
- ✓ Do they use strategies to promote communication and social interaction?
- ✓ Can they implement behavior management techniques based on ABA?
- ✓ Are they able to appropriately handle a crisis?
- ✓ Do they have appropriate credentials in their profession?
- ✓ Do the teaching and therapy assistants receive direct instruction and supervision?
- ✓ Are staff members provided with regular inservice training on educating young children with ASD?
- ✓ Are consultants available to the program?

3. Is the curriculum appropriate for children with ASD?

- ✓ Are educational objectives, methods, and activities based on a written curriculum?
- ✓ Do staff members adapt the curriculum to meet children's unique abilities, challenges, ages, and learning styles?

✓ Does the curriculum focus on important areas for learning, including communication and language, fine and gross motor skills, toy play, imaginative play, and social skills?

✓ Do children have opportunities to interact with typically developing peers?

4. Are the teaching methods effective?

✓ Are the methods EBPs?

✓ Do the methods help children participate in appropriate activities?

✓ Do the instructional methods take advantage of naturally occurring rewards?

✓ Do they encourage children to use learned skills spontaneously in different environments?

✓ Does the staff analyze data collected on each child's challenging behaviors, use a functional behavioral assessment,* and support positive behavior to reduce challenging behaviors?

5. Does the program involve the family?

✓ Does the program involve parents and family members as active participants in all aspects of the child's evaluation and education?

✓ Does the program give parents information about the educational philosophy, curriculum, and instructional strategies?

✓ Does the program staff respect differences in culture, language, values, and parenting styles among families?

✓ Does the program help parents understand child development and support parents' efforts to apply the teaching methods at home? Does the staff meet regularly with parents and inform them about their child's progress?

✓ Does the program work with families to find family support services?

✓ Does the program help the family transition the child into the next phase of education?

---

*Functional behavioral assessment** is an EBP, a technical procedure for identifying the functions of challenging behaviors such as aggression. It involves collecting data about the frequency and severity of the problem behavior and identifying the immediate factors that preceded and followed each occurrence of the behavior. It leads to an intervention approach designed to minimize contributing factors; make environmental accommodations to prevent or reduce the challenging behavior; and build alternative, appropriate skills that address the identified function of the behavior.

with how to assess and treat the medical issues that your child may be facing. If your child is uncomfortable, tired, or in pain because of a medical issue, your child may start to become aggressive, have a tantrum, or become lethargic. These "problem behaviors" may be viewed by the physician as "just part of the autism." If you suspect that your child has an underlying medical condition, work closely with your child's physician to find the answers. Your child's doctor may need to refer your child to a physician who specializes in autism for appropriate medical assessment and treatment. Such specialty

> *Common medical issues that children with ASD experience include sleep disturbances, such as difficulty falling asleep and frequent wakening; eating difficulties, such as finicky eating and food aversions; gastrointestinal problems, such as constipation and diarrhea; and seizures.*

physicians are typically available at university medical centers and children's hospitals, which often have entire autism clinics. Ask your child's doctor if this type of referral is needed for your child. You can also look for a physician in your area by visiting the "Family Services" section of the Autism Speaks website.

Sleep Difficulties

Sleep problems are extremely common among children with ASD. In fact, it is estimated that over half of children have at least one frequent sleep problem. This means that over half of parents of children with ASD have sleep disruption, since parents' sleep is inevitably disrupted when their child has a sleep difficulty! Among the sleep problems that parents report are delayed sleep onset, night waking, early awakening, obstructive sleep apnea (difficulty breathing when asleep), and reduced need for sleep. Research suggests that ASD may be associated with differences in genes that regulate the sleep cycle and the production of melatonin. Melatonin is a chemical secreted by the pineal gland in the brain that helps regulate the circadian (daily) rhythms, including the sleep cycle. Occasionally, sleep problems are caused by seizure activity that is occurring during the night.

> *Fact: Over half of children with ASD have sleep difficulties, with insomnia the most common problem reported by parents.*

If your child is struggling with a sleep problem, he will not be able to take full advantage of early intervention. Studies have shown that sleep disruption in children, including children with ASD, is associated with poor attention, memory difficulties, and behavior problems, such as tantrums and aggression. The most common sleep problem parents of children with ASD report is insomnia. Often insomnia in a child with ASD can be helped substantially by establishing a more consistent bedtime routine (this is often referred to as good **sleep hygiene**). In an

Criteria for Measuring the Quality
of a Home-Based Intervention Program

If the answer is yes to each of the following questions, you can be confident of the quality and experience of the intervention group.

- ✓ Does the program manager have an educational background appropriate for working with young children with ASD, including a graduate degree (master's degree or PhD) in a field like behavior analysis, special education, or psychology?

- ✓ Have the program manager and therapists been trained and certified in an intervention method with scientific evidence to support it? What is it?

- ✓ Have the program manager and all home therapists passed a criminal and educational background check?

- ✓ Does the program manager spend time regularly supervising the home therapists, observing them at work with your child, reviewing your child's progress and working with your child directly, and adjusting teaching strategies to improve progress?

- ✓ Do the home therapists you have met appear well trained, competent, professional, and motivated?

- ✓ Do the program manager and home therapists encourage you to observe and join their treatment sessions with your child and explain what they are doing?

- ✓ Does the program manager consult with professionals in other disciplines (such as occupational therapy, speech–language therapy, and pediatrics), when needed?

- ✓ Does the intervention program use a curriculum that identifies the specific objectives your child is working to achieve?

- ✓ Do the home therapists collect data on your child's progress daily and review the data regularly with the program manager?

- ✓ Does the program manager meet regularly with you and other professionals who are part of your child's intervention team?

- ✓ Do you feel that you are a respected part of the intervention team, and that your program manager listens to you?

- ✓ Does the manager help you prioritize what to focus on with your child? Does he or she show you how to help your child make progress on his or her objectives in your interactions with your child at home?

article on sleep hygiene for children with developmental disabilities published by the American Academy of Pediatrics, the following recommendations[5] were offered for helping children with developmental disabilities sleep better:

1. Provide a sleep environment that is comfortable for the child, in terms of temperature, lighting, mattress, textures of blankets, and so on.
2. Provide a relatively dark sleep environment, because even low levels of light inhibit melatonin production (a night light is okay if necessary).
3. Establish a regular sleep–wake schedule, including regular times for naps, going to sleep, and awakening. In general, there should not be more than an hour's difference in bedtimes and wake-up times during the week and weekends.
4. Plan bedtime activities carefully to help calm your child before sleep, because children with ASD can easily be overstimulated. Avoid new and unexpected activities, excessive noise, vigorous play, and large meals close to bedtime. Bathing, lullabies, presence of a familiar toy or blanket, and looking at books together are usually calming. Other calming activities include light massage, brushing hair, and soft music.
5. Do not have a TV in your child's room. Do not play movies or TV as a way to help your child fall asleep.

If your child has a sleep problem, the first person to consult is the psychologist on your child's early intervention team. There are excellent behavioral methods for parents to use that can improve children's sleep enormously. V. Mark Durand has written two excellent books to help parents improve their child's sleep based on good science: One is called *Sleep Better* (1998), and the other is *When Children Don't Sleep Well: Interventions for Pediatric Sleep Disorders: Parent Workbook* (2008). Full details on both are listed in the Resources section at the back of this book. If these techniques are not effective, check with your pediatrician, who can provide more information about help for sleep. Melatonin is sometimes given orally to assist in establishing a regular sleep–wake cycle, but this should be done under the supervision of your family pediatrician.

Gastrointestinal and Feeding Problems

Another common medical problem experienced by many children with ASD is gastrointestinal (GI) distress. Parents frequently report that their child with ASD has abdominal pain, diarrhea, gas, and constipation. The most common problems reported by parents are diarrhea and constipation, which can alternate in the same child. Although these problems are fairly common in all children, there

---

[5]James, E. J., et al. (2008). Sleep hygiene for children with neurodevelopmental disabilities. *Pediatrics*, *122*, 1343–1350, 2008.

is some evidence that they occur more frequently in children with ASD. Such GI problems cause pain and discomfort and, like sleep problems, can result in problem behaviors and difficulty paying attention. These problems in turn can result in failure to benefit fully from the intervention program.

Because children with ASD have difficulty communicating, it may be challenging to know whether or not your child is experiencing abdominal or other types of pain. Be observant of abrupt changes in your child's behavior, excessive crying or whining, self-injurious behavior, holding her stomach, and other nonverbal indicators of pain. If you are suspicious, take your child to the pediatrician to have her evaluated. GI problems are treatable. Depending on the type and severity of the GI problem, treatments can include dietary interventions, nutritional supplements, and medications. There currently is no scientific evidence that special diets, including elimination of casein and gluten, improve the behavior of children with ASD; however, some parents have anecdotally reported significant benefit from such diets, including improved attention and fewer behavior problems.

> *Fact: Feeding problems are common in children with ASD and can show up during infancy.*

Eating problems are also common among children with ASD. A recent study published by the American Academy of Pediatrics[6] found that children with ASD often start to have feeding difficulties as infants. They are more likely than typical infants to start eating solid food at a later date, for example. By 1 year of age, children with ASD are more likely to be described as "difficult to feed" and "very choosy." As toddlers, children with ASD have a less varied diet. Although this study did not find any differences between children with ASD and typically developing children in terms of nutrition, other studies have found that children with ASD sometimes have deficiencies in certain nutrients, perhaps because of their picky eating or the use of special diets.

If you have concerns about your child's eating patterns, bring this up at your next pediatrician visit. Also, discuss this with your case manager, your behaviorist, or the psychologist on your child's early intervention team. There are many ways you can help your child eat a wider range of foods, and your therapists should be able to help you a great deal. If your doctor is concerned about your child's nutrition, he or she may refer you to a nutritionist. Sometimes at university or hospital clinics, there is a nutritionist on the team who can provide specific suggestions regarding how to help your child eat better or how you can make sure your child is getting the nourishment he needs. There are different reasons a child may have eating difficulties, including having trouble chewing and swallowing, sensory sensitivities related to different food textures, food intolerances

---

[6]Emond, A., et al. Feeding symptoms, dietary patterns, and growth in young children with autism spectrum disorders. *Pediatrics, 126*(2), e337–e342.

or allergies, and avoidance of novelty. Your early intervention team and doctor, working together, can help you determine whether you should worry about your child's nutrition, help you understand why your child is having eating difficulties, and help you improve your child's eating habits.

Seizures

Although seizures are not usually a problem in early childhood, approximately one out of every four individuals with ASD will develop seizures at some point in life. Seizures typically develop for the first time in adolescence or even adulthood in ASD, though occasionally they appear early in life. It is important to have seizures treated, because the seizure activity can affect how the brain functions and develops. Thus, if your child has a seizure or has symptoms (described below) that suggest seizure activity, seek medical attention as soon as possible.

There are many types of seizures: seizures that involve staring spells (absence seizures), seizures that involve repetitive movements (partial complex seizures), and seizures that involve convulsions (grand mal seizures). Mild symptoms may be difficult to detect because some of the symptoms, such as staring into space and not responding when called, are also typical symptoms of ASD. Symptoms of an absence seizure may include "blanking out" or becoming unresponsive to sounds and sights for 10–20 seconds, blinking repetitively, eyes rolling up a bit, mouth movements, muscle stiffness, jerking movements, rubbing fingers together, and staring spells. If you have concerns about possible seizure activity, check with your pediatrician, who may refer your child to a child neurologist for an evaluation.

Putting It All Together

As you can see, there are many different parts to early intervention, including the basic intervention program (either group or one-on-one), and sometimes additional therapy from a speech–language pathologist, occupational therapist, and/or physician. Over time you will learn about the choices that are available in your community, decide what you feel is best for your child, and voice your preferences so that your child gets the best services available in your community. You will need to encourage the different people working with your child to talk to each other and share information. These things need to happen, but they don't happen automatically or all at once. They happen step by step because parents make them happen.

Many parents find it helpful to have regular "team meetings" with all the professionals involved in their child's care. The team meetings help keep all the team members on the same wavelength—focusing on similar goals, handling behavior problems in similar ways, learning from and listening to each other.

You have the right to ask for a team meeting at any time, to review your child's IFSP or IEP, and to discuss progress. Other ways to help your team work together include these:

1. Have a notebook that stays with your child throughout the day, so that teachers, therapists, and family members can make notes about your child's behavior and progress.
2. Ask your child's intervention team to send you information about your child's progress each week.
3. Some "tech-oriented" families even set up a blog or website on which different team members as well as the parents can communicate what they are working on, describe what has been effective (or not), and offer tips that can be helpful for the other providers. This is a place to share problems and victories as your child begins to develop new skills.

In this chapter we have provided basic information on setting up an intervention program for your child. For further reading, we have provided lists of excellent websites and books on the topics covered in this book (see the Resources section at the back of this book). Up to this point we've been focusing on your child. But what about you? Like your child, you and your family need special attention as you meet the challenges ahead. By doing so, you will be less likely to experience "burnout" and will be better able to meet the needs of your child with ASD and the rest of your family. The next chapter provides strategies for making sure that you and your family stay healthy and balanced, in spite of the stresses that come with raising a young child with ASD.

2

Taking Care of Yourself and Your Family

As Carmen and Roberto scrambled to put together the best intervention plan for Teresa, their 3-year-old with autism, several weeks flew by in a flurry of phone calls and appointments. Luckily, Carmen worked the afternoon shift, 3:00 to 11:00 p.m., so she was home during the morning and could make phone calls. All the focus was now on Teresa. Roberto worked the early shift, 6:00 a.m. to 2:00 p.m. The parents saw little of each other except on the weekends. When they had any time together, Carmen tried to tell her husband what was happening with Teresa—all the appointments, all the new people, the advice others were giving her about how to handle Teresa's tantrums and how to help her communicate. It seemed as if Teresa was all they were talking about now, and Roberto felt distant from it. He wished this would all pass, like a bad dream, and life would go back to when he had a happy wife, a close marriage, and a life that was smooth and easy. He worried about his ability to take care of his wife, son, and daughter in the face of this new, unknown, and scary future.

Carmen was living this new life, every waking moment. There was little time to talk about anything else, even 5-year-old Justino, who had just started school. Carmen soon started to have trouble sleeping. She lay in bed worrying about Teresa. Would the intervention program they had found really help her? Would their health insurance cover the expenses? Would she need to quit her job to focus on Teresa and Justino? How could they afford that? Her mind was swimming with questions and worries, and her eyes filled with tears. She looked over at Roberto and felt far away from him. He had become quieter and quieter. They rarely laughed and had fun together any more. He was staying late at work more often. She couldn't blame him for wanting to avoid the challenges they were facing, but she needed him more than ever now.

And what about Justino? He went to kindergarten in the morning, and

Grandma picked him up afterward, since Teresa had therapy until noon far away from Justino's school. Grandma brought him home at 1:00 P.M. and stayed with the children until Roberto arrived home at 3:00 or so. Carmen felt as if she hardly saw Justino any more except to send him off in the morning.

> "I completely relate to this. Even though I worked in the special education field and had colleagues, no one understood what I was feeling, and I felt completely helpless and alone. It's a devastating feeling."

She pulled the covers over her head and buried her face in the pillow. She wished she had someone to talk to about all this, but it was difficult to talk to her family and friends. They told her that she was overreacting, that the doctors were wrong, that she was spending too much time with Teresa. No one knew what she was going through. She needed advice from her mother, help from her family, and love from her husband. She needed all the energy she could muster. For the first time, she was going to have to draw a lot more people into her family circle. Would she be able to find people who understood what they were going through—people who could help with Teresa and even give them a break now and then?

Adjusting to Caring for a Child with ASD

The feelings that Carmen and Roberto were experiencing are the feelings of many parents who are adjusting to having a child with ASD. Research has shown what families of children with ASD have been telling us for years: Caring for a child with ASD can be very stressful! But many parents have also told us that it can be rewarding and fulfilling—not in the first few worried, hectic months, perhaps, but after that, as new routines get set, as children start to progress, and as the future becomes brighter.

During the first several months or even years after learning that your child has ASD, it is tempting to put aside your own needs and those of other family members while you focus on your child with ASD. It is, however, very important to take some time to consider the needs of your whole family, including yourself. It's tempting to put yourself at the bottom of the priority list. Don't do it! Taking care of yourself is the only way you'll be able to take care of everyone else. Therefore, it's important that you frequently take stock of how you are doing and take steps to ensure that you are healthy, both physically and mentally.

The prospect of taking care of yourself, your spouse or partner, and your other children may seem overwhelming when you feel that you're devoting every minute of the day to your child with ASD. We won't pretend it will be easy, but our experiences with numerous parents who have faced the same challenges have taught us some tips for adjusting to having a child with ASD. In every way we can, we try in this chapter to describe some strategies that may make it a little easier to handle all that's on your plate: from the daily management hassles, to the tough balancing act of staying close as a family, to finding some of the rewards and fulfillment that lie along this new path you are taking.

Taking Care of Your Family

Everyone in your family will be affected by the new path that ASD has carved out for you, but the impact does not have to be negative, especially after you've gotten through the initial adjustment period. For most parents, especially during that adjustment period, the biggest impediment to maintaining healthy relationships and keeping the family strong and united seems to be time—time to spend with each other and time to communicate. Of course, finding the same amount of time for your other family members now that you're trying to help a child with ASD is challenging. Fortunately, parents who have been through it have shared ideas that can help.

Fostering Your Marital Relationship[1]

Does the challenge of raising a child with ASD have a negative effect on marriage (above and beyond the effects of having a child without special needs)? Not necessarily! In fact, research[2] based on hundreds of families of children with ASD from early childhood until young adulthood showed that there was *no* difference in divorce rates of couples with and without a young child with ASD. (As the children reached late adolescence and adulthood, couples of children with ASD were somewhat more likely to divorce, but it is unclear why this was the case.)

The added pressures of taking care of a child with ASD often result in less time for your primary (marital or long-term) relationship—time that has already been reduced by the needs of young children. You may feel as if you have no choice here. The needs of your child with ASD may have to come first right now, but if you leave your partner on the sidelines, you're denying yourself a critical member of your social support network. Additionally, managing this huge new challenge outside of the partnership can start to distance the two of you at one of the most significant points in your relationship. A few guidelines are particularly important to follow at this early stage after your child's diagnosis.

---

[1]"Marital relationship" in this chapter refers broadly to your relationship with your partner or significant other, whether you are officially married or not.

[2]Hartley, S. L., et al. The relative risk and timing of divorce in families of children with an autism spectrum disorder. *Journal of Family Psychology, 24*(4), 449–457, 2010.

Communicate!

Talk to each other. Because you are so caught up in the issues involving your young child with ASD, it is hard to think about, or talk about, anything else.

> *Roberto felt as if Carmen was living the new life that had been thrust upon them and had completely left the old one. He himself felt caught between two lives. The old one was gone, and a new one, seemingly much less satisfying, was on the horizon— unknown, stressful, and scary. While Carmen was living it, he was only hearing about it—and not much else from his wife. For Carmen, this was all she could think about. She wanted to share it with her husband, but he didn't seem very interested. It made her angry that he was not joining her in all the decision making and stress she now faced, and she felt distant from him in a new way.*

It's important to share other parts of your lives in your communications. When you see each other after your separate daily routines, make a point of asking about the other things that matter to each of you: "How was work today?" "What do you think we could do for fun this weekend?" "Do you still have a cold?" "Did you talk to your mother on the phone today? What's new with her?" Really listen, and try to join your partner in his or her life when you talk. Try hard to spend just a few minutes each day together, focused on each other, before launching into the subject of the children.

> *"Spending a little time focused on each other is crucial! As I reflect on the past, we never did this. Everything was about the kids and their disabilities and therapies. Nothing about us any more, like we didn't matter. At the time I felt that we didn't—nothing was more important than the kids—but in retrospect, you always need to find time for yourself and your relationships with your other children, spouse, and family members. Everyone is important to the family dynamic, and happiness is key."*

Listen

When your partner is talking, listen quietly. Don't interrupt or judge. Try restating what your partner has said to make sure you've understood his or her perspective and feelings. For example, if your partner tells you about a problem he or she experienced that day, refrain from criticizing and telling your partner what to do. Instead, it's more helpful to restate the highlights of your partner's message and offer support, saying something like this: "It sounds like you really had a rough day. You sound tired and upset. How can I help?"

It's very common for parents to have disagreements about their child with ASD. They may have different opinions about the diagnosis, what type of intervention to use, discipline, and expectations. For these kinds of disagreements, the first step is choosing a good time to talk them through, so you can really hear what your partner is thinking. The second step is really listening to the other's point of view and taking it seriously, rather than thinking that your partner doesn't know or understand. For example, if your partner makes a suggestion about a new treatment that you disagree with, try to respond by eliciting more about why your partner thinks it's a good idea, rather than dismissing the idea or criticizing your partner. Listen closely to hear each other's reasoning, and search for a midpoint or convergence between your two views, or another solution that works for both of you. If coming to a decision requires information about your child that one or both of you need, see if you can find a time to sit down together with your service coordinator or a team member to ask questions and gather the information you need. If you are having trouble hearing each other or finding a common ground, see if you can meet with a psychologist or social worker on your child's team to come to a more shared point of view. But before you seek others' help, try hard to hear each other out openly and respectfully.

> **Helpful Tip**
>
> Avoid placing blame at all costs. It's human nature to try to find someone to blame for your child's diagnosis, for the dreams that you may feel have been dashed, for the sadness you feel right after a diagnosis. *But there is no blame. No one caused this. There was nothing anyone could have done to prevent this. You and your family are the solution, not the problem.* Blaming yourself is destructive and unproductive. Blaming your partner will undermine his or her self-confidence, weaken your shared trust, and lead to feelings of estrangement. You need each other more than ever now. Your partner can be the most helpful person of all in this new challenge. When you start to feel blame or guilt, recognize the feelings and remind yourself that *no one is to blame for autism.*

Show Your Partner That You Care

Showing acceptance of and empathy for your partner's feelings, and expressing interest in what's going on in his or her life, are important ways to show that you care. Dr. John Gottman, a renowned marriage expert, stresses the importance of the small day-to-day interactions that we have with our partners. These everyday exchanges are the foundation on which strong marital relationships are built. See

Helpful Tip

If you need reminders of how to communicate in positive ways and show your partner you care in the midst of the stress of this new path, try a simple device we'll be offering at the end of each chapter in Part II (Chapters 4–13). That is, write reminders to yourself to help you remember the importance of nurturing your relationship in these hard times. Write whatever reminders are particularly helpful for you, whether it's "Don't say, 'YOU ALWAYS . . .'" or "Remember to tell her 'I love you' before hanging up the phone" or "Remember to greet him when he first gets home, no matter what." We call these reminders "refrigerator lists," but you can post them wherever you'll see them regularly: on your phone, in a drawer you open every morning to get dressed, in your closet near your clothes, or any other place that works for you.

if you can find some way to do or say things that are thoughtful, caring, and supportive daily. Dr. Gottman's research has shown that these ordinary but loving gestures act as deposits in your "emotional bank account." Having a full emotional bank account can help each of you now, during this ongoing stress, and when inevitable conflicts arise. You have something to draw upon. Take what you need, and deposit as much as you can.

Keep Your Sense of Humor

Marriage experts have long recognized the benefits of maintaining a healthy sense of humor. Laughter reduces stress, feels good, and increases a sense of intimacy. Especially during an argument, humor (as long as it doesn't attack or put the other person down) can relieve tension and lighten the situation. As silly as it might sound, even watching funny movies together helps bring people together and relieve stress. Seek out ways to laugh. Consider a "Friday Family Comedy Night," when you take turns picking out a comedy film to watch together.

> "I personally have found it really easy to find humor in situations that others can find scary or weird about autism with other parents who are going through it with me. Networking with fellow caregivers about the trials and tribulations can often bring not only comfort but much needed humor, and these people are empathetic and not judgmental. (For example, if I want to talk about how my daughter smeared poop on the dog, I think a fellow autism mommy may get that a lot more than a neurotypical mom.)"

Make Time for Your Relationship

Is making time for your relationship easier said than done? Definitely—but it's not impossible. Try to carve out some regular time that is devoted specifically to being (1) together with your partner, (2) free of the distractions of children, and (3) enjoyable for you both. Spending just a few minutes each day involved with each other can really help connect you after a tough day and open you to hearing about each other's lives—both the joys and the sorrows—in a caring, nonjudgmental, and honest way. When friends or family members ask what they can do to help, ask them to come over to give you a little "couple time," or ask if you can drop the children over for a little while with them. Making time for your relationship involves finding help with the kids that you trust. If there is no one to help, ask your service coordinator or a team member for ideas. In some places, respite care is available for children with ASD, and there are a number of resources you can turn to. We describe these next.

Use Respite Care

Respite care is a term for babysitting or other short-term care provided to an individual with a developmental disability (or other chronic medical condition), so that the family members can get some time away from the daily routines of caring for the individual. Respite care can be very helpful in relieving stress and providing an opportunity to take a break and spend time by yourself, with your partner, or with other family members. It's a time to recharge your batteries, relax, and take care of yourself and the rest of your family. You can find a respite care provider through the National Respite Network and Resource Center (see *www.archrespite.org*). The website offers a National Respite Locator Service that will help you locate respite care services in your state. Services are provided by trained, sometimes licensed, employees of these agencies. Many programs are provided by local organizations such as churches, school, and other nonprofit organizations. Respite care can be provided in or out of the home. Respite care programs often offer training for friends and family members in how to care for a child with ASD, so you can call upon a friend or relative to care for your child.

In addition to respite care, there are resources to turn to for the occasional night out. Ask people at the local autism association or parent group for references. Ask other parents that you meet about child care. Many parents have experienced, skilled people working with their children with ASD who might provide babysitting for you. If you have no other leads, call a college near you; ask for the psychology, social work, or child development department; and ask if there are students who would be willing to babysit for a child with ASD. Have a prospective sitter come over to play and meet your child ahead of time. See how the student interacts with your child. Ask for references. Then slowly let the student provide some care while you and your partner get some time together.

Leaving your young child with ASD with someone else for a little bit is not neglecting your role as a parent. It provides something positive for your child. First, it gives your son or daughter a refreshed parent. Second, it provides benefits on its own. It is quite important that all children learn to accept care from other adults. It helps them learn that the world is a place to be trusted. It helps them get ready for preschool. It is a growing experience for children and for parents, and it is a superb learning experience for the students involved. Two of us (S. J. R. and G. D.) got into this field through babysitting experiences we had as teenagers. Help others learn about ASD by sharing your child with them.

What about Your Other Children?

Carmen was losing a lot of sleep worrying about whether she was neglecting her other child, Justino. And she missed the time they used to have together before Teresa was born, just the two of them. She had so much fun playing with Justino. He made parenting so rewarding. Now everything she had to give—all her energy and all her time—seemed to go to Teresa. She missed time with Justino, and he was talking about missing time with her. She didn't want him to suffer because of his sister's diagnosis.

Brothers and sisters of children with ASD have special needs. Being sensitive to these needs will help all your children make a positive adjustment. Many studies have documented the concerns of brothers and sisters of children with ASD. Often they feel a sense of loss and loneliness when their parents' attention is consumed by their sibling with ASD. They may also experience feelings of resentment toward their sibling with ASD, and older children will feel guilty about feeling resentful.

Schedule Time to Spend Exclusively with Each of Your Other Children

It helps a sibling to spend some time alone with parents. This special time can be as simple as going to the store, washing the car, having a bath, or reading a book together. Use the time to listen to this child—to hear about friends, school, interests, problems, feelings. Let the sibling know how special he is to you and how much you enjoy time with him. Also, let him know that you know the child with ASD takes a lot of your time and attention, and that the sibling can tell you if he needs some time with you. Younger siblings may not be able to ask for time and attention, but they express it through their behavior or misbehavior (e.g., crying, clinging, developing fears, or misbehaving to get attention). The important thing during these times is for a sibling to feel that this is his special time, when your attention is focused on him.

Teach Skills That Will Help Siblings Interact in Pleasurable Ways with Their Sibling with ASD

Siblings may feel bad or rejected and unloved when their sibling with ASD won't play with them. Fortunately, research has shown that siblings can be taught skills that will help their relationship with the child with ASD. This can be helpful for all of the children. Help each sibling understand that ASD makes it very hard for children to learn to play, and that the sibling with ASD does not know how to play now, but that over time the child will learn. Teach siblings how to give simple instructions that their sibling will follow, how to engage in simple games, and how to reward the child with ASD for appropriate play. Be sure to help the child with ASD follow through. These simple interactions help promote a bond and social relationship between siblings. "Parallel play" activities where the siblings are all playing with similar materials—at the kitchen table with art materials, or puzzles, or snacks, should be encouraged. Be sure to include activities such as swinging outside on swings, playing chase, or watching a DVD together. These activities don't require the child with ASD to share or to engage in complex, back-and-forth interactions.

Talk about It!

Studies have shown that siblings benefit from talking openly and frequently about a child's ASD. A sibling may not understand why the child with ASD does not play and talk with her. When you explain what ASD is and how it affects social and language development and other behavior, the sibling will be less likely to interpret the child's behavior as dislike. As the sibling gets older, her understanding and perspective will become more like yours, with more and more questions and worries, so it is important to have an open line of communication about ASD with your children. Use words and concepts that your children can understand. Provide simple explanations and phrases that a sibling can use to explain ASD to her friends, so she has ways to deal with other people over the ASD-related differences that take the "sting" out of teasing or questions. Model this by letting the sibling hear you explain ASD to others.

Explaining ASD to a sibling will take different forms, depending on the age of the sibling. A preschool-age child won't be able to understand what ASD is, but will notice that a sibling is behaving differently. Elementary-school-age children are likely to be very aware that their sibling is different and to be embarrassed about their sibling's behavior around friends. Talking openly about these differences with your children from the time they are little will enable them to voice their feelings instead of being ashamed of them. If a sibling doesn't want to have friends come over, ask about it. See if there are ways you can help this sibling be more comfortable. Siblings may also worry that ASD is contagious or that they too may develop ASD. Siblings may feel guilty about their negative feelings toward the child with autism. They can even feel guilty that they don't have autism! Some wonder if they somehow caused their sibling's ASD. Talk openly with your child about these fears and worries so you can provide facts and reassure your child. You will probably have these conversations many times, because it is unlikely that your child will understand everything that you say the first time you explain it. Different questions and concerns will arise over time. Make ASD an open subject in your household. If your child never asks about ASD, it's most likely because it seems to be an unacceptable topic. Bring it up yourself, the sooner the better, and the more frequently the better. Ask your child what scares him about his sibling's ASD, what worries him, what makes him angry, what he thinks about, and how it affects his life.

Some siblings feel they must try to be "perfect" to make up for the child with ASD; they may feel pressure to achieve in academic or sports activities. The pressure may come from inside them, or it might be coming from you. Have your expectations increased for your other children because they do not have a disability? Not having autism does not make them "super-children." Help your child voice these feelings, and listen quietly, as you do with your partner. Acknowledge and restate the feelings rather than rejecting them, interrupting them, or denying them. (Some of them will be hard to hear, so be prepared.)

Your child may have some painful observations about you—about your absorption in the sibling with ASD; about the lack of family time; about your increased expectations for your child for greater maturity, responsibility, child care, household care, or emotional support. Listen! Take it in. Try hard not to deny, not to become defensive, and not to get angry. Listen to what your child is saying; provide the information your child is asking for; correct any misconceptions; and reassure your child of your love, your acceptance of the child's feelings, and your appreciation for the child's honesty and trust in you.

If your child's behavior has changed significantly (acting out, not seeming like herself for a long period, withdrawing from activities and relationships); if your efforts to talk to your child or provide more support are not helping; and if your child's functioning at school, at home, or with friends is suffering—talk to your child's doctor. Signs that a sibling may be having difficulty include these:

- Needing to be perfect
- Eating too little or too much
- Frequent complaints of headaches or stomachaches
- Loss of interest in everyday activities
- Frequent crying or worrying
- Withdrawing from social activities
- Increased aggression
- New problems at school
- Signs of anxiety or depression (see page 41)

Take Advantage of Books and Other Resources Specifically for Siblings

Increasingly, the special needs of siblings of children with ASD and other developmental disabilities are being recognized. Numerous books written about and by siblings, including those with ASD, are available. We've listed some of these at the back of the book (see the "Further Reading" list in the Resources). Also, look for special programs, websites, and workshops for siblings of children with ASD. These programs offer siblings an opportunity to talk with other children who have a sibling with ASD, and especially to share their feelings and concerns with other children who understand the challenges and rewards of having a sibling with ASD. The Sibling Support Project (*www.siblingsupport.org*) is a national program dedicated to the brothers and sisters of people who have developmental disabilities and other special needs. The project's website offers information about workshops, conferences, publications, and opportunities for siblings to connect with one another. Autism Speaks (*www.autismspeaks.org*) also lists resources for siblings in the "Family Services" section.

> *Studies have shown that being a sibling of a child with ASD can have benefits! Siblings often grow up to be people who have insight, empathy, and compassion; are mature, accepting, and self-sufficient; and are loyal toward their siblings with ASD and their families.*

Dealing with Your Extended Family: Help or Hindrance?

Extended family members can be among the greatest parts of a support system for a family with a newly diagnosed child with ASD, and they can also be one of the biggest challenges for young parents. If both your and your partner's families are there for you, supporting your concerns, aware of the evaluation process, sharing all the emotions that occur after diagnosis, providing comfort and reassurance—then rejoice! They are a strong part of your support system and will help immensely in the adjustment process. Provide them with all the information that they want and you have. Let them help you. Let them care for your child. Let them join you in appointments, meetings, evaluations, as you and they wish. The more the extended family shares the challenge of autism, provides ongoing love, support, and encouragement for you, and appropriate optimism for your child, the better the adjustment process goes.

However, extended family members go through all the same emotional processes that parents do. They may not want to see the problems your child has and may deny your observations. They may tell you that you're worrying too much, you expect too much, boys don't talk until later, an uncle didn't talk until age 3, or you're spoiling your child and doing too much for him. This makes it harder for you to move ahead, and young parents sometimes move away emotionally from their families during this period to get through it.

If this is happening to you, there are several things you can do. First of all, trust yourself and your partner. You live with your child every day. You are not crazy, you love your child, and your worries are real. Proceed as we have suggested, by calling your doctor. Don't feel guilty about distancing yourselves a little from your family members if you need to get through this. Tell them as much as you can about each step in the process so they know what is going on, but make the decisions you know in your heart are right for you and your family and child.

Second, turn to other people in your support system. Talk to friends and others who are sharing your concern and providing you with emotional support. Lean on them right now, so you don't feel so alone. You need support to get through this period, and the more support a young couple has, the easier the process can be. Third, ask others who are part of the process to talk to members of your extended family. Your service coordinator, a parent from the autism advocacy group, one of your child's therapists or evaluators, or your child's doctor may be very willing to have a family meeting and answer members' questions. It is much easier to have another person providing the information than to do it alone when your family is not "ready" for the diagnosis. Take others up on their offers of help!

Finally, continue as you need to for your partner and your children. Keep your extended family members aware of what is happening. You might provide them with copies of reports that people give to you, treatment plans, home programs. If they sometimes take care of your child, show them how to implement basic treatment routines that help your child. At some point, your family *will* come around to accepting the diagnosis and supporting you. However, family members all have their own timetables of acceptance and have to move at their own pace. Families come around, and seeing a child they love making progress is a big part of what brings them around. Occasionally some family member will not adjust to your child's special needs and may even undermine what you are trying to do. If this happens, it's okay to limit the time your child spends with this person until he or she comes around.

Taking Care of Yourself

Now it's time to talk about you! No time to take care of yourself now that you're devoted to helping your child with ASD? Ask yourself this: If you are tired, preoccupied, and stressed, how can you optimally care for your child—and the rest of your family? Even though you may feel like your needs come last, they can't, or all will suffer. Your needs are as important as your children's and your partner's, and you need to monitor and care for yourself—your physical well-being and your emotional well-being—daily, just as you monitor and care for everyone else, so that you can continue to do so.

Physical Health

We don't have to tell you what you've heard a thousand times before: Physical and emotional health are built upon adequate nutrition, sleep, and exercise, and these are even more important when you are faced with stresses, such as learning that you have a child with ASD. When you're caught up in caring for a child with autism, it's easy to make these fundamental healthy behaviors a low priority. It's easy to forget to eat until going through a fast-food drive-through seems like your only option. It's easy to pretend you can maintain your energy on 5 or 6 hours of sleep a night. And it's easy to forget how good you used to feel after a walk, bike ride, or trip to the gym.

So let's review the fundamentals. You know the importance of good nutrition—whole grains, lots of fruits and vegetables, low-fat milk products, lean meats, poultry, and fish, as well as nuts, seeds, and beans—for protecting you from illness, maximizing energy, and enhancing your mental capacities. How can you manage that for you and your family, when fast food, soda, and snack foods are quick when time is short? Try these ideas:

- Buy and put fresh fruit and ready-to-eat veggies out on a table or counter, to help you and your family learn to turn to fruit instead of rooting around in a cabinet for high-calorie snacks. Substituting fruit and veggies for some of the snacks and cookies doesn't cost any more.
- Try to eat home-cooked meals (not necessarily cooked by you!) as often as you can. Try to find a weekly time to cook, and when you do, make a big stew, or soup, or a big platter of grilled chicken to go in the fridge so you can use it for dinners for a few days. Buy salad ingredients and veggies that are already washed, cut, and ready to use. It may seem more expensive, but you will eat more veggies and end up with less waste (the most expensive food is the food that gets thrown out!).
- When others ask what they can do to help, ask them to make and freeze a healthy dinner for your family. It will make them feel better to be able to contribute, and it will help you with a big and important task—feeding yourself and your family well.

Are you uncomfortable accepting or seeking help from others? Asking for a cooked meal is a good way for you to get used to accepting the help that is offered to you and identifying the sources of support among the people outside your immediate family that you're going to need.

Sleep can feel like a rarer commodity than ever if you're occupied with your child all day and then kept awake by worries at night. Here are a few ideas for better sleep that you probably already know but might need help remembering:

- Consider your bedtime sacred. Go to bed at a reasonable hour, even if you feel that your to-do list is endless.
- Help yourself ease into sleep with things that make you sleepy, not stressed. Don't watch the news in bed, use your computer or phone right before retiring, or try to plan tomorrow's agenda in your head while you lie there. Take a hot bath or shower, read something innocuous, listen to relaxing music, or imagine the most restful moments of your life as you ease yourself into sleep.
- If you're suffering from insomnia, don't wait for weeks to see if it will pass. Talk to your doctor soon! There is much he or she can do to help.
- If your children are sleeping with you and you wish they were not, move them into their own beds. If you need help with this, consult your pediatrician or your child's team. There are also excellent books for parents on helping their children sleep independently and through the night.
- There are excellent self-help books available to you on improving adult sleep.

Consider your own nutrition, sleep, and exercise as part of the treatment for a family with ASD, rather than a luxury for you that you can't afford right now. Not convinced? Check out the list of benefits in the sidebar on the next page. Getting 20–30 minutes of exercise a day can improve your heart, your lungs, your sleep, and your mood. Here are some exercise opportunities that can work for parents with young children at home:

- Regular walks around the neighborhood with your child in a stroller
- Regular trips to the park with two adults—one watching the children and the other getting in a good walk, then switching
- Trading off times and days with your spouse to go for a walk or ride or to a gym or dance class
- Trading child care with friends so you can get in exercise time, maybe even as a couple

"I know I hated taking my daughter to the park. I was so worried about all the stares and questions about her behaviors or peculiar sounds. So I took baby steps to that point. I started with 5-minute stroller walks, then 10, then 15; then we found a nature trail; and finally we could end at the park for a few minutes at the end of our walk. The fresh air was good for all of us, even on days I didn't feel any energy to leave the house."

According to medical research, regular exercise can . . .

- Improve your mood
- Reduce stress
- Boost your confidence
- Prevent heart disease
- Increase your energy level
- Help manage your weight
- Promote better sleep

Research has shown that exercise can also ease depressive feelings and anxiety. One study showed that people reported feeling less tense and had improved energy after only a 10-minute brisk walk!

Emotional Health

Because you now have more responsibilities and challenges, paying attention to your emotional health is more important than ever. Emotional health has many facets: giving yourself time to deal with the emotional impact of your child's diagnosis; cultivating your supports; spirituality; and problem solving. We touch on a few key points here.

Dealing with Grief, Sadness, and Anxiety

Even when you are doing all you can to cope with the challenges of raising a child with ASD, you're likely to find yourself feeling waves of grief and sadness, depression and anxiety.

Grief. During the period after first learning that your child has ASD (or any other chronic medical condition, for that matter), it is not uncommon to experience a period of grieving. All parents form an image of their "imagined" child (often even before birth). But part of the typical parenting process is gradually coming to know and love our children as they are, rather than as we imagined or hoped them to be. The athletic father who imagined playing baseball with his son comes to accept and appreciate the child's emerging preference for music, and the musical mother who dreamed of singing in the choir with her daughter learns to play basketball with her when she shows no interest in music. However, when parents find out that their child has a long-term medical condition, such as ASD, their "imagined child" is changed very suddenly.

As with any other grieving process, it may take time to feel better. And even when the strong feelings of sadness subside over weeks or months, they may resurface temporarily, especially during events such as birthdays and holidays. Fortunately, these feelings don't supplant the love you feel for your living, breathing child. This is still the same child you loved and treasured before the diagnosis, with unknown potential and a future that has yet to unfold. Your child's learning, success, and happiness in life are as much in your hands as they were before the diagnosis. The future may look different than you had imagined it because your path is a new path, but there is still an unwritten future for your child.

Depression and Anxiety. Grief is a normal condition, and feelings of anger, sadness, depression, and low self-esteem are all part of the grief process. However, for some people, these feelings do not resolve but deepen into chronic depression. According to the National Institute of Mental Health, symptoms of depression can include difficulty concentrating, fatigue, feelings of guilt and hopelessness, insomnia or excessive sleeping, irritability, loss of interest in pleasurable activities, overeating or appetite loss, persistent aches and pains, chronic sadness, and suicidal thoughts. Temporary, mild to moderate depressive symptoms can feel debilitating for the short term while you are adjusting, and you will need the help of friends and family as you go through these first few weeks or months after your child's diagnosis. If, however, you find that your feelings of sadness, irritability, or anxiety are so intense that you cannot cope with daily life—can't get out of bed, do the basics, care for the children, eat or sleep, stop crying, or have images of hurting yourself—tell your partner and your closest friends or family members, and call your doctor and let him or her know what you are experiencing. Your family doctor will be able to help you by providing medication and/or a referral for counseling. These are *very helpful* for dealing with depressive and anxious feelings. Don't resist getting help. It is not a sign of weakness or being crazy. Everyone in your family needs you, and you need to be able to use your own personal resources to cope with your new path. Depression and anxiety can block you from using your own strengths and talents. If your chronic sadness or anxiety has lasted over 6 months, or if you have had thoughts of suicide at any point, we urge you to call your doctor and get help now.

Parents of children with ASD are more likely than other parents to experience anxiety, perhaps because of the worries and the unknowns that come with parenting a child who has this diagnosis. Anxiety has several faces. It may include constant feelings of worry and fear (generalized anxiety); it may trigger repetitive, irrational, upsetting thoughts (obsessions); it may trigger repetitive actions linked to coping with irrational anxiety (compulsions); and it may take the form of panic attacks, which to some people feel like a heart attack. If you find that one or more of these symptoms is becoming part of your life, call your doctor. Anxiety disorders are very treatable with medication and behavioral strategies. Again, both anxiety and depression can prevent you from having the energy and creativity to do what is needed for yourself and your family. By voicing these feelings to your partner and others closest to you, and getting help from your doctor, you will be much more able to help your child and family.

Building a Strong Social Support Network. Decades of research have shown that one of the most helpful things you can do to combat stress is to build up a strong social network. Building and using a network of family and friends *who genuinely care about you* will help buffer you from the negative effects of stress and give you people to turn to for help and support.

> *"Being in the special education field for 14 years, I thought I would be equipped to handle my daughter's diagnosis. I wasn't. What has given me great relief and peace is surrounding myself with other parents who are going through what I am going through. I network with families on the Internet; I volunteer as a walk chair at Autism Speaks; I engage with families through the local resource center. Helping other people and having others understand me have been a great comfort."*

Ironically, sometimes when a big challenge arises in our lives, we avoid turning toward our friends and family for support. We feel that others may not understand our problems, that they will be judgmental, that we are weak and should be able to take care of our problems by ourselves, or that we will become a burden on others. However, people who love you want to help you. It gives them an opportunity to show you that they love you. They will feel honored that you trust them enough to tell them about your feelings, fears, and problems and to ask for their help. It is a gift to a loved one to confide in him or her and ask for help. Give close friends and family the gift of being included. Few things feel worse than to learn that a person you love dearly has gone through a difficult time and you did not know and did not help. Give those closest to you the opportunity to be part of this new aspect of your life and your feelings. You will not feel so alone, and they will cherish being included.

Cultivate and nurture your circle of friends and family by staying in touch however it works best for you: phone calls, emails, Facebook, or social gatherings. If you find that someone in your inner circle is adding to your stress by being negative, critical, or judgmental, or by refusing to accept the reality of the situation, avoid spending so much time with that person. Turn to the people who help you feel better—by listening and really hearing you without denying or rationalizing, by boosting your confidence, by providing sound advice, by accepting you for who you are, by being trustworthy, and by encouraging you to engage in healthy behavior.

Do you have a strong social support network? Here are some questions adapted from the RAND Corporation Medical Outcomes Social Support Survey[3] that can help you assess your resources. For each question, consider whether this is true all or most of the time, true some of the time, or never true.

- Do you have someone you can count on to listen to you when you need to talk?
- Can you turn to someone to give you good advice in your current situation?
- Do you have someone to confide in or talk to about yourself and your problems?
- Do you have someone with whom you can share your worries and fears?
- Can you turn to someone who shows you love and affection?
- Do you have someone who hugs you?

If the answer was yes, all or most of the time, for many of these questions, then you have a strong social support network. If the answer indicates that you could use more support, keep reading.

Parents of children with ASD often find it extremely helpful to talk to other parents of such children. Other parents who are more experienced can help mentor you and provide invaluable advice and information. Most U.S. states have an organization called Parent to Parent USA (*www.p2pusa.org*), which is a national nonprofit organization that provides parent-to-parent support and training. Parent to Parent USA is committed to providing emotional and informational support to families of children who have special needs by matching each parent seeking support with an experienced, trained "support parent."

> **Helpful Tip**
>
> Building and relying on a network of family, friends, peers, and acquaintances *who genuinely care about you* will help buffer you from the negative effects of stress. If you don't currently have a strong support network or find it is difficult to turn to friends and family at this time, build up a social support network.

Another way of finding a support group of parents who are in the same place you are is to visit the Autism Speaks website. Click on the "Resource Guide" section under "Family Services." Then click on the state you live in on the map that is provided, and you will find a list of community and support networks, including support groups in your area. Support groups for parents of children with ASD and other special needs are often sponsored by local schools, intervention programs, churches or other religious institutions, and medical institutions. These

---

[3]Based on the RAND Medical Outcomes Study Social Support Survey. Available at *www.rand.org/health/surveys_tools/mos/mos_socialsupport_survey.html*.

are often listed in the newspaper and on the web. Try a computer search with "autism," "parents," and the name of your city as keywords; local parent groups are very likely to come up.

If you can't find a support group close to where you live, you can also consider joining an online social network. Autism Speaks offers the Ning Community, which hosts groups and discussion forums, as well as the ability for members to share information with one another within an active community of other parents of children with ASD. Another site sponsored by Autism Speaks is FriendFeed, which sponsors discussions and sharing of information about autism among parents and others concerned about ASD. To get information on both, click on the "About Us" tab on the Autism Speaks home page, and then on "Social Networks."

The bottom line is this: However you do it, cultivate and nurture a strong social network where you experience a sense of belonging, self-worth, and security, and where you can ask for and get help and support. Don't hesitate to lean on the people who care about you during your time of need. You, your family, and your child with ASD will reap the benefits both now and in the future.

Helpful Tip

The Autism Speaks website offers opportunities for forming a social network with other parents of children with ASD, including the Ning Community and FriendFeed.

Spirituality. Spirituality also improves emotional health and can help people cope with difficult circumstances. In fact, spirituality is now considered by many doctors to be an essential part of medical care. In 2001, it was reported that nearly 50 medical schools offer courses in spirituality and medicine[4] to new doctors in training. Spiritual practice can take many forms, including attending religious services, praying, meditating, doing yoga, taking a nature walk, singing, reading inspirational books, and listening to music. Because spirituality has been found to improve physical and emotional health, we encourage you to take a moment to identify things or activities in your life that give your life meaning and that provide you with inner strength and comfort. Then consider including spiritual activities with your partner as a regular part of your new journey.

In this chapter, we discussed some of the stresses and strains that come with parenting a child with special needs. We also want to emphasize that recent studies have shown that many families adjust quite well to having a child with special needs. Families are often very resilient and respond with strength and

---

[4]Anandarajah, G., et al. Spirituality and medical practice: Using HOPE questions as a practical tool for spiritual assessment. *American Family Physician, 63,* 81–89, 2001.

determination. They don't just survive the challenge but actually thrive. A review of studies on family adjustment by Hastings and Taunt[5] found that parents often had very positive attitudes about their child and the new situation they were facing. Parents reported that they derived pleasure from parenting their child and saw their child with special needs as a great source of joy. Learning to help their child gave them a sense of accomplishment and purpose in life. Parents sometimes reported that their marriage was strengthened. Finally, they said that having a child with special needs had led to a deeper awareness of spirituality and greater perspective on what is important in life. We hope that some of the suggestions in this book will promote resilience in you and your family.

To conclude this section, let's review the suggestions for taking care of your emotional health. These suggestions are based on studies[6] of parents of children with special needs who have developed effective strategies for coping with stress and have continued to thrive and experience happiness:

- ✓ Identify a specific goal or challenge and start working to achieve it. Research has shown that addressing stress by defining specific challenges and developing a plan for addressing those challenges helps reduce stress and create a sense of confidence and self-esteem. The goal could be as simple as spending 10 minutes of interactive time with each person in your family most days, or getting your child into an intervention program in the next 12 weeks, or finding a babysitter who can give you a night out once or twice a month.
- ✓ Take control. Studies have shown that stress results when you feel your life is unpredictable. You may feel that you have no control over your life right now—that everything depends on someone else—but that's not true. Recognize that you have some control over your life right now. Figuring out what you have control over, setting goals in those areas, and acting on them will not only solve some problems, but will also prevent you from feeling powerless. What if you make a mistake? It's not the end of the world. You can make a different decision. Think it through, look at the results, get some advice from people you trust, and if you made a mistake, then undo it and make a different decision. Mistakes are fixable. Action feels much better than doing nothing, and action leads to outcomes.
- ✓ Take a break. You may feel that you must spend every waking minute focused on your child and others in the family, but taking a moment to

---

[5]Hastings, R. P., & Taunt, H. M. Positive perceptions in families of children with developmental disabilities. *American Journal of Mental Retardation, 107*(2), 116–127, 2002.

[6]Murphy, N. A., et al. The health of caregivers for children with disabilities: Caregiver perspectives. *Child: Care, Health and Development, 33,* 180–187, 2007.   Raina, P., et al. Care-giving process and caregiver burden: Conceptual models to guide research and practice. *BMC Pediatrics, 4,* 1–14, 2004.

focus solely on yourself will help recharge your energy and help you keep perspective. Even if only for a short period, taking time to do the things that give you pleasure and are restorative will reap benefits not only for your emotional health, but for that of others in your family as well.

✓ Share caregiving responsibilities with others. Find others who can help with these responsibilities, whether these persons are family members, day care providers, other parents, or friends. Studies have shown that parents whose children participated in a day program that the parents trusted and had confidence in felt happier and were less stressed.

✓ Reach out to others. As we have discussed earlier in this chapter, establishing a reliable, loving, accepting group of people who care about you and are willing to listen and offer support is a key to maintaining emotional health. Research has shown that forming relationships with other parents who are experiencing similar stressful situations improves the emotional health of those parents.

✓ Pat yourself on the back frequently. Take a moment now and then to think about all you are accomplishing, and give yourself some positive feedback! Pride yourself on reading this book, seeking an evaluation for your child, balancing the needs of your family, and so much more you are doing. You will learn about inner strengths that you and your partner have that you had never seen before. You will experience joys that you never would have shared. You are on a different road from the one you expected, but it is taking you to new opportunities for learning, sharing, and building relationships. Jot down some of the things you are learning from time to time—to see where you have come and how you have grown in the face of stress.

Of course, you will need some new skills to build your sense of control and competence in your new role as a parent of a young child with ASD. We have written this book to provide you with skills that should help you in your new role. We hope the strategies you'll learn in Chapters 4–13 of this book will help you see what a difference you can make to your child with autism by building on the ways you already interact with your child during your typical routines, without having to add hours of work for yourself. Combining this with the experience-backed advice of the professionals who help you with your child's intervention program will give you the skills and confidence you need for the challenges of your daily life.

3

How Your Early Efforts Can Help Your Child Engage with Others and Boost Your Child's Learning

Terell, age 2, was recently diagnosed with ASD. His parents, Patricia and James, are meeting with the doctor who conducted the evaluation, and they mention that one of the most frustrating things for them is Terell's difficulty communicating. They find it very hard to know what he wants or needs and are always guessing why he is upset. Is he hungry or tired? Uncomfortable or in pain? If only he could just point to what he wants, instead of erupting in a tantrum that seems to come out of the blue! When his mother tries to talk with Terell, he seems to ignore her and often pulls away. Patricia and James are feeling helpless and frustrated.

No doubt you're having experiences something like these. In this case, the information in this book should give you some very useful tools to help your child with ASD communicate and learn, and in turn to lessen your (and your child's!) frustration. That's because it's based on decades of research and clinical practice with young children with ASD—experiences that have informed us about how and why good early intervention works. Your use of our techniques will be enhanced when you know what's behind the strategies, so this chapter is intended as a foundation for the rest of the book.

How Young Children Learn

In most cases the communication difficulties associated with autism begin very early, long before speech develops. Sometimes a child will begin to communicate, but then loses those skills in the second or third year of life. Young children with ASD are often unaware that messages can be sent between people, from one mind to another, through thin air, by using our eyes, body movements, and speech sounds. The child with autism sees these movements and hears the speech sounds, but doesn't know there is meaning behind them—a message to be read.

If you think back, you might have seen the beginnings of your child's autism when your child was still a baby. For some children, the differences in behavior are easy to notice; for other children, the differences are subtle and easily missed. Still other children with ASD don't seem to have any difficulties during their first year of infancy, but develop autism symptoms later. Studies by one of us authors (G. D.) examined parents' home videotapes of babies who later developed autism.[1] These videotapes showed Dawson and her colleague Osterling that by 8–12 months of age, these babies as a group spent less time looking at other people, responded less when their parents tried to get their attention (by calling their names), and did not use the early gestures (like pointing) that babies typically use before words develop and that help them progress into speech. Thus the way these babies experienced their environments was very different from that of most babies; they spent less time focused on other people and had much less experience with communication. This is important, because during the infant–toddler years a baby's brain is changing rapidly, soaking up information and being shaped by that information. Babies' brains are not fully programmed by their genes. The brain is developing quickly, and every experience a baby has affects his brain's wiring and builds more circuits that can carry more information, more efficiently. As scientists put it, there is a great deal of **brain plasticity** early in life.

> "I knew at 9 months of age something was going on with my daughter. I could leave her in her bouncer for hours, and she would just zone out and watch TV. What baby does that? She was perfectly content having no interaction with me. She would flip through books, watch TV, and had a completely flat affect. I knew at that moment my daughter was either deaf or autistic."

Language learning especially depends on brain plasticity. We are all amazed by the ability of very young children to learn languages—whatever languages are around them—and speak them like natives. In contrast, many of us have tried to learn a new language as adults and found it virtually impossible to sound like native speakers. This is one of the best examples of the special capacity for learning in the first 5 years of life. For young children with autism,

---

[1]Osterling, J., and Dawson, G. Early recognition of children with autism: A study of first birthday home videotapes. *Journal of Autism and Developmental Disorders, 24,* 247–257, 1994. See also Palomo, R., et al. Autism and family home movies: A comprehensive review. *Journal of Developmental and Behavioral Pediatrics, 25*(2, Suppl.), S59–S68, 2006.

beginning intervention as soon as we possibly can allows us to capitalize on the tremendous plasticity and learning ability during the infant and toddler years. The more progress made in the preschool years, the fewer disabilities children with autism have later.

> **By beginning intervention as soon as possible, we are able to capitalize on the tremendous plasticity of the infant period and minimize the disabilities that often characterize ASD.**

Research shows that early intervention increases children's play skills, their cognitive abilities (IQ), their speech and language, and their desire for social interaction. It increases their social abilities and decreases their ASD symptoms and their behavior problems. It helps them learn faster and participate better in all aspects of life—at home, at school, and in the community. Some studies have found that even the diagnosis changes for some children as a result of early intervention: Children who receive intervention may show lessening symptoms of autism. This allows many children to go on to a typical preschool, kindergarten, or first grade; develop greater conversational and play skills; and develop more complex peer relationships. Positive changes don't just happen for a few children who get early intervention. *All* children who receive early intervention benefit, though the changes are faster and greater for some than for others.

How Does Early Intervention Work?

Studies on infant learning have helped us understand why early intervention is so effective. Here are some facts about how babies and toddlers learn.

In the past 30 years, scientists have learned that even very young infants are highly engaged in learning and know much more than we believed. Young infants are like little scientists: They develop ideas of how the world around them works, and they test these ideas through their body actions and their senses. They take in information from all their experiences, and they use this information to improve their ideas about how the world works. For example, scientists have learned that infants have a rudimentary knowledge of physics, number, and other physical properties, and use this knowledge to experiment on the world around them. At birth, infants actually have the capacity to hear and produce all of the different speech sounds that make up all of the spoken languages in the world—a capacity that is lost over time for those languages a child is not exposed to (this explains why we have an accent when we learn new languages as adults). Right from birth, infants can recognize familiar voices and faces. They come into the world prepared to interact with things and people, and to discover and learn from the world around them. Because of the active nature of infant learning, it is important to consider the following:

- What opportunities for learning are available in the various daily activities of your young child with ASD?
- What kinds of activities does your child actively attend to and find rewarding?
- Does your child have the basic skills for learning from others, such as paying attention to others, imitating them, playing with them, and watching what they do?
- Does your child exhibit any problem behaviors that interfere with learning from others, such as frequent tantrums or overly repetitive behaviors?

The typical infant learns during every waking moment of the day. When she wakes up, she begins babbling and playing with her hands, or toes, or toys in the crib. She examines how they work, what happens when she throws the toys out of the crib, and how her parents respond when she coos or when the toys make a loud crashing sound on the floor. When she hears the crashing sound, she may call out, imitating the loudness of the sound. She remembers that the last time she made a loud sound, a parent arrived. Chances are that she notices the sound of Mom or Dad opening the bedroom door. She turns quickly toward that sound and focuses intently on her parents' facial expressions and words as they approach her. She's been awake for only 5 minutes, and she has already learned something about cause and effect, gravity, emotions, and words!

Now let's compare this child to a young child with ASD. She wakes up and also begins to play in the crib, but her play is different. She may ignore the toys and instead be fascinated with the way the light is shining through the crack in the curtains. She may tilt her head back and forth to experiment with the light, noticing how it changes with her head movement, watching her hand and fingers move in the light. She may spend a long time rocking her head back and forth, watching the light. She is quiet, not making many sounds. When her parents come to get her up, she does not look to see their expressions or turn to their voices. The light patterns still hold her attention. She too is learning, but instead of learning about toys, speech sounds, faces, and people, she is learning about patterns of light and movement. She has missed important opportunities for learning how to communicate, socialize, and play, because she didn't call for her parents or watch them come in and because the light was more interesting to her than the toys. Her long attention to the light and to the movements of her fingers and head has interfered with her attention to other learning opportunities available to her. Some of the key differences between most young children and those with autism are shown in the box on the facing page.

A central goal of early intervention is to help young children with ASD pay attention to key social learning opportunities like speech, faces, and gestures, and to "boost," or make more salient, their attention to people—their actions, sounds, words, and faces—so that the children can more readily make sense of the information that is essential for typical language and social development.

Some Learning Differences between Typical Children and Many Young Children with Autism

	Most young children	Many young children with ASD
Opportunities for learning	Engage in a wide range of learning opportunities by actively exploring both the social and nonsocial environments.	Tend to be less focused on the social environment, and more focused on the nonsocial environment; this limits social learning opportunities.
Rewarding activities attended to	Are naturally interested in other people, including their facial expressions, movements, gestures, and words. Find social activities very rewarding. Seem more interested in people than objects.	Are naturally interested in objects and explore them in unusual ways, such as smelling and looking at an object at an angle. Seem more interested in objects than people.
Basic skills of learning	Readily imitate what others do; understand that others respond to their movements, gestures, and sounds; use many ways to explore objects.	Don't readily imitate and understand that their behavior affects the behavior of others; tend to play with objects in limited ways.
Interfering behavior	Engage in some repetitive play, but easily shift attention to other activities.	Engage in repetitive play for long periods of time, and have difficulty or become upset when others try to direct them to other activities.

Developmental psychologists use the term *scaffolding* to describe the way parents aid their children's learning by drawing their children's attention to the most important learning opportunities in the environment. When parents scaffold their children's attention in learning opportunities, parents increase or decrease stimulation as needed, provide appropriate toys, repeat and exaggerate certain actions, slow and simplify their speech, and so on, so that the children can learn more readily. When you, as a parent of a young child with ASD, use early intervention strategies to scaffold your child's attention, you will use the same scaffolding strategies that other parents use, but you will build a stronger scaffold for your child—one that is tuned to your child's individual learning characteristics (his favorite activities, experiences, and sensitivities), as well as the learning challenges that are seen in most young children with ASD.

When you begin using specific early intervention techniques with your child, like those described later in this book, you will learn techniques for doing these things:

1. Drawing his attention to the people in his environment
2. Making social play more enjoyable and rewarding
3. Teaching him the basic skills of learning:
   - Attending to others' faces, voices, and actions
   - Imitating others
   - Using his voice and body to communicate
   - Sharing emotions, needs, and interests with others
   - Understanding that others' communications have meaning for him
   - Playing with toys in typical ways
   - Learning to use and understand speech
   - Reducing any behaviors that interfere with learning

With these special intervention techniques, you will be able to open up a world of learning opportunities for your child during the period when your child's brain is still developing very quickly, and this will maximize the impact of early intervention.

The Unique Learning Challenges Associated with ASD

Many studies have shown us the unique ways in which children with ASD interact with the world, and have thus helped us better understand some of the learning challenges associated with ASD. These challenges are what early intervention is designed to target. These are some of the common challenges to learning associated with ASD:

Attention	Rather than naturally paying attention to people, including their faces, gestures, and voices, children with ASD tend to pay a greater amount of attention to objects and other types of nonsocial information (lights, patterns, etc.).
Social motivation	Rather than frequently seeking out others for interaction and being motivated to share experiences with others, children with ASD may prefer to spend time alone, or to play near but not with others.

Use of gesture	When attempting to communicate, children with ASD often don't use gestures to share their experiences with others, such as pointing and showing things to others. They tend not to understand or respond to other people's communicative gestures, either.
Imitation and turn taking	Instead of readily imitating the sounds and actions of others, children with ASD don't often imitate others and don't often engage in back-and-forth toy play. It doesn't seem particularly enjoyable to them.
Toy play	Rather than exploring lots of objects and using them in creative ways, children with autism can often be overly focused on a small set of objects and repeat the same action over and over. They may become distressed when this pattern of play is disrupted by others. They tend to play alone with toys, rather than with others.
Babble	Rather than making lots of sounds and paying attention to other people's sounds, young children with ASD may be unusually quiet. They may make only a small number of sounds. Their sounds may not sound much like speech, and they tend not to use their sounds to send messages to others.
Arousal and sensory sensitivities	In contrast to other children, children with ASD may seem easily overstimulated or may seem underresponsive to various sensations. They may have unusual sensitivities to touch, sound, or light.

Why does a child with autism have these unique challenges? It has to do with how autism affects brain development. There are areas of the brain that are specialized for aspects of social learning, such as eye contact and emotional responses. When these areas are functioning properly, a child is naturally drawn to social experiences and easily learns language and social interactions. Research has shown that these key areas of the brain specialized for language and social interaction are underfunctioning in young children with autism. There also seem to be fewer connections than is usually the case between certain regions of the brain—such as between the sensory areas that are specialized for sound, vision, and touch, and the thinking areas that are specialized for comprehending and making sense of the sounds, sights, and touches we experience. This suggests that a child with autism experiences the people and objects in the environment but has difficulty making sense of those experiences, especially those related to social learning and communication.

Where do these differences in brain function come from? Science has shown that these differences in autism as a whole appear to be caused by a combination of genetic and environmental factors that influence very early brain development. The evidence for a genetic influence is based partly on studies of identical versus fraternal twins. Identical twins share all of their genetic makeup, whereas fraternal twins (and nontwin siblings) share half of their genetic makeup. If one identical twin has autism, the chance that the second twin also has autism is about 70%. In contrast, for fraternal twins, the chance is only 35%. So, clearly, genetic risk factors are influencing the cause of ASD. However, given that only 70% of identical twins (who share 100% of their genes) both have autism, other factors must also be playing a role. Research on environmental risk factors is still in its early stages, but studies thus far point to factors that influence fetal development during the prenatal period and around the time of birth. Such factors include older parental age at conception, maternal infections (especially flu) during pregnancy, birth complications (such as respiratory distress), and premature and/or underweight birth. These factors, by themselves, do not cause autism; they are related to higher risk of many kinds of developmental problems. However, autism may be more likely if there is already some genetic risk. For more information about the causes and other research on autism, we encourage you to visit the Autism Speaks Official Blog (*http://autismspeaks.org/blog*) and click on "Science."

Fortunately, as mentioned earlier in this chapter, the brain has great plasticity early in life. A great deal of brain development is still in the future for a young child, so by providing specialized experiences that stimulate social and communication development (like those described in this book) and using other kinds of early intervention, it seems possible to steer your child's brain development back onto a more typical path.

Young children with ASD are highly capable of learning. They form social attachments to their family members, and they respond well to teaching strategies that take into account their unique learning styles. Young children with ASD can overcome many of their challenges and become socially engaged, motivated, and creative learners. The remaining chapters in this book will show you how to help this happen for your child.

Parent-Delivered Intervention for Young Children with ASD: What Is the Evidence?

Over the past 20 years or so, many, many studies have shown the benefits of early intervention for young children with ASD when the intervention is delivered by trained therapists. For example, in 2011, the federal agency that evaluates the evidence base for treatments (the Agency for Healthcare Research and Quality) published a systematic review of early intensive intervention for ASD.[2] It included 34 clinical trials of early intervention in its review. The agency concluded that the evidence shows that early intensive behavioral intervention results in improved cognitive and language outcomes. One finding from many of these studies is that children had better outcomes if their parents learned to use strategies at home with the children that were similar to those their therapists were using in early intervention.

> *Studies have shown that parent-mediated therapies can increase children's nonverbal and verbal abilities and play skills, and can improve parent–child relationships.*

This makes perfect sense. Parents know their children better than anyone else; they are strongly motivated to help their children; and they spend more hours with their children than anyone else. Parents who scaffold their children's learning by using specific teaching strategies, in addition to the hours their children are receiving other interventions, are adding many more learning experiences for their children every single day. This should help their children learn more!

Lately, research has begun to look more deeply into the effects of parent-delivered intervention. Various studies show that parent-delivered interventions can increase children's communication and play skills, and can increase the amount of success and fun that both parents and children have interacting with each other. When parents learn to use intervention techniques at home, young children with ASD are more likely to remember and use the skills they have been taught by teachers or therapists. Furthermore, parents who use intervention strategies report feeling happier, less stressed, and more optimistic and empowered.

> *"Empowerment is key. I remember while working as a service coordinator before I was a mother of a child with ASD, we were going to fade an ABA in-home program for a 7-year-old boy who was making minimal progress over the years. His parents were panicking. They kept saying over and over, 'We don't know what we are doing—you are the experts, not us!' It is vital to teach these skills to the parents, as they will be parents for life and will need to be comfortable and proficient in teaching in a way that the child learns best. Parents cannot become dependent on therapists, just like children can't. We need to strive for teaching and independence at all levels."*

---

[2]Warren, Z., et al. A systematic review of early intensive intervention for autism spectrum disorders. *Pediatrics*, *127*, e1303–e1311, 2011.

A recent study conducted by two of us with a coworker[3] looked at how parents learned the intervention techniques included in this book and how their children benefited from them. The study involved eight families of 1- and 2-year-olds with ASD who had just been diagnosed. The families volunteered for a parent intervention program of 12 weekly sessions lasting 1 hour each. Parents learned to use a number of teaching techniques that focused on building their children's attention, communication, social interactions, and play. The parents learned to do these things:

1. Create fun and satisfying exchanges between their children and themselves
2. Help their children's language develop by emphasizing the social power of the early sounds that children make
3. Increase their children's nonverbal communication and imitation skills
4. Build up their children's interest in a wide range of toys, and skills in social toy play

Parents learned to use these intervention techniques during their typical playtimes at home and during their typical caregiving routines. Parents did not create hours of special teaching time. These were working parents who already spent as much time as they had taking care of their children and playing with them. They learned to use their existing time with their child in a more focused way.

Were parents able to learn the intervention techniques? Yes! The study actually found that even before they were taught the techniques, parents naturally used many of these techniques between 40% and 60% of the time during their typical play activities with their children. However, *after only a few hours of coaching and a few weeks of using the techniques at home, most of the parents were using the techniques over 90% of the time.*

The study then examined how parents' use of the techniques affected the

> "The thing that I liked most about this approach is that it felt so natural, like high-quality play that all parents would want to do with their child. Once I learned the basics, it felt easy to incorporate them throughout everything. This provided many, many opportunities for learning, while also giving us new ideas for creative ways to have fun together. Instead of being overwhelming and draining, it was fun and easy. I could see my son respond, which was motivating and encouraging."

---

[3]Vismara, L. A., et al. Can one hour per week of therapy lead to lasting changes in young children with autism? *Autism, 13*, 93–115, 2009.

children. Before parents began to learn the techniques, the children in the study were using almost no word-like sounds. However, once the parents started to use the intervention techniques regularly at home, most of the children began to try to say words to communicate, not just to imitate or echo. The same thing was found for children's imitation. It increased steadily once parents started to use the intervention techniques at home.

Furthermore, parents were just as skilled as therapists in helping their children learn to use words and imitate. This shows that parents who learn to use intervention skills can be as effective as trained therapists in teaching their children critical new learning skills and scaffolding their children's use of their new skills.

There are several different parent-delivered intervention programs available to the public, and several of these are currently being studied in ongoing research. Some examples include Hanen More than Words; the Early Start Denver Model; Pivotal Response Training; Responsive Teaching; and Social Communication, Emotional Regulation, and Transactional Support (SCERTS).

In this book, we describe a set of easy-to-use strategies that parents and other caregivers can use throughout their regular daily activities with their children to help their children engage, communicate, and learn. You can use these strategies during playtime, bathing, mealtimes—really any time you are with your child. This ensures that, like typical children, your child with autism is learning every minute of the day, not only while participating in an intervention program. The strategies we offer in this book are based on the Early Start Denver Model.[4] They focus on helping children become actively engaged in learning and communicating by building up their core social learning abilities: imitation, sharing attention, initiating communication with gestures, using their voices and bodies to talk, and learning to play with other people in varied ways with toys. The strategies we offer in this book are ones that help parents and other caregivers (and therapists as well!) develop these skills by being play partners with their children during child-preferred play activities and during typical caregiving routines. Parents and their children develop joyful, back-and-forth play during these activities and routines. The strategies we will teach you will help you find fun play activities that both you and your child enjoy. We will teach you how to scaffold your child's attention and learning during play and caregiving activities by following your child's interests and helping your child experience more learning opportunities. In the remaining chapters of this book, we go through these intervention techniques, one by one, for you.

However, before we end this chapter, let's review some of the key points that we have covered here:

---

[4]Rogers, S. J., and Dawson, G. *Early Start Denver Model for young children with autism*. New York: Guilford Press, 2010.

- The brain is very plastic during early development and is shaped by learning experiences. As learning occurs, connections between brain cells are formed.

- Infants actively explore the world, develop ideas about how the world works, and test to see if their ideas are correct.

- Typical infants are learning during almost every waking moment and spend most of their time interacting with people. Children with autism tend to spend less time focusing on people and more time focusing on objects than other children do. This limits their opportunities for social learning and communication.

- Parents can help their child with ASD learn by drawing their child's attention to important learning opportunities by exaggerating their actions and speech and providing appropriate toys, which is called *scaffolding*. This helps provide many learning opportunities.

- Early intervention with young children with autism can improve learning, play, communication, and social abilities. It can also help with problem behaviors, such as tantrums and aggression.

- Studies have shown that children with autism are emotionally attached to their parents and other members of their families but may demonstrate this in different ways than typical children.

- Children with autism have trouble talking and have difficulty using gestures and facial expressions to communicate their needs and wishes to their parents. They usually need to be taught how to use gestures such as pointing.

- Children with ASD don't readily imitate others, but they can be taught to imitate, which opens the door to learning about others.

- Although children with autism are drawn to objects, they may not be adept at playing with toys in varied and appropriate ways. They may be very good at operating their toys, but their play with toys tends to be overly repetitive. Intervention helps them learn to play with lots of toys in functional, social, and creative ways.

- Parents can learn to use intervention strategies with their children; in fact, they are able to master the techniques as well as trained therapists.

- Children whose parents use intervention strategies at home tend to retain the skills they learned. When parents use intervention strategies at home, this reinforces their children's learning in other intervention programs, so children are able to remember the skills they have learned and use them in many different settings.

- Parent-delivered interventions can help parents feel happier, less stressed, and more optimistic. When parents learn to use intervention strategies with their children, they have a more positive outlook, feel empowered, and are less likely to be depressed.

- Parent-delivered interventions don't require special equipment and hours of special "teaching" time spent working with a child. The materials required for carrying out interventions at home are simple toys and other play materials. The strategies are carried out during everyday activities, such as bath time, meals, and indoor and outdoor play.

- Most parent-delivered interventions stress the importance of positive emotions and a happy relationship between parents and children for promoting learning. Studies have shown that the parent–child social relationship is the foundation for learning and communicating.

Part II

Everyday Strategies
to Help Your Child Engage,
Communicate, and Learn

4

Step into the Spotlight

Capturing Your Child's Attention

> **Chapter goal:** To teach you how to increase your child's attention to you, so that your child's opportunities to learn from you will increase. Learning requires paying attention to people.

Why Your Child's Attention to Others Is So Important

There are many things that young children cannot do yet, but one thing they do very well is pay attention to their environment and learn from what they see. Babies see fairly well very soon after birth, and they learn a lot about the world, people, and objects around them by watching objects and people in action. They are also surprisingly good at seeing patterns in the actions of people and objects around them. They learn to expect people to move and act in typical ways and are surprised and intrigued by unexpected events. In fact, they pay more attention to the unexpected than to the routine and predictable so that they can figure out new things.

Watching and listening to people are very important learning activities for young children—perhaps the *most* important learning activities, because they learn so much from interacting with other people. Most babies and toddlers prefer watching people and interacting with them over any other activity. Their brains are wired in such a way that looking at and interacting with other people are the most pleasurable activities of all (assuming that they are not hungry, fatigued, or uncomfortable).

What's Happening in Autism?

However, young children with autism spectrum disorders (ASD) do not show as strong an interest in watching and interacting with people as other children do. Why would that be? There are two different possible explanations that you may read about. One suggests that children with autism have more difficulty than others understanding complex and unpredictable sights and sounds. Social interactions are certainly complex and sometimes unpredictable: They require a young child to make sense of facial expressions, speech, sounds, and gestures. Objects, on the other hand, are more predictable and generally less complex than people. When a young child acts on an object, it tends to respond in a reliable and predictable way. The child can make the object repeat the same action over and over. People act spontaneously and more variably than objects; they do not respond the same way every time. People who are trying to engage a young child can sometimes be very stimulating. They may speak very quickly and with a lot of emotion, creating a lot of sounds for the child to process at once. People may also move and gesture during interactions, talking with their hands and changing their facial expressions quickly to fit the mode and tone of the conversation. All of this information may be at times too stimulating for the child, whose response in such instances may be to fuss or to withdraw. This used to be a very popular way of understanding autism, but research suggests that this view is not the most accurate way to understand young children's decreased attention to others.

The other line of thinking suggests that young children with autism are less tuned in to others from the start. This line of reasoning begins with the finding from scientists that children typically come into the world built to favor watching and interacting with people over anything else. As with any other trait, some children have less of this built-in "attraction" than others. In autism, this innate preference for people seems to be lessened. Because people are not so interesting, the physical world may compete more strongly for their attention than it would in a child who has a very strong built-in attraction for people. Notice that the end result of both of these theories is that children with autism find interacting with objects somewhat more interesting, and interacting with people somewhat less interesting, than most children do.

Why Is It a Problem?

When young children don't pay much attention to the people caring for them, they miss out on very important learning opportunities. Children need to attend to everything that other people do—their physical movements, body language, facial expressions, and words—in order to learn. What very young children learn about communication, emotions, language, and social interaction comes from having lots of individual experiences with watching, imitating, and interacting with people. If they're not spending much time tuned in to their parents or others—that is, if they're not spending a lot of time focused on others' faces, voices, and actions—their learning may be slowed, especially their learning about social communication and play. To increase their rate of learning, their attention to other people has to increase. Attention throws a spotlight on others that lights

"As a parent, this was the single most motivating part of the [Early Start Denver Model] approach. It makes sense that a child can make better progress if taught to pay more attention to others as early as possible, giving more chances to learn things through those observations. Additionally, it's encouraging to work with a child who is looking at you and paying attention. Of all of the things that I learned, the techniques in this area were the ones that I used the most and found the most helpful."

them up and highlights their actions, speech, and emotions, which are so critical for social learning. *In short, more attention to others equals more opportunities to learn from them.*

⇒ What You Can Do to Increase Your Child's Attention to People

How can you as a caregiver step into your child's attentional spotlight? There are five specific steps you can carry out to increase your child's attention to you:

Step 1. Identify what is in the spotlight of your child's attention.

Step 2. Step onto the "stage"; take your position.

Step 3. Eliminate the competition.

Step 4. Identify your child's social comfort zone.

Step 5. Join in by following your child's lead.

In the following pages, we describe how to carry out each of these steps, give you some ideas for activities to try, and suggest what you can do to solve problems that may come up.

Step 1. Identify What Is in the Spotlight of Your Child's Attention

Most young children with ASD are interested in objects and toys, and spend much of their time manipulating and playing with them. If this is true for your child, then it will probably be easy for you to find interesting materials for play. Young children are often very motivated to obtain objects, to handle favorite objects, to create interesting effects with objects, and to get help with objects they enjoy. Most also enjoy lively physical games their parents create—roughhousing, moving in time to music, running, bouncing, and swinging. By including materials that relate to your child's interests and preferences (whether it be a favorite toy such as trains, a favorite cartoon character, or a preferred activity such as tickling), you can create learning situations in which your child is likely to attend to you and interact with you, thus learning from you. In addition, building social interactions into your child's interest in specific objects will allow you to increase your child's social skills. Social interactions will become linked with favorite activities and become more rewarding for your child.

Rationale. Highly appealing materials and play activities motivate children to interact with their parents. A motivated child is a happy child, attentive to his parents and ready to learn. Strong motivation supports active learners rather than passive observers, and active learners show initiative and spontaneity—two important characteristics to nurture in young children with autism. A motivated child also wants to continue an activity, which gives you as the parent the chance to embed many learning opportunities into the activity. The longer the activity goes on, the more learning opportunities you can create. This is why you want to know what objects and activities your child really enjoys—so you can create learning opportunities for your child. The following activity will give you tools for identifying your child's preferred activities and materials. The questions will help you focus your own attention on your child's attentional spotlight.

 ## Activity: *Figure Out What Your Child Likes*

Spend time over the next few days really observing your child during the following six types of activities:

1. Toy or other object play
2. Social play
3. Meals
4. Caregiving (bathing/changing/dressing/bedtime)
5. Book activities
6. Household chores

Here are some ideas for learning about what your child is interested in and paying attention to:

● In each of the six types of activities just listed, notice what your child is interested in and pays attention to. For each one, make a list of the objects, materials, toys, or physical games that your child seems to seek out and enjoy. (We have provided a form for you to keep your list right in this book, if you want to. It's on page 89.) If your child does not naturally seek out objects or physical games, set out a few materials or toys, and encourage your child to manipulate or play with them to see what your child might like.

● Next, answer these questions from your observations of your child when he is engaging in the activities listed above. For each of the six activities:

  - What objects or activities does my child search for?
  - What objects does my child like to watch, grasp, or hold?
  - What activities does my child come to me or another family member for help with or to do?
  - What makes my child smile and laugh?
  - What calms my child when upset or cheers my child when cranky?

● If your child does not have much interest in traditional play objects, then focus on your child's response to other daily activities. There are very few young children who do not approach anything or anyone or who do not act on any objects without being guided. It happens, but it's very rare. When your child moves independently, what is she moving toward or away from? When your child touches or holds anything, or watches anything, what is it? When you physically play with your child—tickle, cuddle, squeeze, spin around, whatever games you play—what are your child's reactions? What does she seem to enjoy?

● Sometimes children's favorite objects are rather unusual for their age or are used in a repetitive, limited manner.

> *For instance, 26-month-old Pablo spends his day with the TV remote in his hand. He keeps the TV on and switches channels as he stands in front of the TV or lies on the couch. Most of his awake time is spent in front of the TV, and efforts to turn it off or to take the remote away from him lead to big tantrums.*

"One mistake I made was trying to get more and more interesting toys, hoping my son would learn to play with them if I found something that caught his attention. It was much easier and more effective to take whatever he was using as a toy and create a game around that. We developed games as simple as 'Tickle the body part with a duster' that were great fun and much more effective than imploring my son to meet his goals by obediently pointing to a body part on command. Some of my son's favorite games included 'Spin!' (being held while we went in circles), bouncing in and out of the crib, and running cars around. All of these built simply on everyday activities and then let us add more and more learning opportunities."

Three-year-old Matthias likes to lie on the back of the couch and watch out the window, for hours at a time. He shows very little interest in toys, people, or any activities going on in his household, even though there are toys and interesting activities around, thanks to his 4-year-old sister and the family pets.

● Even if your child's interests are unusual, they are interests, and you can add them to your list. There are a few young children who are not very interested in any objects or activities. For these children, we will teach you how to create more social games (also called **sensory social routines**) or other types of face-to-face routines, and, later, how to build your child's interest in playing with toys. We describe strategies for creating those types of activities with your child in Chapter 5.

Summary of Step 1

If you have followed along and carried out the preceding activities, you will have learned quite a lot about your child's interests, preferences, and the objects and activities that capture your child's attention. See if you agree with most of the statements in the following checklist. If so, you are now armed with important knowledge about your child's attention—knowledge you will use for **Step 2**. If not, start experimenting to find out what your child likes in each of these categories.

Activity Checklist: What Does My Child Like to Do?

_____ I know a number of toys or objects that my child likes to play with.

_____ I know several social games (games without toys, like tickling or roughhousing) that make my child smile.

_____ I know some outdoor activities my child likes (playing on swings, walking, etc.).

_____ I know some objects and activities that help make my child happier when he or she is in a bad mood.

_____ I know some songs or sounds that my child likes to listen to.

_____ I know some activities or toys I can use while I am involved in meals or caregiving activities (meals, bathing/dressing/changing/bedtime) that can make my child smile or laugh.

_____ I know what my child likes to do with books.

What about Pablo? *As described above, Pablo's only interest in objects was holding the remote control. Pablo's mother initially offered a wide selection of toys to see* *whether he would trade the remote control for another item she offered, but he didn't seem to care about the other objects. Instead, Mom started thinking about what effects or actions she might use to capture his attention herself. She had seen Pablo smile briefly when tickled by his older sister, so she tried that first. To her surprise, Pablo laughed. She didn't worry at this point about taking the remote control out of his hands; instead, she held up her hands and wiggled her fingers each time she said the word "tickle." Pablo didn't pull away, but in fact leaned in toward his mother in anticipation of the next tickle. As Pablo relaxed into the game, he loosened his grip on the remote control and his mother was able to gently take it out of his hand while continuing to tickle him. Once out of his reach, she placed it behind her so it would remain out of sight and not distract him from the game.*

Pablo's mother also found other ways to tickle him, such as blowing raspberries on his neck and belly. She showed him how to pull up his shirt before tickling him on his belly, and she made sure to respond right away each time Pablo did this. When Pablo tired, she offered other objects he might want to hold and showed him how they operate, such as banging the wooden spoon on the table or pushing the buttons on a toy phone. With the remote control out of sight, Pablo was more open to exploring new things. He still tended to repeat the same action with the object, but now Mom knew she could get him away from the remote control and engage him in activities more appropriate for learning.

What about Matthias? *Matthias was the child who had very little interest in objects. He preferred to lie on the back of the couch and look out the window most of the time. His dad could not figure out how to interest him in his toys, and after each attempt Matthias returned to the couch. So Matthias's dad tried a different approach to interact with Matthias. The next time Matthias walked toward the couch, his dad lifted him up and dropped him onto the couch. He repeated this game a few times— helping Matthias climb off the couch, lifting out his arms to pick Matthias up, and dropping him onto the couch. Now Matthias started to understand the game, and, after falling, he walked over to Dad to be picked up and dropped again.*

In trying to figure out what Matthias enjoyed, his dad realized that Matthias enjoyed more than just the couch, and smiled and came back for more when he was tossed into the air. So Dad experimented a little with some other "movement" games. He found that Matthias loved being flipped up onto his shoulder and "airplaned" around the room, loved being bounced actively on the big exercise ball; loved having his dad flip him onto the bed and push on his chest with a pillow; and loved being dried roughly after his bath with a big towel and a lot of action. During these kinds of activities, Matthias was much more likely to laugh, smile, look at Dad, and pull on Dad to repeat the game.

Matthias's dad discovered that he could also bring a stuffed animal into these physical games on the bed and use the stuffed bear to tickle and push. Matthias would reach out to the bear for more play—the first interest he had shown in his stuffed animals. Matthias enjoyed it when Dad sang, "Head, shoulders, knees, and toes," as he dried those body parts with a towel. And he enjoyed it when Dad stood in front of him, instead of behind, to swing him at the park, swinging him strongly and then catching him in his arms. Matthias would laugh, wiggle, and look at Dad expectantly for the next push. Dad's detective work and experimenting have helped him identify many activities that Matthias enjoys.

Step 2. Step onto the Stage; Take Your Position

Rationale. Social communication occurs especially through eyes, faces, and bodies. We want children to look at us; to make repeated eye contact; and to have clear views of our faces, expressions, gaze patterns, and mouths as we talk. In general, having children sit down when we play with them helps us get in their spotlight or focus of attention. Sitting down helps focus your child's attention, because the chair provides support and keeps your child from moving away easily. Sitting in front of your child to read a book or play with a toy may seem like an odd way to position yourself, but holding a child in your lap to read won't allow you to engage in face-to-face interaction and limits social exchange. Once you get used to reading books and playing in front of your child, it will become a habit, and you won't have to think about it any more. If you use a bean bag chair or any chair that has arms and provides support, your child will be more likely to stay focused on the interactive activity.

> *"Think of yourself as a preschool teacher, not Grandma. You need to get the child's attention, not cuddle during this time."*

♟ Activity: *Find Positions That Put You in the Spotlight*

When you are playing with or caring for your child, start to position yourself in such a way that your child has a very clear view of your face and eyes. As much as possible, try to be close up, on the same level, and face to face with your child during both play and caregiving activities. We can't overemphasize the **importance of positioning** to increase your child's attention to people and learning opportunities.

Here are some ideas for positioning yourself and your child so that learning occurs more easily:

- Positions in which your child is lying down on his back and you are seated while leaning over him are wonderful for social games, finger plays, and little songs and routines. Diaper-changing time, whether on the changing table or on the floor, is a great time to be positioned face to face and to talk to your child and sing some little songs or finger games as part of the diaper change.

● Sitting on the floor with your legs out in front of you, with your child on her back on top of your legs or between them, is also a great position for tummy tickles or creepy fingers and for playing social games like "This Little Piggy," peekaboo, pattycake, "Round and Round the Garden," and "Where Is Thumbkin?"

● Physical play routines on your bed or a couch provide excellent face-to-face positioning, both when the child is lying down and when the child is standing.

● Seat your child on your lap, facing you, or on a small chair, bean bag chair, high chair, or corner of a living room chair or couch while you are sitting on the floor in front of him. This is a terrific face-to-face position for songs, finger plays, toy play, and reading books, as well as for dressing routines (shirts, pants, socks, and shoes). Keeping a face-to-face position is easier when you use some supports—a bean bag chair or pillow for your child to lean on or sit against; a couch, chair, or your knees for your child to lean against; a small table or chair for sitting or standing play. Social games and even book activities can be carried out face to face, with the book held in front of your child, your hands pointing to pictures, and your eyes and face in front of and close to your child's face, ready to make eye contact, facial expressions, key words, and sound effects.

● When seating your child, make sure her back and feet are well supported, so your child is comfortable and can attend to you rather than in an uncomfortable position. Her back should be against the back of the chair, her feet flat on the floor. Think about right angles. In a chair that fits your child, your child's hips, knees, and ankles should all be at approximately 90 degrees. Feet should not be dangling in the air. For toddlers, a little stepstool is often a perfect height, and if you push it against the wall, there is also back support. Children (and adults, too, as you know from experience!) are more comfortable when a chair fits them well, and they will stay in it longer.

● Bean bag chairs are very helpful. We recommend them for all families. They allow you to seat your child in front of you with good support. Children also like to lie in them, and you can play many social games in that position.

● Some young children want to move so much that they do not want to sit for very long. However, standing can also be a good face-to-face position, and for this a coffee table or child table is a great asset. Many youngsters like to stand at a table and play with toys, and it is easy for you to go to the other side of the table and be there, face to face, to join in. It will help if the table is heavy, so it will not slide when your child leans on it, and it should be low enough that your child can lean against it at the waist and have arms free to handle objects and reach to you. Your position can be across from your child or at the corner, where the two of you can face each other across the corner of the table. Avoid playing with your child side by side; it's too hard for your child to see your face that way.

♟ Activity: *Take Advantage of Mealtimes*

Mealtimes in a high chair or toddler seat provide easy opportunities for a face-to-face position at the kitchen table, especially if they are set up as social times. It's tempting to have young children feed themselves while parents finish preparing food, rather than having a social meal. However, for children with autism, each mealtime and snack time at the table presents a rich opportunity to work on social attention and interaction.

Here are some ideas for increasing your child's attention to you during meals:

- Instead of giving your child the finger food on his tray, pull the high chair right up to one end of the dinner table and orient your chair so it is facing the high chair tray, so you can easily face your child and have a meal or snack with him. Place your child's food on the table, and provide a little on a plate for your child and a little on your plate for you. Have fun talking about the food.

- When your child has finished the small portion you gave her, offer more, but don't hand it to her until your child has signaled in some way that she wants it. It can be any subtle behavior—a brief look to you, a reach toward the food, a point, or a sound or word—but wait for your child to do something, and then treat that behavior as an attempt to communicate with you. Once you hear or see it, quickly hand over the food while saying something like this: "More? Sure, you can have more."

- Offer your child a bite, and then encourage your child to give you a bite by leaning toward your child with your mouth open.

- Place your child's cup on the table out of reach but within sight, hold it up in front of your child, and ask if he wants it before handing it to him. Put just a little in the cup, so he will quickly finish and need more. Then, when your child has finished it and wants more, offer another pour, but wait for that communication before you provide it.

● As the meal is ending, sing a little song or two with finger plays before you finish; help your child make a gesture that goes with the song by moving her hands through the motion. Songs are great language builders. Sitting face to face like this at the table is a great position for gaining social attention, and managing the food for the child brings your child's "beam of attention" to you.

Summary of Step 2

If you have followed along and carried out the preceding activities, you will have found a number of ways to step into the spotlight of your child's attention. See if you agree with most of the statements in the following checklist. If so, you are now armed with important skills for stepping into your child's attentional focus. You will use this knowledge for **Step 3**. If you have not quite mastered using these skills, start experimenting with each of these, one at a time, during play with your child until you have found some ways to accomplish them.

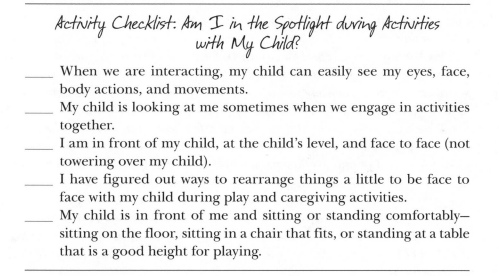

Activity Checklist: Am I in the Spotlight during Activities with My Child?

_____ When we are interacting, my child can easily see my eyes, face, body actions, and movements.

_____ My child is looking at me sometimes when we engage in activities together.

_____ I am in front of my child, at the child's level, and face to face (not towering over my child).

_____ I have figured out ways to rearrange things a little to be face to face with my child during play and caregiving activities.

_____ My child is in front of me and sitting or standing comfortably—sitting on the floor, sitting in a chair that fits, or standing at a table that is a good height for playing.

What about Pablo? *After completing the checklist for Step 2, Pablo's mom realized that she spent a lot of energy following after Pablo, rather than creating the right social zones for play. One of her habits was offering Pablo objects when he was walking away from her or not looking at her. She decided that an important step to help Pablo learn was rearranging the play area to make it a better fit for Pablo's size and focus of attention. She pulled the coffee table closer to the couch, so that when Pablo stood at it, his body was more supported by the couch. It was also an easy way to "wrangle" him in without forcing him to sit in a chair—a task that was difficult for Pablo except during mealtimes. Pablo also liked pillows, so she brought in some from* *the bedroom and propped them against the wall to create a soft, plush seating area without having to buy a bean bag chair.*

Finally, Mom thought about other opportunities throughout the day at home where she could create a better spotlight of attention. During dinner, it was difficult for her to remain seated, because her other children always needed things from the fridge or help with cutting their food. During the day at snack time, though, when she and Pablo were alone, staying seated was more manageable. Mom decided that she would seat Pablo facing her while she drank her morning coffee as a way to interact and engage with him.

She also realized that when Pablo became tired, he usually wanted to be held. She decided to hold him in her arms with his face looking up at hers, rather than seated with his back to her and maximize this face-to-face time by singing his favorite songs.

What about Matthias? *After completing the Step 2 checklist, Dad thought of more ways to enter Matthias's spotlight of attention. Since Matthias already enjoyed lying on the couch, Dad was able to lean over him and establish face-to-face contact as he started and continued more active games. Dad created other games to do on the couch that required Matthias to sit upright, such as bouncing on the couch, being lifted up for "blastoff" like a rocket ship, and falling forward and into Dad's arms.*

As Matthias sought out these games, his tolerance for sitting improved, and Dad introduced books to Matthias and encouraged him to look at books with Dad while seated on the couch. He made sure to add fun sound effects and exaggerated motions to keep Matthias amused. Dad also brought a child-sized table and chair into the family room, and gradually started placing a few books and other toys he thought Matthias might enjoy on the table. The two started transitioning to the table and chair when coming into the family room and before going to the couch. Over a few weeks, Dad was able to increase their time interacting together at the table.

Also, any time Matthias needed help that involved an object (taking something out of a container, opening a snack item), Dad took Matthias over to the family room or kitchen table and had him sit down before helping. Matthias started to learn about other locations in the house besides the couch where fun and enjoyable things could happen.

Step 3. Eliminate the Competition

Rationale. The physical environment can be a powerful pull for your child's attention. Observing your child will tell you what the attentional magnets are in a particular space. Video or computer images, mechanical toys, and moving objects can compete strongly with parents who are trying to capture their children's attention. You may need to control and engineer the environment so that you have less competition for your child's attention.

♟ Activity: *Notice Distractors and Manage Them*

As you join your child for a face-to-face play or caregiving activity, observe your child's attention and identify the objects in the environment that take your child's attention away from you. Once you notice one, take steps to minimize it.

Here are some ideas for managing distractors:

- During toy play, put loose toys away on shelves or out of sight, so that toys you are not using are not attracting your child's attention. Toys can go into cabinets with doors, into toy boxes, or even on open shelves covered with a blanket.

- Turn off the TV unless someone is actively watching it. Keeping a TV running is a powerful attention magnet for little children with autism.

- During playtime, try to turn off the computer and TV screens.

- During social play, if the environment is busy and keeps distracting your child, go into another room. A big bed is often a great place for social play.

- During bath time, give your child with autism a bath without others in the room (if it's possible), so you can engage more with him.

- During mealtimes, if several children are having meals at once, see if you can intersperse the food routines for your child with ASD (described earlier) with mealtime chat with your other children and adults at the table. However, don't feel that you need to feed your child alone. The social mix of a family table is a very important experience for your child, as long as she is attending to others as well as to food.

> "I found that moving toys into bins was helpful in many ways. Not only did it remove distractions, but it gave me opportunities to teach cleanup skills and to push for more words to ask for specific boxes and toys. Having boxes of different colors can help to teach colors, while having clear boxes can help to provide motivation to request the toys inside. My son was reluctant to ask for things, but would eventually request his favorite cars when he could see them inside of a box (helping us teach more and more complex phrases, although this would also help teach pointing skills)."

What about Other People?

When your child with autism is just beginning to learn how to interact and pay attention to others, having several people try to interact with your child at the same time you are trying to can be distracting. It's wonderful when several family members want to play together, but it's also important to think about your child's attentional spotlight. Children without ASD are highly skilled at switching back and forth between different people and activities, but children with ASD have difficulty attending to even one person, and you are actively working to build that capacity to help your child learn. Social interactions are the most important teaching tools you have, and you need to protect and increase your child's interactions and attention to parents, siblings, and important others. In the beginning, it will be helpful to keep the spotlight on one person at a time. If other people are trying to interact with your child at the same time you are, your child's attention will be diverted from you. When no one commands the spotlight, no learning can occur. So try to encourage everyone to interact one at a time with your child and not to interrupt your child's attention and interaction with another person in the group. Later, as your child's ability to pay attention to others improves, you should check to see if he can switch attention from one person to another and interact with both. This is an important skill too; it's how families interact as a group.

However, for now, here are some ideas to manage multiple interactions:

- Help family members understand the idea of your child's attentional spotlight and the importance of your child's focusing her attention on a person for increasing learning opportunities.

- Ask others to wait for a turn rather than interrupting the child's interaction with you. (This is just good manners, like waiting for a pause or an invitation to join in rather than interrupting a conversation between two people.)

- The same idea can be applied to other children who want to join in, as long as they are old enough to learn the idea of not interrupting others.

- "Turn about is fair play": when another person is engaging your child, be sure not to interrupt or vie for your child's attention. If you interrupt others and try to show them "how to do it," you risk discouraging them from interacting with your child. All the people who are in a position to interact with your child will find their own way to do it or will ask for help when they want it.

Summary of Step 3

If you have followed along and carried out the preceding activities, you will have found a number of ways to eliminate distractors and increase your child's attention to you and your shared activities. See if you agree with most of the statements in the following checklist. If so, you are now armed with important skills for increasing and supporting your child's attentional focus on you—knowledge you will use for **Step 4**. If not, start experimenting during play and caregiving activities until you have found some methods that work for you.

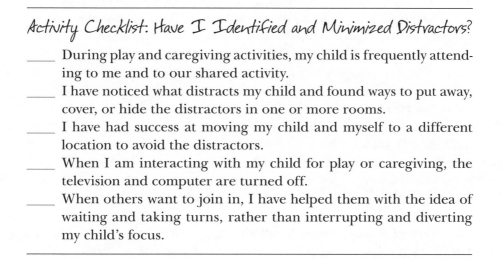

Activity Checklist: Have I Identified and Minimized Distractors?

_____ During play and caregiving activities, my child is frequently attending to me and to our shared activity.

_____ I have noticed what distracts my child and found ways to put away, cover, or hide the distractors in one or more rooms.

_____ I have had success at moving my child and myself to a different location to avoid the distractors.

_____ When I am interacting with my child for play or caregiving, the television and computer are turned off.

_____ When others want to join in, I have helped them with the idea of waiting and taking turns, rather than interrupting and diverting my child's focus.

What about Pablo? *For Pablo's parents, the remote and the TV were the distractors. As much as they tried to interest him in his toys or physical activities, his attention to the TV prevented them from stepping into the spotlight of his attention. However, they noticed that during bath time he enjoyed squeezing his bath toys and making them squirt water. He also liked it when his parents put shampoo bubbles on his hands and belly. They added a couple of bath toys that wound up and swam, and he loved these and handed them back to his parents to rewind when they wound down. They tried blowing bubbles toward him when he was in the bath, and he loved this too, batting excitedly at the bubbles and looking right at them with a big smile, waiting for more.*

His parents also found that Pablo enjoyed being seated on the counter to be dried off after his bath, and they began to "rough him up" with the towel, play peekaboo with it, and play games like "This Little Piggy" with his toys as they dried them off. His mother turned him around toward the mirror, and as he watched, she put her face next to his and made silly faces and noises in the mirror. He enjoyed this, patting at the mirror and then at her face.

All of these observations made Pablo's parents realize that he did enjoy playing games with toys and people, so they decided to take more control of the TV and remote. They made a point of having the TV off during meals, during bath time, and early in the morning. They also began to dress him and change him on the bed in the room he shared with his brother (instead of in front of the TV), first thing in the morning and in the evening before his bath, and they used these times for play on the bed. In addition, his dad sat with him at the table at breakfast, and his mother sat beside him at dinner. They took more control of his food and drink, giving him little bits so he needed to request them more frequently. They also spent social time interacting during meals—having him help pass things, having him give them little bits, and having him help wipe the high chair tray before he was finished.

Having the TV off during these activities cut down the amount of time Pablo was focused on it and increased his attention to them. However, Pablo still spent hours in front of the TV. Finally, after a few weeks, his parents took a huge step. One night, after he was asleep, they put the remote high up in a cabinet. They took more control of the TV, turning it on for 1 hour in the morning, 1 hour before dinner, and 1 hour in the evening before Pablo's bath. They set a kitchen timer at these times. When the timer went off, they plugged in and turned on the TV and reset the timer for 1 hour. When the timer rang again, they turned the TV off and unplugged it.

The first morning, Pablo searched and searched for the remote. He was very upset when he couldn't find it. His mother turned the TV on after breakfast for an hour, while she got dressed and ready for the day, and when the timer went off, she was ready with the stroller and his coat. She turned the TV off and put his coat on him immediately, and they headed off to the park. Pablo cried when the TV went off, but he was distracted by the trip to the park, which also provided some good playtime on the swings. When they got home, his mother changed him on the bed, then put him in his seat at the table for a snack, and she sat down for a cup of coffee. She provided some toys at the table while he was eating—a puzzle, a book—and she managed to hold his attention with these for more time than she expected. He fussed for the TV, but she just ignored the fuss, and after the snack they went into his room for some roughhousing on the bed and then some toy play on the rug.

This was the new routine of the household, and in a few days Pablo stopped

"My son never had great affection for television, but when he was 3 years old I found it useful in certain ways. I had big picture books showing objects, people, facial expressions, and other things that we used often to practice pointing. It seemed a natural complement to watch carefully chosen television segments and talk about what emotions the characters were showing, with comments like 'Is she happy?' and 'Which one is sad?' and, later, 'Why is she sad?' The reward for being engaged and talking was getting to watch a favorite show!"

searching for the remote and began to show much more interest in playing with his parents—with toys, at the table, and in the bath. Mom and Dad had worked very hard to figure out how to eliminate the competition from the remote and the TV, but soon realized that they couldn't actually compete directly with these powerful draws; they had to remove the competition altogether. They also had to put up with the fussing and crying that they knew would occur in the first few days, but by substituting other activities their son enjoyed, and getting him out of the living room, they got through the roughest part. And, day by day, Pablo adjusted to the new routine.

Step 4. Identify Your Child's Social Comfort Zone

Rationale. All people, including children, have different reactions to the physical closeness of other people. Some people need more social distance than others. Others love to be close. To attract your child's attention to your face and body, it's important to determine your child's comfort level with physical closeness.

♟ Activity: *Learn Your Child's Signals about How Close Is Comfortable*

You are going to carry out a little experiment here: learning from your child where he is most comfortable watching and enjoying your company. That space is your child's social comfort zone. Wherever your child seems comfortable looking at you establishes the right distance for learning for your child. It may well be that after a while, when you and your child have developed a number of familiar, enjoyable social routines, your child will be comfortable with your coming in closer. But it's not really so important how close or far out you are; what's important is increasing your child's attention to you and being close enough that you can still touch the materials and your child.

Here are some ideas for learning and responding to your child's signals about how close is comfortable:

- During the face-to-face activities you are using from Step 2, pay attention to how close you are to your child and how she reacts to your closeness. Most parents playing with a young child find themselves within arm's length of their child's face, able to touch their child's face with their hands. This is a natural place to be when talking to a young child and sharing play and emotions. Most young children with ASD can handle this level of closeness comfortably, though your child may need a little time to get used to a closer distance if it is different from the typical way you interact with your child.

- If your child shows marked head turns and looks away from you (this is called **gaze aversion**), back up and observe how your child responds!

Backing up goes against most people's instincts; the natural tendency is to get closer or to touch the child's face or do something to draw attention. However, some children need more distance to enjoy face-to-face interaction. If you see your child look away as you come in closer, then back up to where you were before the child looked away. See if you can resume your interactions without eliciting gaze avoidance. If not, back up a little more and try again.

● Some children are more changeable than others and may change their reactions very quickly during an activity. They may appear to enjoy your closeness during an interaction one minute and then suddenly shift to a less positive mood, even if the activity and your involvement remained the same. If your child's mood changes rapidly from happy to unhappy, or the opposite, or the child takes a little longer to "warm up" to an activity, you may want to move around a little. Think about what actions or effects your child may enjoy most about the activity, and show these to your child from a slightly greater distance.

Summary of Step 4

If you have followed along and carried out the preceding activities, you will have found the boundaries of your child's social comfort zone in several different activities, and will have used this to help your child attend to you and your shared activity. See if you agree with most of the statements in the following checklist. If so, you are now armed with important skills for adjusting your position to maximize your child's comfort and attention for **Step 5**. If not, please return to the start of the section, review it, and try again. Seek some advice from another person who knows your child very well.

Activity Checklist: Am I in My Child's Optimal Social Comfort Zone?

_____ My child is not actively looking away from me or leaning back.
_____ My child is looking up at me and my actions sometimes.
_____ I am in front of my child and close enough to touch my child and the objects between us.
_____ My child seems comfortable—playing with objects, smiling at times or focused on play, calm, interested, or happy/excited.

What about Matthias? *When we first met Matthias, his main interest was lying on the couch to stare out the window. Dad developed several physical, active games to* *interact with Matthias, but it still required a lot of effort from Dad to keep the inter-action ongoing. Matthias smiled and laughed when he was thrown onto the couch or "airplaned" around the room, but he did not always persist or actively seek out Dad to continue the game. Dad felt that he could at times take it or leave it. So how could Dad elicit more excitement from Matthias?*

To figure out this next step, Dad started to experiment with the social comfort zone to see how slight changes in his own positioning might affect Matthias. Dad started by observing differences in how Matthias responded when Dad's face was up close versus farther away while he was bouncing Matthias on the couch or circling him around the room. When up close, Matthias at times pushed Dad's face away, but when Dad placed Matthias down and leaned or sat back from him, Matthias tended to follow Dad with his gaze. Matthias's attention to Dad was most apparent when Dad took a few steps back from the couch to sit on the floor. Matthias got off the couch and ran over for Dad to lift him up in the air. Dad continued experiment-ing with the physical distance between himself and Matthias, and realized that for physical games, having more distance worked better. It seemed to ignite more effort in Matthias to seek out Dad and continue the game. This was the same for playing an airplane game or swinging him around the room. When Dad stopped to place Matthias on the ground and took a few steps back, Matthias was more likely to look at or lift his arms up in response to Dad's open arms than when Dad crouched down right in front of Matthias's face and asked him. The same was true when Matthias was tired of an activity. Dad saw that a little extra space helped him interpret when Matthias was truly finished with a game, because he did not pursue Dad but instead looked elsewhere in the room. Dad was then able to confirm that Matthias was "all done" with an activity and follow his eye gaze to the next play idea. Dad felt more successful in understanding his son's attempts at communication and in building more interactive games for participation.

Step 5. Join In by Following Your Child's Lead

It is very common for parents to interact with their child by creating a new activ-ity and offering it when the child is already attending to something else. The child with autism might be engaged in opening and closing a door or rolling a car back and forth, and when Mom or Dad interrupts to propose an unrelated activity, the child might ignore the parent or even become angry and upset. This can make the parent feel like a failure, or at least feel frustrated by the child's lack of attention or interest in the new activity. Instead of trying to direct your child's attention to something, in this step you will practice *following* your child's attentional focus.

Rationale. Following children's attention as a way of teaching them may seem "unnatural" or "backwards." We are very used to teaching by instructing and direct-ing our children. However, many studies have taught us that children, especially young children in the language-learning years, learn language more easily if parents and others follow their children's attention and talk about what the children are already attending to. Redirecting their attention breaks their concentration and runs the risk of losing it altogether. The following activities use the four main techniques that we employ in ESDM to follow children's attention. These are major teaching skills that you will use again and again as you follow these chapters along, so practice them until they come easily and naturally to you.

The watchword for Step 5 is this: "Where you lead, I will follow." Instead of trying to change your child's activity or focus of attention, try to *follow* your child's attention into her current activity and *join* your child in it. You can use the objects, toys, or activities your child is focused on to build an interaction.

♟ Activity: *Use Active Listening*

A great place to begin is with ***active listening***. You may know that phrase from other contexts, and if so, you know that it means listening, really listening, to what the other person is saying and working hard to understand the person's intended meaning. With other adults, we try to understand by listening and by asking questions for clarification, by restating what we have heard, and by giving supportive comments. When we are active listeners of a young child at play, we position ourselves in front of the child so it's easy to share gaze, watch what the child is doing to understand his goals, narrate his actions, make admiring comments, and add sound effects or drama (drum rolls, cheers). We might help the child—picking up a toy that has been dropped, pushing something closer that the child wants. We also might imitate the child's actions with another object.

This kind of active listening and commenting can occur in many situations with your child. It creates a situation in which both of you are sharing attention to the same thing, and sharing attention is a powerful tool for child learning. It makes language meaningful, and it puts you into the child's attentional spotlight—on center stage, engaging and responding to your child's play (without interrupting or changing your child's focus). Active listening can also help to *maintain* your child's attention to the activity, so you can add more learning opportunities. It communicates to your toddler: "I'm here, I'm interested in you, I see what you are doing, and I'm doing it too." As you join and follow your child and become more active—with comments, approval, sound effects, and mirroring actions—your child will attend more to you.

♟ Activity: *Narrate*

Joining your child begins when you share your interest in her activity by watching, smiling, nodding, and gesturing (***active listening***). It's easy to proceed from actively and approvingly watching your child's actions to *being your child's narrator.* As you watch actively, add simple single words or short phrases to describe what your child is doing. (The reason for using simple language is to help your child begin to hear individual words and associate them with objects and activities. If your language is too complex, then your child may not understand which word or phrase describes the object you're holding or the action you're demonstrating.) For example, if the child is picking up a toy train on the floor, you might say, "It's a train!" As the child rolls it, you might say, "Chugachugachug!" and help the child roll it. If the child pokes at the wheel, you might say, "That's the wheel!" The chart at the very end of this chapter provides ideas for narrating other kinds of activities.

> ### Helpful Tip
>
> If narrating doesn't come naturally to you, pretend you are a sportscaster calling the play-by-play while observing your child in play. Comment about the objects and actions you and your child are using as you play. Use short phrases! Have fun!

Describing your child's play without interrupting or changing your child's focus can help to maintain your child's attention to you and the activity while you provide opportunities for learning language. *Remember to position yourself in front of your child in such a way that your child can have a very clear view of your face.* It helps your child to be more aware of your attention and your speech.

Activity: *Offer Help*

Another way to increase your child's attention and engagement as you watch and narrate is to offer help. Hand your child toys during play or changing and bathing times after your child indicates an interest, rather than simply placing them within the child's reach. Name them as you give them. Hand over bits of food one by one, rather than putting all the food on the high chair tray during meals, while you are seated in front of your child and narrating what's happening. When your child reaches for an item slightly out of reach, say, "You want banana? Here's the banana," and hand it to your child. Or you can divide something into several pieces (like breaking a cookie into bits or handing over one block at a time). Using more pieces means more learning opportunities for your child to communicate with you and take in the words you say and the actions you do. Assist your child when he is struggling to reach a goal (like trying to stack a block), and make sure that your help is obvious to your child. Being the deliverer of desired objects and needed help makes you a part of the activity and helps your child attend to you and your language. Have the desired object ready, waiting and in plain sight, and deliver the object dramatically to be sure your child attends to you as you join in.

"My child never needs help!" Some children are so determinedly independent that they never seem to need help. If you have a child like this, you will have to engineer some situations in which your child needs your help. You can create a situation in which your child needs your help by sometimes putting a favorite toy or food item in a clear plastic baggie or a jar with a lid, so that your child can see and touch the bag or jar but cannot open it. Then you can offer help by extending your hand and asking if your child needs help, opening the bag or jar, and giving the child the desired object. When your child recognizes the object in the bag or jar, he may indicate interest in getting it and may look from the bag or jar to you and back, or make a sound while looking at it, or pat it with his hands, or hand it to you. Even if you're unsure whether your child wants the item inside the bag or jar, you can open it and give him the object. As you repeat this game over time with a few different materials, a game may develop.

You can also offer enticing toys with special effects that the child needs your help to produce, such as winding up a toy that spins.

Activity: *Imitate Your Child's Actions*

Another way of increasing attention to you and creating interactions is to *imitate* or *mirror* your child. While facing your child, play with the same toy or object, taking turns—or use a second identical toy or object to imitate her actions, so you don't have to take the toy away from your child. For example, if your child begins to roll a car back and forth, you might use a second car to roll back and forth, imitating the speed with which your child is rolling the car. Imitation can also extend to noises or verbalizations your child might produce.

Helpful Tip

Refer back to your list of actions, sounds, and movements your child performed when you observed the child's play. Either take turns with your child's toy, or use a second, similar toy to create these actions. Remember to narrate or give a label to the objects and actions you're using, keeping the language as simple and short as possible. If your child does not imitate you back, go down your list and try another action.

Helpful Tip

Some children may become upset when you first join them and handle their materials in play. They are used to playing in a certain way, and they may resist the change that comes when another person joins in. If your child reacts negatively to your attempts to join in, don't worry! Your child just needs to get used to your involvement. Reestablish facing your child within your child's social comfort zone, and use only the techniques of active listening and narrating for a few days. Stay with these techniques until your child seems quite comfortable. Then begin the next technique of helping. Stay with helping for a few activities, and then begin to imitate occasionally.

Positioning yourself in front of your child and imitating her will almost certainly attract your child's attention. If your child is trying to put a block in a box, hand blocks over one by one (helping), and also put some in yourself (imitating). If your child is banging a spoon on the high chair tray, get another spoon and bang in rhythm in front of your child, while saying, "Bang, bang, bang" (narrating). You are very likely to see your child's attention come your way. This strategy of imitating your child's play helps to *shift* her attention and builds awareness of you as a social partner. By joining your child's ongoing activity and narrating as you go, you are turning a solo into a duet.

Final Activity: *Mix It Up—Combine Listening, Narrating, Helping, and Imitating*

We have just discussed four techniques for following your child's interests and activities: active listening, narrating, helping, and imitating. These four techniques typically occur together when people play with very young children. Even though you have been focusing on one or another of the techniques as you were practicing them, you have probably found that you often used more than one at a time. Now that you've practiced each of these during your play and caregiving activities, take some time to practice following your child in many of your activities during the day. Do this with as many of the six types of activities listed earlier under Step 1 (page 66)—toy or other object play, social play, meals, caregiving (dressing/changing/bathing/bedtime), book activities, and household chores—as you can over the next few days.

You will probably have to make a conscious decision to practice during an activity (though this will become more and more automatic for you as you practice and see the results). You will get an activity going or join your child in an already-begun activity, and once you are positioned well, consciously begin to *follow* your child. Spend about 5 minutes in the activity, and at the end, take a few minutes to think about when you listened and narrated, when you helped, and when you imitated. Try to take some notes, perhaps by using the form on the next page. We have put an example in the form to show you one way that might be helpful. The example comes from 18-month-old Landon, playing ball with his mom on the living room floor. The form shows the ways his mother followed his interest in the ball and joined him in ball play without redirecting him. Read it through, and then imagine your child's favorite toy or object play routine. Think about how you could use narration, helping, and imitating with your child in that routine. Then think through a caregiving routine, like bath time. How could you use these strategies during bath time?

Summary of Step 5

If you have followed along and carried out the preceding activities, you will have found a number of ways to follow your child's interest into an activity and join

Combining the Four Techniques in an Activity

Example	Listening	Narrating	Helping	Imitating (you may want two objects, one for each of you)
Toy or other object play Playing ball	Looks at ball Drops ball Picks up and throws ball Watches while I roll it to him Lifts his arms up as I offer ball Drops arms down Catches ball I throw to lap Drops ball accidentally Ball goes behind him He gestures for me to throw ball to him	"Ball" "Bounce" "Throw" "Roll" "Up" "Down" "Good catch" "Whoops" "Oh, no" "Here it comes"	Gives the out-of-reach ball to Landon Roll to Landon to start game Roll it back to Landon Throw it into Landon's arms Hold Landon's hand to help him kick ball Hold ball so Landon can kick Fetch the ball from under the chair and give it to Landon	Landon's action with ball: rolling, kicking, or throwing Sounds or squeals Landon makes Gestures Landon makes
Toy or other object play				
Social play				
Meals				
Caregiving (bathing/ changing/ dressing/ bedtime)				
Book activities				
Household chores				

From *An Early Start for Your Child with Autism*. Copyright 2012 by The Guilford Press.

him or her without redirecting your child to a different activity. After you have carried out one of these practice activities, look at the following checklist and see if you agree with most of the statements. If so, you are now armed with important skills for increasing and supporting your child's attentional focus on you—knowledge you will use for the rest of the chapters in this book. If not, go back through the chapter again, following along and trying each new activity multiple times with your child over the next week or so. Take your time to master these skills. There is no rush! You and your child will both enjoy your interactions a lot more when you can incorporate these skills easily into your play.

Activity Checklist: Am I Following My Child's Lead?

_____ I followed along with my child's interest for a few minutes and did not try to redirect it to other activities.

_____ I was face to face with my child, and my child was well positioned to notice me.

_____ I watched my child's actions and narrated what my child was doing or looking at for a little while before I touched his or her toys.

_____ I joined in by imitating what my child was doing, including making sounds.

_____ I helped my child by making it easier for my child to reach his or her goals, by repeating the activity, and/or by handing over objects he or she wanted.

_____ My child looked at me from time to time.

Here is an example of "mixing them up."

Two-year-old Dominique and her father, James, are playing on the floor with toys. They have a bag of blocks in front of them, and as James watches (active listening), Dominique reaches into the bag and pulls out a block in each hand. "Oh, you like those blocks," he says (narrating), and James hands her another one (helping) and says, "Here you go," as he holds out his other hand. Then he says, "Here, Dommy, can Daddy have a block?" She takes the offered block and releases one to his hand. He has two and puts them down in front of her (helping), stacking them up and adding a few more to the stack. She looks at the stack, and he begins to add sound effects (whistles) and make a bigger "display" of stacking the blocks, hamming it up and making it a fun spectacle. As she watches him, smiling at his sound effects, he offers her another block (helping), and she puts one of hers on the stack and takes the offered one. He immediately puts one on the stack (imitating). James and Dominique each add blocks to the structure (imitating) while he narrates, "Another one, and another one, and another one," until they crash. He says, "Crash!" in a big voice (narrating), and they share looks, smiles, and laughter. Dominique begins to build the tower again, and he follows along, narrating, helping, and imitating, while the game is repeated.

In this example, James uses active listening, narrating, helping, and imitating to follow Dominique's interest in blocks. He does not try to change the activity or direct her to something else. He stays with blocks and follows her interests and reactions as he tries one thing and then another to see how she will respond. He is a great playmate! They create a fun game, and he has her full attention as he sits across from her, helping her create fun routines with the blocks. Her attention lasts a long time, and they have lots of back-and-forth interactions with the blocks, each one a learning opportunity for her. She has not stacked blocks before—look at how fast she learns this from him!

Chapter Summary

We have been discussing ways to increase your child's attention to you and foster face-to-face interaction. **Watching** your child to see what he is paying attention to will tell you where the spotlight of his attention is falling, so you can join your child on the stage, inside that spotlight. **Carefully positioning yourself,** so that you and your child are facing each other without too much distance between you, gives your child a very clear opportunity to look at your eyes, face, and expressions and to learn about all the social information that comes from faces. Although at first this may seem awkward, you will find that it becomes easier and easier with practice. This kind of face-to-face interaction is great for play, but it will also help you provide many more learning opportunities for your child during daily activities. Remember the six main activities described for Step 5 (toy play, social play, meals, caregiving, book activities, and household chores), and try to use these techniques in each of them.

We have also described some ways to increase your child's attention to you during activities. The most important of these are the **"big four."** The first two of these are **(1) active listening** while interacting with your child, by watching what she does and commenting on it; and **(2) narrating her activities** in short phrases and single words, while joining in and following rather than trying to redirect or interrupt your child's activities. We have added the activities of **(3) helping** and **(4) imitating** as other important ways of joining your child and increasing your child's attention to you. We know that it is more natural for some parents than for others to chat and interact with their young children face to face during caregiving and play routines. For young children with autism, increasing the amount of time they have people inside their spotlight of attention is absolutely crucial to their progress. You will be joining your child in things that your child already loves to do, and joining a happy child is a fun activity for most parents. Have fun practicing these steps!

Games, Activities, and Objects That My Child Enjoys

Activity	Objects	Physical games/ social interactions	Sensory play
Toy or other object			
Social play			
Meals			
Caregiving (bathing/dressing/ changing/bedtime)			
Book activities			
Household chores			

From *An Early Start for Your Child with Autism.* Copyright 2012 by The Guilford Press.

Refrigerator List

Goal: To increase your child's attention to you.

Steps:

✓ Identify your child's attentional spotlight.

✓ Find your position in that spotlight, face to face with your child.

✓ Eliminate the competition for your child's attention.

✓ Find your child's social comfort zone and stay inside it.

✓ Follow your child's lead: Use active listening, narrating, helping, and imitating.

5

Find the Smile!

Having Fun with Sensory Social Routines

> **Chapter goal:** To help you increase your child's smiles and laughter during face-to-face social games, songs, and social exchanges. The more fun your child is having, the longer your child is attending and interacting with you, and the more learning opportunities you can provide.

This chapter assumes that you feel comfortable and successful with the skills from Chapter 4. If you have started spending more time interacting with your child during play and daily routines, and have been rewarded with more eye contact, more gesturing, and even some smiles from your child—and if you've been checking your Refrigerator List and also reviewing the Activity Checklists to help you remember the strategies—you are ready to add to what you've learned. In this chapter and each chapter that follows, you will add a new set of ideas and strategies to the previously learned skills that you will continue to practice.

> ### Helpful Tip
>
> If you don't feel very secure yet with Chapter 4's skills, spend some more time practicing them before using this chapter. Try using the Activity Checklists right after a playtime and after a child care activity. Give yourself a pat on the back for those skills that went well, and then practice the ones you were less comfortable with a little more in the next few days. *We are providing you with the same tools that we use ourselves.* When we provide therapy to children with ASD, we use checklists after sessions, score ourselves, and zero in on those skills or behaviors that didn't go as well as we wanted, so the next time we can enhance the learning opportunities embedded in our interactions with children.

Why Having Fun Together Is So Important

This chapter focuses on increasing the *fun quotient (FQ)* of the activities you and your child do together. Fun is an important part of helping your child learn for numerous reasons, especially these six:

1. *More fun = faster learning.* People of all ages want to continue activities they're enjoying. This seems so simple—but fun keeps both you and your child at an activity, and for your child more practice leads to faster learning.
2. *More fun = more learning opportunities.* The longer the two of you interact, the more learning opportunities you will provide for your child.
3. *Adding fun to a learning activity aids the learning and memory process.* Pleasurable activities result in much faster and durable learning than carrying out activities that do not have any emotional meaning.
4. *Your child's cues that tell you she wants you to continue a fun activity are the basis for your child's learning to communicate.* Looking and anticipating, smiling, reaching, or bouncing with excitement can all be developed into clear gestures, words, and eventually sentences! This is one of your most powerful communication-teaching opportunities as a caregiver.
5. *A favorite activity is its own reward!* Repeating an enjoyed activity after your child communicates wanting more provides a strong reward for your child's communication. The power of teaching through play is built on this natural reward system.
6. *Being a very frequent source of fun and pleasure increases your child's attention to you at all times.* As your child learns what kinds of fun activities the two of you can do together, your child will be looking for more and more opportunities to do them with you, which means more engagement, more communication, and more learning opportunities.

What's Happening in Autism?

Children with autism do not seem to experience as much natural reward in social interactions as other children. Based on research conducted by one of us authors (G. D.),[1] we think that one of the basic biological differences underlying autism is this decreased internal reward from social interactions and engagement. The good news, though, is that this biological system is moldable and responsive to experience. Through enjoyable play experiences, you can increase your child's experience of pleasure in social interactions and his internal motivation to seek

---

[1]Dawson, G., et al. Brief report. Recognition memory and stimulus–reward associations: Indirect support for the role of ventromedial prefrontal dysfunction in autism. *Journal of Autism and Developmental Disorders, 3*(31) 337–341, 2001.

out and enjoy social engagement. This paves the way for more interaction and more learning opportunities.

Why Is It a Problem?

Not finding social interaction as rewarding as most other children means that children with autism are not seeking out as many opportunities to interact with others as other children do, and that's a problem, because humans learn so much from these interactions. We learn communication, language, object use, imitation, play, friendship, pretending, emotional intimacy—all aspects of mental and emotional life—not so much from school or other organized educational activities, but in the ebb and flow of daily family life. We think that this reduction in learning opportunities day in and day out, which results from fewer interactions, adds to the social-communicative delays in autism. Let's consider this example of a little boy with autism:

> *I (S. J. R.) met 17-month-old André at his home, with his new baby sister, 4-year-old brother, and parents all together. The parents had just recently recognized his ASD and had received a diagnosis that week. As I entered the house, all of the family members were in the main room except André, who was alone in his parents' darkened room, holding three figures from* Toy Story. *His parents told me that when he could, he spent his time either there or in a closet, and they had to keep all the doors closed to keep him in the main room. He held the figures in his hands, then dropped them together onto the carpet and circled around them, watching them, then picked them up and held them together in his hands, and then dropped and circled again. He noticed me but didn't really look at me, and his handsome little face was quite serious. This went on until his father led him by the hand out of the bedroom.*
>
> *I asked his parents to show me André's play routines. His father carried out a lively roughhouse game involving flipping André onto his shoulder, "airplaning" him around the house, and then somersaulting him down to the floor. André smiled delightedly during this game, and when it was over, he lay on the floor, smiling and looking at his father with his big brown eyes. Dad scooped him up again, and the game was repeated. His mother also had play routines that André enjoyed. She sang "Itsy-Bitsy Spider" to him as he lay on the floor, using some hand motions and creeping her fingers up his chest when the spider went "up the water spout." He smiled happily, looked directly at her, and waited eagerly for her to repeat it when she finished.*
>
> *So here was the fun quotient (FQ): The parents had some great tools to work with. They instinctively knew the power of these games. André did not try to leave to play with his figures. He stayed with these games until his parents and I began to talk and the parents stopped initiating the games. Then he took his figures and returned to the bedroom. André's parents and I talked about how to increase the number of fun social games they played with André each day.*

*When I walked into the house 1 week later, I was amazed at the difference. The figures were up on a shelf and out of the way. André was on the floor with his father, completing a puzzle when I arrived. His parents reported that they had tried to engage him frequently during the day, and the more they tried, the more he responded. As I watched each of them take turns playing with him, I saw André playing happily with his parents, using his eyes, hands, **and voice** to continue games when his parents paused. What's more, when they stopped playing for a minute to talk, André directly approached one of them to start another game. He initiated social interactions again and again. His face was lively, and he was highly motivated to interact throughout the hour.*

A few weeks later, André had a whole repertoire of songs and social games. He was reaching and communicating with voice and eyes. He could imitate the motions in some of his mother's songs, and when I came to the door and knocked, he was right there, opening the door with his mother, smiling and looking right at me. I asked his mother about his play with the figures. She told me that he was no longer interested in them. She hadn't seen them for a while, and he no longer spent any time in the bedroom or closet; he was now underfoot and wanting to be engaged with them constantly.

This chapter is all about this kind of social play between two people—a kind of social play that promotes touch and gaze, fun and excitement, for both you and your child! We refer to these early games that are designed to be fun, engaging, and pleasurable for your child as *sensory social routines*—*sensory* because they often involve stimulating sensory experiences; *social* because the primary focus of these games is the social experience of another person, not playing with objects or teaching cognitive or other self-help skills (although sometimes this happens as a by-product of the games); and *routines* because these games become familiar and ritualized for the child—a feature that makes them easier for your child to learn, so the child can quickly come to initiate and request these games.

⟫⟫⟫➡ What You Can Do to Increase the Fun Quotient

Three straightforward steps can help you find the smile to boost your child's learning during sensory social routines you do together:

Step 1. Find the rhythm of sensory social routines.

Step 2. Build a repertoire and refine the routines.

Step 3. Optimize your child's energy level for learning.

In the following pages, we describe how to carry out each of these steps, give you some ideas for activities to try, and suggest what you can do to solve problems that may come up.

Step 1. **Find the Rhythm of Sensory Social Routines**

Sensory social routines are activities in which you and your child are happily engaged face to face in highly social activity. These activities are marked by *reciprocity*. That is, you and your child are taking turns and communicating with words, gestures, or facial expressions to keep the "game" going. Neither of you is "directing" the other (though you often need to start the game). Each partner leads, and each partner follows. You can see your child's leads when you pause or end one round of the game; your child will do something to continue it. That is your child's turn, or lead. Finally, sensory social routines typically do not involve manipulating objects (though there are exceptions). It is not object play. It is people play. In sensory social routines, each play partner's attention is intensely focused on the other, and they cue each other back and forth. There is a clear rhythm to this—a kind of balanced exchange in which both partners are engaged, in a back-and-forth manner. You start, you pause, your child cues, you continue, you pause, your child continues, and so on.

Rationale. Sensory social routines teach your child that other people's bodies and faces "talk"—that they are important sources of communication, and that people can send and receive emotions face to face. In sensory social games, you will share smiles, make silly faces, add sound effects and expressions to all kinds of games, and draw your child's attention to your face. Creating fun routines will motivate your child to communicate that he wants to continue the activity, which will form the basis for expressing other meanings, like "Don't do that again" or "I'm not sure about this." These routines can also help regulate your child's emotions, energy, and arousal levels, so that your child is as alert and attentive as possible to you and ready to learn from you.

Activity: *Pick a Sensory-Rich Activity and Find the Smile!*

First, pick an activity—a physical activity like tickling, bouncing, flying through the air, or swinging; playing "This Little Piggy," or using finger plays or songs; playing face-to-face games like peekaboo or pattycake—any games that capture your child's interest and attention and bring forth big smiles. Try to find an activity that doesn't incorporate a toy or other object. At the end of this step, there is a list of sensory social games that may give you some ideas.

Here are some ideas for finding the smile:

- Do something inviting to get your child's attention focused on you. Approach your child at a time when she's not engaged in anything. Join her on the floor or couch if she is sitting, or if she is walking around or standing somewhere, join her, greet her, and touch her, maybe pick her

"At first, I had a great deal of trouble trying to think of good activities to use as sensory social routines. I liked the idea of making the social interaction its own reward, but felt lost at actually developing one that worked. Just trying those I'd seen wasn't enough; my son didn't always seem interested in the game that I thought looked like so much fun! So I used ideas about following my child's lead [Chapter 4] to come up with ideas. We developed spinning games, bouncing games, tickle games, and all sorts of others just through expanding on any little activity that happened to seem fun. Going in and out of a crib seems like a mundane activity, but I happened to put my son down with a bounce once, and he loved it. A game was born; I'd bounce him on the way in and fly him through the air on the way out, while he learned more and more words to request what he wanted. At first, it seemed very intimidating to come up with these routines, but it became easy and natural after only a few tries."

up and give her a squeeze or two, spin her around, or do something else that will be fun.

- While you have your child's attention, and the two of you are face to face and close, begin a brief game with your child. Repeat it two or three times quickly if it's short, like spinning, and then pause and wait, looking expectantly at your child and positioning your body to play the game again. If the game you picked is long, like a song or finger play, start with the first line and finger movements. Do that a little bit once or twice. Then stop, look expectantly, and see if your child seems to want you to continue.

- Pause right before the *big event*. The big event is the most dramatic moment of the game. If you are playing chase, the big event is the moment you are positioned and ready for the chase. If you are playing tickle, it is the moment that the fingers are ready to descend. If you are playing peekaboo with a blanket, it is the moment before you pull the blanket off your head or your child's. Pause right before the big event and look expectantly at your child. Get your child's attention, then GO! After the big event, be sure to pause, smile, and laugh to accentuate the fun of the big event.

- At the end of the big event, stop, look at your child excitedly, place your hands and body as if you are about to do it again, and *wait*. Wait for some action or sound from your child that invites you to begin again. Any small indication—a wiggle, a brief look, a quiet sound—will do. Wait for a signal from your child that tells you your child wants the game continued. (Your child's expectant looking or waiting is also a cue for you to continue.)

Once your child signals, finish the game and then pause again, waiting for another signal. Keep it going until either your energy or your child's attention starts to lag. Waiting for your child's cues brings your child into the game and **balances the interactions**. Now it is a two-person game, with two active participants, rather than an actor and an observer.

● Once either you or your child is starting to lose interest, say, "All done with [airplane, or whatever game you played]." Give your child a hug and be finished.

Helpful Tip
Don't discount expectant looks and waiting from your child as signals that your child wants the game to be repeated. As long as your child's attention is on you, even subtle nonverbal communication is communication.

● What should you say during the routines? Songs are easy—just sing the songs, with motions! If you don't know any motions, try making some up. For games like swing, tickle, and chase, invent a simple narration that goes along, like "I'm gonna get you" for chase; "Where's [name]?" and then "Boo!" for peekaboo; "One, two, three swing!" for a spin-around. Use the same words day after day. These little chants will help your child learn the game and learn language. Often children's first words are spoken in games like this.

> *Nancy begins a sensory social routine with 2-year-old Devon, who is sprawled on a bean bag chair in front of her. She begins to sing "Itsy-Bitsy Spider" and combines a gesture that fits each phrase. When Nancy sings, "The itsy-bitsy spider crawled up the water spout," she creeps her fingers up along Devon's chest. She pauses, and he looks intently at her. For the next phrase, "Down came the rain and washed the spider out," she brings her hands down his chest repeatedly, brushing against his chest with her fingers. She pauses, and he smiles expectantly with great eye contact. Then she raises her hands to her face and frames her face as she sings, "Out came the sun and [moving her hands like water down through the air] dried off all the rain." Finally, she positions her hands to creep her fingers up his chest for the last phrase, "And the itsy-bitsy spider—" She waits in position (her pause), and he looks at her, smiles, and reaches for her hands—at which point she finishes "crawled up the spout again" (fingers up his chest).*
>
> This is a lovely sensory social routine that many parents instinctively use to engage their young children—and most children seem to love it. Devon smiles, gives great eye contact, and reaches toward his mother in those pauses, taking his turns on cue. And why wouldn't he? It's a kind of mutually enjoyable conversation—each partner taking a

turn and pausing for the other: a balanced interaction; both of them on the same "topic"; each clearly enjoying the other and showing it with smiles, actions, eye contact, and happy voices and movements. The feelings are genuine and positive between them, and they are speaking the same emotional language: "It's fun to play together."

>  **Helpful Tip**
> Repetition is key here. The more familiar a game is, the more it becomes a "routine," the more the child can participate as a full partner (as Devon did when he communicates that he knows what is coming after his mother's pauses), and the more the child learns.

- When you introduce a new sensory social routine, your child may look dubious. Present the activity in brief segments, by starting and stopping the activity several times, so that your child learns the routine and what to expect. Children do not always show immediate pleasure in a new routine. It may appear that they are not even interested in the game. It is all right to persist in the three quick repetitions of a new game even if your child does not seem to like it very much, as a way to introduce the game. However, if your child is wary, be gentler on the next repetition—softer and slower—so your child can get to know what is coming and does not start to avoid the routine. Over several repetitions, the game may become more and more interesting. However, if your child is clearly uncomfortable (backing away, still, serious face, avoiding contact, or protesting), stop the routine and shift to a familiar, happy one.

If there are no routines your child enjoys, you will need to start to build them up. Here are some ideas:

- Bath time: Use bubbles in the tub to place on your child's arm; then rinse away by pouring water; repeat; dry your child with extra little tummy rubs; pour water from a cup over your child's hands while in the tub.

- Changing or dressing: Try a little peekaboo with a diaper or pieces of clothing. Try a few toe tickles or "This Little Piggy" before putting on socks, or after taking them off, or while washing feet in the tub.

- Try massaging a little lotion on your child's hands and arms. Does that feel good to your child?

- Try squeezing your child gently in a bean bag chair, bouncing your child on your bed, or putting a pillow over your child's tummy as you play on your bed.

Some Sensory Social Games to Consider[2]

Games and Songs without Objects	Silly Faces and Noises
Pattycake (with hands and also with feet)	Pop your cheek with your finger
Peekaboo	Make a raspberry noise with your lips
"The Noble Duke of York"	Kissy face and kissy noises
"Where Is Thumbkin?"	Fish face
"This Little Piggy"	Blow raspberries on your child's feet, hands, or belly
"Round and Round the Garden"	Hide your face in peekaboo
Chase/"I'm gonna get you!"	Yodel
Swinging through your legs	Whistle
Airplane	Stick your tongue out and wiggle it
"So Big"	Pull on your ear: "Honk, honk"
Creepy fingers	Tongue machine: Pull on your ear and stick out your tongue, then push on your nose and pull in your tongue—make sound effect for each
"Itsy-Bitsy Spider"	
"Open, Shut Them"	
"London Bridge"	
"Twinkle, Twinkle, Little Star"	
"Ring-around-the-Rosy"	
"The Wheels on the Bus"	
"If You're Happy and You Know It"	
"Way Up in the Sky"	
Dancing to music	

Summary of Step 1

If you have followed along and carried out the prescribing activities, you will probably have an idea of what kinds of sensory social routines your child prefers, and you can build on those in the days ahead. Some children enjoy more physical or roughhouse games—being chased and caught, somersaulted in the air, swung around, or spun. Others may favor games involving touch: "Round and Round the Garden," creepy fingers, tickle, having their bellies soaped up in the bathtub or having raspberries blown on their bellies, or foot games like "This Little Piggy." Then there are the songs and finger plays your child likes to hear you sing and do, or silly faces and noises that your child enjoys watching you make.

---

[2]For more ideas and descriptions of games, see *www.parents.com/baby/development/intellectual/classic-games-to-play-with-your-baby*.

You have probably also experienced the rhythm of these activities—the back-and-forth nature of the starts, pauses, cues, and continuations that make the games reciprocal. Over time, build up your child's repertoire of sensory social routines from 5 to 10, to 20.

See if you agree with most of the statements in the following checklist. If so, you have learned how to create sensory social games with your child and are ready for some additional techniques involving these games. If not, continue to try different routines; your child might need more exposures to them to learn the pattern and what to expect.

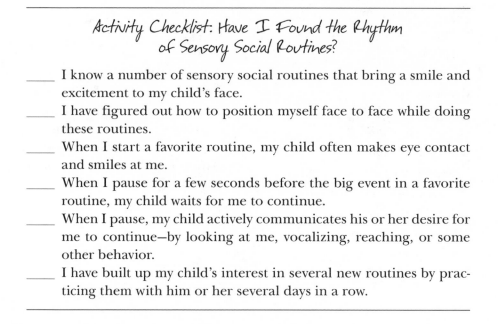

Activity Checklist: Have I Found the Rhythm of Sensory Social Routines?

_____ I know a number of sensory social routines that bring a smile and excitement to my child's face.

_____ I have figured out how to position myself face to face while doing these routines.

_____ When I start a favorite routine, my child often makes eye contact and smiles at me.

_____ When I pause for a few seconds before the big event in a favorite routine, my child waits for me to continue.

_____ When I pause, my child actively communicates his or her desire for me to continue—by looking at me, vocalizing, reaching, or some other behavior.

_____ I have built up my child's interest in several new routines by practicing them with him or her several days in a row.

Step 2. Build a Repertoire and Refine the Routines

Once you've identified at least a few sensory social routines that your child enjoys and that allow you to find the smile, you're ready to add to this skill.

Rationale. These are repetitive activities, and once your child has learned them, they can lose their excitement. Early signs that a child is losing interest during a sensory social routine include lessened responding in between your pauses, looking away during your turns, and changing her body language (from active to passive or from passive to overactive). To make sure you don't completely lose the benefits of sensory social routines, be alert for the need to add to your repertoire, promote your child's participation as a full partner, vary the routine enough to keep it interesting, pick the best times and settings, and add objects judiciously if that seems likely to help.

Activity: *Get Creative in Building and Varying Your Sensory Social Repertoire*

Here are some ideas:

- Keep your turn short, so your child has more opportunities to respond. Ideally, your child will have an opportunity to respond every 5–10 seconds. If you do too much, the interaction is not balanced. Your child isn't a full partner and will become bored, or at least won't communicate enough to get the full benefit of the activity.

- **Caution!** Avoid the situation in which you are making your child happy by simply entertaining your child, and your child is happily but passively observing and enjoying watching you do all of the work! Rather, you and your child should be in a balanced, back-and-forth communication throughout, via movements, gestures, eye contact, sounds, words, or other actions. The goal is for your child to actively attend and communicate with you in some way, even if only through gaze, to initiate, respond to, or continue the sensory social routine. You will need to start, pause, and wait often, to give your child a chance for her communicative turn. Be patient during your pauses, and wait for a response from your child.

- As soon as your child has shown enjoyment, participation, and recognition of one familiar routine, go ahead and add another. Simple songs that involve simple hand movements are especially important to develop, for many reasons: the repeated language, which makes it easy for the child to predict; the shared social meaning that the games have for both of you; and the gestures that eventually build your child's ability to imitate gestures. A good goal is to build up your child's repertoire to 10–20 different sensory social routines that he enjoys and can play with various people.

- Try to find a variety of times during the day to build in sensory social routines. Put them in all six activity types. Besides bath time and dressing, mentioned above, diaper changing is a great time for playing belly games, toe games, pattycake, peekaboo, and creepy fingers. Try to work a sensory social routine into regular diaper changes or potty times. Mealtimes can also provide a great setting for making silly faces and noises, with food and drinks as props, if you can make time to sit with your child at the table during a meal or snack. If it's feasible for you, try sitting with your child at the table, getting as close to a face-to-face orientation as you can by positioning your child's chair and your chair. Give you and your child the same food, and each of you have a drink. When your child takes a bite or a drink, imitate your child and add sound effects: drinking sounds, eating sounds, "Mmm-good," "DEElicious!" See if your child starts to enjoy your big displays. If you see signs of enjoyment, do it again. Ham it up! Offer your child a bite of your food. Try to get your child to feed you a bite. Make fun noises and other reactions when your child does. Some children think it is very funny when a parent picks up a child's bottle and pantomimes drinking from it—as long as the child gets it back quickly! Be sure to repeat all these routines several times, so your child begins to see the pattern in them and knows what to expect. Exaggerating your reactions, your sounds, your silliness—this is often the "attention draw" that children with autism (and those without autism too!) need to attend to you and the game, learn the patterns, and find the humor.

● Once it starts to feel repetitive to you, add some variation! Surprise your child by adding a new verse, new sound effects, new steps to the routine, or maybe some props or another person. Variation will keep the game going longer—and that means more learning opportunities for your child.

> *Alexis and her dad are playing "Ring-around-the-Rosy" on the floor. She initially likes the fall-down part and does a few rounds with Dad, falling down first (her communication), then laughing and looking when he falls down too (sharing the fun), then standing up again and reaching for his hands (her communication to begin again). However, after a few rounds, she stops falling down on her own and stops reaching. Dad thinks she is getting bored, so, rather than stopping the game, he says, "Let's get your sister!" Eight-year-old Tessa rolls her eyes, but Dad takes Alexis to Tessa (who is on the couch reading), takes her hand, and pulls her into the circle. He helps Alexis take Tessa's hand, and the three of them play a couple more rounds. This is very exciting to Alexis, who watches Tessa intently as they both fall down, and takes Tessa's hand to restart. Tessa says, "Get Daddy," and motions to her father. Alexis looks at him and reaches her other hand for Dad, and the three of them repeat the game.*
>
> This variation—adding another person—is enough to increase Alexis's interest and motivation for the game, and it results in a number of new learning opportunities. Dad could also add a big stuffed animal as a "person" in the game, or he could put a small object (like a stuffed animal or pillow) on the floor between them to circle around. These types of little variations can add interest for your child, and also for you, as you try to think of variations that will work!

● Know when it really is time to end the game. If your child's responses diminish, and you cannot revive them through variations, it is time to be "all done" and to offer a different choice of activities. If you are bored, it's time to change. If your child's responses increase and get disorganized and overactive, it's time to calm things down. Slow down the game, lower your voice, or decrease the intensity. If that does not help your child calm down during the game, then end the game, say you are finished, and help your child transition into some quieter play with toys.

Activity: *Know When to Use Objects in Sensory Social Routines*

Sensory social routines often involve activities without any objects at all. In songs, finger plays, social games, and physical games, your ability to position yourself and your child for face-to-face interaction is crucial for capturing your child's attention to your face and to your directed communications.

But you can also incorporate certain kinds of objects into sensory social routines. The object has to support the goals of a sensory social routine—to draw your child's full attention to your face and body—so that there will be smiles and expressions of pleasure, and the child will communicate repeatedly for the routine to continue. If you carry out a sensory social routine with an object, the object has to be a special kind of object that will support your child's attention to you, instead of pulling it away from you and toward the object. *For this reason, one rule of using objects in sensory social routines is that only you can handle them.* The child does not get to handle and operate them (because this pulls your child's attention away from you).

> ### Helpful Tip
>
> Try to choose objects that your child does not know how to use alone. This way, you can keep hold of the object, because your child needs your help to start and continue the game.

Objects like bubbles, balloons (***never** let the child have control of the balloon; it's a choking hazard!*), pinwheels, noisemakers, tops, flutes, and pompoms can be woven into powerful sensory social routines. Other examples include wind-up toys, party blowers, Slinkies, rocket launchers, spray bottles with water in them, lotion, and scarves.

Here are some ideas for using objects in sensory social routines:

- When you use an object in a sensory social routine, you will *not* take turns with your child in operating the object. You are the sole operator. You will begin the routine by doing something with the object to make a big effect. Watch your child: You want to see smiles, pleasure, and an approach to you or to the object. If your child freezes, looks worried, backs up, or moves away, stop and wait. Try to repeat the action, but *very gently, and aim it away from your child's face and body* the second time. Watch for your child's reaction. If you continue to see worry, freezing, or moving away, put the object away and do something else.

● If your child smiles, approaches, and looks interested or excited, operate the object again, and then *pause*. Wait for your child to communicate in some way that she wants you to do it again. When you get the communication (which might be a look, smile, gesture, approach, sounds, or words), say, "More? You want more bubbles?" or something like that, and then operate the object again. Keep this going several times if your child maintains interest. This is also turn taking: communicative turn taking. You do something, your child communicates, and you answer.

● Ideally, your child will come right up to you, touch the toy, look for the repetition, touch your face or hands, or otherwise be very excited. If your child doesn't, offer the toy and entice him to come closer. This is a close-in activity that should be a great source of fun and pleasure for both of you! It is also a powerful communication frame for your child, and in subsequent chapters we will give you many ideas for helping your child learn more ways to communicate his desires in sensory social routines.

● What should you say? Just as before, develop a simple narration that goes along with the activity. A few words and sound effects are important to add. For a bubble routine, a typical narration might be something like this: "Want more bubbles? Want me to blow? Blow! [then blow]. Get the bubbles. Pop, pop. See the bubble? Get it—pop," spoken as your child does the various actions. Use a similar narration each time you play a specific game. Emphasize the names of things, the actions you are making, sound effects, and little chants like "One, two, three" or "Ready, set, go." Add sound effects, gestures, facial expressions, and anything else that makes

---

Helpful Tip

We can't stress enough how important it is for you to maintain control of the object. If the child requests it, treat the request as a request for you to activate the object, rather than hand it over. Don't get into a struggle over it. It's better to end a sensory social game by putting it away or with your child holding the object than to have a big upset over control. There is always another opportunity to repeat this in the next few hours or days.

the routine fun and playful for you and for your child. Be dramatic; ham it up! Use your child's reactions to tell you what creates energy, fun, and excitement for your child without becoming overstimulating—a point we will return to soon.

Games and Songs with Objects

Blowing bubbles

Balloons—blow one, count "One, two, three," and let it go flying around the room (again, though, be careful, because children can choke on balloons)

Pinwheels—blow to make them turn

Pompoms—shake, put on your head, throw, and so on

Clothes to put on each other: beads, glasses, hats, bracelets, or watches

Lotion—put a small amount of lotion on your child's body, rubbing, and massaging

Filmy scarves—throw, hide under, prance around with

Blankets or mats—roll your child up in one like a hot dog

Peekaboo with props

Squeeze and wiggle games with a bean bag chair

Bouncing your child by his hips on a little trampoline or the bed

Bouncing and rolling belly down on a big exercise ball

Swinging the child through your legs

Rocking the child on a rocking horse (from the front, to stay face to face)

Rocking chair—rock fast, rock slow

Spinning in a swing

Splash games with water in the bath

Bubbling with straws in the bath

Noisemakers—party favor blowers, flutes, tambourines, and the like

Slinkies

Pushing your child on a swing from the front and catching her to stop and wait

Activity: *Alternate between Sensory Social Routines and Object Play*

Because sensory social routines draw you and your child close together socially and emotionally, they are wonderful parts of all interactions. When you are playing with your child, see what it's like to alternate between object-focused play and sensory social routines. The object-focused play builds your child's skills in thinking, imitation, hand and body coordination, and complex play skills. The sensory social routines build social skills, communication skills, emotional connectedness, and imitation. Alternating between joint activity with objects and sensory social routines ensures:

- Greater enthusiasm, motivation, and energy for learning
- More learning across developmental areas
- Reciprocal turn taking and responding inside typical routines and activities
- More social attunement and engagement

Keep in mind, too, that when it is time for a sensory social game to end, you will probably be wise to move to an object play activity. This will give both of you a little break from the intensity of well-done sensory social routines! Some children will resist ending a sensory social routine; this is good, because it means that they really enjoyed it! However, if you feel it is time to end (you are exhausted, or it feels too repetitive) and your child resists, you can help the transition go more smoothly by introducing an object or another enticing activity (like a snack), diverting your child's attention toward the new object or activity, and then leaving the sensory social routine.

Sensory social routines draw children with autism back into the social world and the pleasure of social exchanges. They are a very important part of our social-communicative approach to early intervention for ASD, and they are used in one form or another by many different treatment approaches.

Summary of Step 2

If you have followed along and carried out the activities described above, you will have built up not only several different types of sensory social games, but also your skill in observing and assessing how and when to use a sensory social routine. You will also know when you need to vary a routine, end it, or transition to an object-focused routine. See if you agree with most of the statements in the following checklist. If so, you're ready to go to the next step. If not, reread this section, try some different routines, and consult with someone who knows your child well if you are having problems trying to come up with some new ideas.

Activity Checklist: Have I Built Up a Bigger Repertoire and Refined the Routines?

_____ My child and I have built up a repertoire of 10 or so fun sensory social routines, including songs and finger plays.

_____ I have worked out one or more sensory social routines for most caregiving and play activities of our day.

_____ My child is active in the games, not just a passive observer or recipient. He or she cues me, one way or another, to continue during pauses in many of our games.

_____ I have learned how to vary routines, or elaborate them by adding steps, to keep the routines from getting too repetitive.

_____ I can narrate and produce simple scripts for these games fairly easily.

_____ I have learned the signs that my child is losing interest and it's time to end the game before my child leaves, fusses, or shuts down.

_____ I have learned to carry out some sensory social routines with objects.

_____ I have experimented with going back and forth between toy/object play and sensory social routines with my child.

Step 3. Optimize Your Child's Energy Level for Learning

The last step in this chapter involves helping your child find her best energy or arousal level for learning from you in these fun activities.

Rationale. Children who are overaroused or underaroused are not in an ideal state for learning. Optimal learning occurs when a child is alert, attentive, and engaged—not when he is passive, spaced out, or tired, or when he is overexcited,

> **Helpful Tip**
>
> Next time you play a game, watch your child carefully for signs of over-excitement, and try to play the game more calmly *before* your child goes over the top. You want a child who is attentive and engaged, but not overaroused, which limits your child's ability to learn from the experience.

agitated, or overly aroused and out of control. It's important to be able to judge when your child is getting too aroused or is not aroused enough, and to take steps within your sensory social routines to optimize your child's arousal level for learning.

Activity: *Learn to Dial Down the Activity When Your Child Is Getting Highly Aroused*

You probably have experienced your child, or other children, getting "revved up" when their parents play with them in a very vigorous way. It's fun to see children become excited and energized by play. But at a certain point they get so wound up that they aren't listening, aren't responding to others, and instead are "over the top." They are overaroused. They have temporarily lost their ability to control themselves and their own behavior. They may start running around, yelling or screaming, and perhaps getting destructive or aggressive. This is a point when parent–child play or play between brothers and sisters can quickly evolve into a conflict situation, with children being corrected and parents being upset.

Here are some ideas for heading off overarousal:

- Make the play gentler the minute you see your child getting overly aroused. You don't need to stop; just get softer, slower, quieter, and less stimulating. You should see your child become less excited quickly.

- You can use sensory social routines to help your child adjust her arousal or excitement levels in many situations. Children who are upset and over-aroused for other reasons often calm down in response to gentle sensory social routines. Children who are very upset because they are angry, frightened, or frustrated may be helped by gentle sensory routines involving rocking, hugging or squeezing, or having gentle pressure on their heads and backs. These may be accompanied by your soft and soothing voice singing a calming song, or saying a little chant like "You're okay, you're okay, you'll feel better, you're okay."

Activity: *Find Ways to Energize an Underaroused Child*

Children who seem sluggish, bored, uninterested in things, unresponsive or underresponsive to your initiations or to events going on around them can't learn any better than children who are overaroused. They tend to sit or lie around rather than move around as actively as most young children, who seldom sit still for very long. Their facial expressions look neutral; it's hard to tell what emotion they are feeling, either in face or in body. They may seem tired. They may do one thing for long periods of time without changing position—watching their hands, staring out the window.

Here are some ideas to "perk up" or activate an underaroused child by using lively sensory social routines:

- Move the child quickly by bouncing, jiggling, spinning, or using fast-paced actions and songs.

- Use stronger touches, more volume, a bigger voice, more emotion.

- Use physical actions involving rapid or rather jerky movements: fast bounces on your lap or on a ball, lively jumps on a mini-trampoline.

- Use sensory social objects that create big sounds or visual events.

● Use touch to "rev up" an underaroused child: rubbing or squeezing limbs; using lotion; giving foot massages on bare feet; rolling up in a mat; squeezing in a bean bag chair; blowing bubbles on hands, feet, or belly. Be careful with tickles: They are very arousing, but can also quickly become noxious. If the child comes back for more or pulls your hands for more, continue once more, but if not, end.

Summary of Step 3

We have been discussing concepts related to your child's level of arousal or excitement during sensory social routines. You may have observed your child getting too excited at times and either crying, getting really overactive, or becoming disorganized in some routines. You have likely tried to experiment with those overexciting routines by slowing them down, calming them down, or ending them sooner, to prevent the overexcitement. Or your child may be a low-key child with a mellow, laid-back disposition, who doesn't get excited about much or show many emotional changes. We hope that you observed your low-key child get more excited in sensory social games—more smiles, more animation, more social behavior, more attention to you, more liveliness, more emotion.

See if you agree with most of the statements in the following checklist. If so, you are ready to move on to the next chapter. If you have not thought much about these concepts with your child yet, spend a little more time observing, playing, and thinking about this. When you see either one of these states (overaroused or underaroused), try to use a sensory social routine that you have developed to help optimize your child's state—to slow down and reorganize an overly aroused child, or to rev up and energize an underaroused child. Doing both of these as needed will optimize the child's ability to attend and learn from you.

Activity Checklist: Have I Optimized My Child's Energy and Arousal for Learning?

_____ I have become much more aware of my child's arousal levels across different activities.

_____ I can see when my child is overaroused, underaroused, or in an optimal state for learning and interaction.

_____ I have learned how to use some of our sensory social routines to help my child become calmer and better organized when he or she is overaroused.

_____ I have learned how to manage our routines to keep my child from becoming overaroused and disorganized during our social play.

_____ I have learned how to use some of our sensory social routines to help my low-key child become more energized and motivated to participate.

_____ I know what it means for my child to be in an optimal state for participating, and I know how to use sensory social routines to help create and sustain that state in my child for several minutes or longer.

Chapter Summary

Sensory social routines help you help your child in several ways—increasing the FQ, or fun quotient—of your child's interactions with you; getting your child engaged for longer periods of time in social exchanges; increasing your child's communications for activities; and optimizing your child's energy levels (arousal levels) for learning and engaging. As these routines become familiar to both of you, putting in pauses so your child can communicate somehow that you should continue allows the two of you to take turns and be active partners in the games. It also fosters your child's intentional communications with you. It sends your child the message that communicating is powerful—it controls other people's actions. It gets your child what he or she wants. Sensory social routines provide you with a wonderful tool for helping your child find this optimal emotional state for learning—energized, engaged, and in tune with you. You can use these routines any time you see your child in an over-aroused or underaroused state. When alternated with object play, they help your child stay connected with you. They are not only fun for you and fun for your child, but powerful tools for supporting communication, for sharing emotions, and for fostering social growth.

Refrigerator List

Goal: To use sensory social routines to increase your child's smiles and laughter during face-to-face games and songs.

Steps:

✓ Find the smile!

✓ Stay in the spotlight, face to face, with your child.

✓ Create fun routines from songs, physical games (roughhousing), and touch.

✓ Accompany them with lively faces, voices, and sounds.

✓ Narrate as you go.

✓ Use stimulating objects to create sensory social routines.

✓ Vary the routines when they get repetitive.

✓ Pause often and wait for your child to cue you to continue.

✓ Use sensory social routines to optimize your child's arousal level for learning.

6

It Takes Two to Tango

Building Back-and-Forth Interactions

> **Chapter goal:** To help you build joint interaction routines and back-and-forth interactions with your child into your daily play and caregiving activities, so your child is more engaged and is communicating more with you.

Why Back-and-Forth Interactions (Turn Taking) Are So Important

One of any child's biggest accomplishments in interacting with others is to learn to take turns. The ability to cooperate in give-and-take exchanges is fundamental to social development and to communication. Think about board games, conversations, the grocery store checkout, religious services, meetings, dancing, children playing pretend—all these social interactions are built on taking turns. Take a moment to notice your social interactions with other people, and look for all of the turn taking that occurs during those exchanges. We are not talking about structured interactions in which one person says, "It's my turn," and the other waits. We are talking about the natural turn taking that occurs in adult conversations, in parent–child social games, and in playful interactions between young children—for instance, where one child picks up a bucket in the sand and puts sand in, and the other watches and then comes over to put sand in the bucket too. Watch two people interacting, and you will see this natural turn taking everywhere.

Even the youngest children have a sense of taking turns, which parents often experience while playing with their baby. A parent may make a silly face, and the baby may then look at the parent's eyes with a delighted smile and laugh. That is the baby's turn, and the parents are likely to respond by taking another turn and repeating the silly face. This kind of turn-taking pattern also occurs in vocal play. The baby makes some sound just for the fun of it, and the parent takes a turn and imitates the sound. Then the baby takes another turn, imitating the sound again or watching and smiling, and the parent responds again in turn. When babies become toddlers, they continue using this turn-taking structure in imitation and interaction games with adults and with other children. In a very familiar kind of play, a 2-year-old watches another child do something and then imitates it, at which point the other child does it again, and so on.

In these interactions, what may look like nothing but light-hearted play is actually serious learning. Each person in the interaction fits his response to the other person's response, and the two partners build their interaction back and forth: Maybe a little boy opens his mouth wide and throws his arms in the air when a block tower topples. His playmate then knocks over a block tower and makes the same gestures. The first child watches this imitation with delight and then builds on it by adding jumping to his feet the next time the block tower falls. Young children use this behavior to learn an enormous amount from other people. They watch a person who is important or interesting to them; they observe the other person's words and actions; and they hold them in their minds to make sense of them and remember them. They may imitate it right then and there or later, to practice and learn what the other person was doing. This kind of social learning is one way that little children learn so much without anyone teaching them directly.

Turn taking also establishes a kind of balance to the interactions. No one is the boss, and no one is the follower. Instead, the two partners take turns directing and following. One leads, and the other follows; then the follower may lead something new, and the previous leader now becomes the follower into the new routine. We refer to this as ***sharing control*** of the play. When partners share control, the activity is balanced. Both partners lead, and both partners follow. This requires each to communicate to the other, back and forth. Neither controls the other or the activity. They share control and trade the lead back and forth. Your child takes control when she makes a choice of objects; acts on a toy; refuses a toy; fusses or reaches; speaks; or communicates with her eyes, body, and facial expressions. You take control when you offer a choice, demonstrate a toy, hand something to your child, or ask a question. Sharing control in turn taking creates an activity that both partners build together—a shared activity. The balance between partners increases the learning opportunities available for the child. It fosters the child's initiative and spontaneity by giving the child some control. It fosters the child's attention to the partner when the partner has the lead by focusing that spotlight of attention on the partner—the leader. Each shift of the spotlight highlights a learning opportunity for the child.

What's Happening in Autism?

The social play routines—sensory social routines—that we have encouraged you to build with your child in Chapter 5 build on turn taking. The back-and-forth interaction of you starting a game, your child responding with indications of enjoying the game and wanting more, and you continuing—this whole back-and-forth dance builds the child's awareness of turn taking and of the whole purpose of communicating. This comes easily to most children, but it is more difficult for children with ASD. They may be less aware of their partner's turns, because they are less tuned in to the subtle communications of eyes, face, and voice that speak volumes to most babies. For children with ASD, the volume of those communications seems to be turned down.

> *Joni wanted so much to play with her 2-year-old son, Jacob. He was her first child, and she had looked forward to being a mother and being a good playmate for her child. She had gathered many toddler toys from garage sales and hand-me-downs, and she had cleared out space in the family room TV shelves for his toys. But all he ever wanted to play with were his little cars, and all he wanted to do with them was drive them back and forth along the edge of the coffee table or carpet. He liked to watch the wheels turn as he ran them along. Joni tried to play cars with Jacob, but he got upset when she touched them, and he wanted them back. She tried to show him how to use the toy parking garage with the cars, but he wasn't interested in it. He just took the cars off and lay down on his side to run the cars back and forth on the carpet in front of his eyes. It made her sad, having him turn away to play alone. She felt like a failure as a mom and didn't know what to do.*

Why Is It a Problem?

When young children with ASD do not tune in to their parents' communications or do not respond to them (take a turn), they miss the opportunity to build critical skills (imitation, sharing emotion) that underlie communication. The risk is that young children with ASD will continue to play mostly alone, rather than to draw parents into their activities or to look for social responses from their parents. They may become more and more removed from the social world around them and from all the crucial learning experiences available within that world. This early lack of engagement not only interferes with their learning, but also occurs during a very sensitive period of brain development, when their brain cell networks are particularly ready to absorb and process social and language information. This sensitive period lasts only a few years during early childhood, and we want to make sure that those developing brain networks are receiving the input information they need to learn to process social communication.

Fortunately, there are lots of ways to turn up the volume of your communication, making the learning opportunities present in your turns stand out for your child. In this chapter, we focus on taking turns in play with toys or other objects and in other daily activities, so your child no longer misses the learning opportunities inherent in social interaction but instead learns to expect your responses, imitate you in play, use gestures and words, and experience the fun of social interaction.

What You Can Do to Increase Your Child's Turn-Taking Skills

There are six specific steps you can carry out to increase your child's participation in taking turns:

Step 1. Understand the four-part framework of joint activities for taking turns.

Step 2. Start to practice—beginning involves setting up the joint activity.

Step 3. Set the theme.

Step 4. Elaborate the joint activity—add the variation.

Step 5. Close the joint activity and start another.

Step 6. Create joint activities during other daily routines, to foster multiple areas of development.

In the following pages, we describe how to carry out each of these steps, give you some ideas for activities to try, and suggest what you can do to solve problems that may come up.

Step 1. Understand the Four-Part Framework of Joint Activities for Taking Turns

There is a specific structure for carrying out play with very young children that is particularly rich in learning opportunities for social communication and turn taking. *Joint activities*, or *joint activity routines*, were originally described and given those names by a very influential language scientist.[1] A joint activity is like a conversation, involving a set of turns between you and your child, based on a shared activity. In Chapter 5 you learned how to build sensory social routines, mainly those that don't involve toys or objects. In this chapter you'll learn to do the same thing with toys and other items, devising joint activity routines that may last for 2–5 minutes for very young children. The framework consists of the

---

[1] Bruner, J. Early social interaction and language acquisition. In H. R. Schaffer (Ed.), *Studies in mother–infant interaction* (pp. 271–289). New York: Academic Press, 1977.

following four parts (each of which is elaborated in one of the remaining steps in this chapter):

1. One of you chooses a toy and begins to do something with it—the *setup*.
2. Then the other joins in on the same activity so that the two of you imitate each other, build something together, or take turns to complete the same activity—the *theme*.
3. Doing the same thing for a while can be boring and repetitive, so after a while you add some changes to the play—the *variations*. During the variations, the turn-taking structure continues, and the two of you go back and forth playing a little differently from the way you started.
4. As your child's interest in the activity wanes, you know it's time to start a different activity, and so the two of you finish the game you have been playing—the *closing*—and move on to something else (a *transition* to a new activity).

The new activity begins with another setup or initiation, and continues through the theme, one or more variations, and another closing.

Rationale. The balance between partners and the structure around a shared theme that are the critical features of joint activities enhance learning opportunities. The back-and-forth interaction of turn taking repeatedly puts each partner in the other's spotlight of attention. Whenever it's your turn, your child's attentional spotlight is focused on you: He sees what you are about to do, hears your words, sees the effect of your actions, and so can learn from it. Then it is your child's turn, and he can practice right away what he has just seen and heard (with your help), so he is an active learner in the process. Following your child's interest into a theme that your child understands makes the purpose of your actions clear to your child, and that helps him extract the meaning of your gestures and words. In the variation, varying or adding new play materials or actions to a game adds interest to the activity; keeps it from getting too repetitive and boring; and so helps your child stay motivated to keep participating in the activity and to continue learning, practicing, and strengthening new skills. Finally, ending and transitioning or moving on to the next activity in an organized fashion help you hold your child's attention through the transition and helps your child learn to anticipate what is coming next. The joint activity structure will allow you to help your child learn a wide variety of early social communication skills: understanding and using everyday language; imitating actions that similar-age children would do; playing flexibly and creatively with others.

> *Jocelyn bought a new toy for 3-year-old Rascheed—a round wooden pegboard that held six fat red pegs and spun around. She thought this would be a good toy for him. The pegs were fat enough for him to hold easily, and the goal for using the toy was*

clear. But it was hard to get her son's attention long enough to show him something new. She decided to show it to him while he was having a snack in his high chair. That was one place where he would sit for a while and look at her. So when Rascheed was finishing his crackers, Jocelyn set up the toy on the kitchen table, right in front of his chair. She put the pegs in the base one by one, while talking about what she was doing: "See, baby, here's a peg. It goes here. And another, and another. They go in." Once they were all in, she spun the base, and they circled around. (This was the setup phase.) Rascheed was watching intently as he finished chewing. Then Jocelyn took the pegs out fast, put the base on his tray, and handed him a peg, He struggled a little, and she helped him put it in. (This was the theme.) Then she handed him another, and another. She helped as needed, so this went easily for Rascheed. After he had done three, she put in one (her turn), and then gave him another. She put in the last two quickly to take a turn and to move the activity along so her son wouldn't lose attention. When they were all in, she spun it for him (variation), which he loved! Then she took out most of them and put them in a plastic container, but she left the last two in for him to take out. She helped him put each in the container (closing). Then she took the base off his high chair tray and got him down. Jocelyn had Rascheed's attention and participation throughout. She felt great about the success of this new play routine!

Step 2. Start to Practice—Beginning Involves Setting Up the Joint Activity

Rationale. The setup phase is important, because this is where you first hook your child's interest. You will use your child's toys as the setup that will allow you to demonstrate the theme, introducing a new action that you would like your child to understand and imitate. For example, the setup might be a group of blocks you know your child enjoys. At a moment when your child is unoccupied, you might set up the activity by getting out the container of blocks ("Let's play blocks; I've got the blocks. Sit down. Block goes on top, another block on top") as you take a few and begin to build a tower. Remember to include in the setup good body positioning, with you and your child situated face to face. Good communication relies on your being able to see each other's eyes, facial expressions, gestures, body movements, and words spoken.

Now the theme is set, and you pass some blocks to your child. Your child's turn could be imitating what you just did, such as stacking the next block onto the tower, or reaching and saying "ba" for "block"—as a way of signaling that she is motivated to continue the activity. Or she might start doing something else with the blocks. If she does, encourage her and help her build onto the tower or start her own. That's the theme. Go back and forth, each taking a turn and adding to the tower. Then make the variation happen—knock the blocks down! That's usually fun for children. Then start up again together. Another variation may be lining them up and then driving a car over the "road," or making them into a square as a "house" for toy animals. When your child starts to lose interest, or you run out of ideas, it's time to clean up. Clean up before your child takes off, by having your child help you put the blocks back in the container and put it back. Then it's time to pick another toy. There you have it: a four-part joint activity, with turn taking throughout.

Activity: *Choose Toys or Objects That Will Be Helpful in Establishing the Setup and Will Become the Theme of the Play*

We generally try to choose the same kinds of objects that other children your child's age typically play with, both toys and household objects (for instance, pans, lids, or other kitchen and bath materials). This way your child will know how to play with these objects when she is with children of the same age. Your child probably already chooses objects to play with without your help. If not, you can choose one or two toys or other objects for play that you think will interest your child.

Here are some ideas for selecting objects or toys for the setup:

- Choose objects or toys that have several pieces or that will allow your child to do several different things with the toy. Toys that involve only one action or one piece make it very hard to take turns or to come up with both a theme and a variation. When there are multiple pieces or multiple actions (or both), you and your child can each have a turn doing something or making something interesting happen; this is the idea of shared control. Examples include building blocks, shape sorters, books, a bucket of play animals, toys in which balls are inserted and roll down a slide, and so on.

- **Caution!** Electronic toys are very difficult to use for joint activities, because children tend to want to produce the same action again and again. This makes it hard to take turns, come up with variations, or capture your child's attention.

- Finally, if your child is already playing with a toy, try to start by joining in, rather than introducing a new toy. As discussed in Chapter 5, joining your child allows you to follow your child's interest, rather than trying to entice your child to shift attention. You will be well positioned—in

> ### Helpful Tip
>
> If your child is already playing with an object, follow all the steps to "step into the spotlight." *The best teaching moments come when we follow children's leads rather than trying to make them switch.* (It's true—there is research on this!)

your child's attentional spotlight, interacting, and ready to join in the theme. You can join into your child's theme, take some turns, and then initiate a variation.

- **Caution!** Avoid using toys that your child covets highly and/or uses for highly repetitive, ritualized actions. It is really hard to develop joint activities out of things your child handles in a special, repetitive, or ritualized way and wants to have all to himself. Sometimes it's possible—it never hurts to try—but if your child resists your taking a turn with it, or will not vary the way he handles it, the pattern may be difficult for your child to change.

> ### ✋ *Helpful Tip*
>
> Sometimes children want to hold little favorite things in their hands all the time, but will put them down to play with other toys. If so, and you can still get joint activities going even with the favorite things present, then the favorite things are not interfering and you don't need to manage them. But if a child spends all his time focused on holding or manipulating the favorite toys, and you cannot draw him into anything else, it is probably a good idea to start to limit the all-absorbing toys. Put the highly preferred toys up and away and allow your child to play with them only at certain times, such as in the car, at bedtime, in the high chair while waiting for dinner, or during the hour that you need to prepare dinner.

- What if your child is absolutely not interested in objects? Go back to Chapter 5 and build up your repertoire of sensory social routines first. Once they are well established, begin to work cause-and-effect object play into the sensory social routines. *Cause-and-effect object play* is play in which you perform an action on a toy or create a "big event" with the toy—you make something interesting happen as a result of an action on a toy. For example, you could play chase (a sensory social routine), but at the end of the chase, pick up a ball, chase your child with it, and then throw the ball in a basket! Use maracas in a dance during a musical sensory social routine that you and your child already enjoy, shake the maracas, and then hand them to your child to shake as part of the routine. Notice that in these descriptions of joint activities with objects, we are breaking the rule used in sensory social routines about not letting children play with the objects. That's because now we are elaborating on the basic sensory social routine to include turn taking and building children's interest in shared object activities. In other words, you can use the familiar sensory social routine as the setup and theme for the play, and then use the object as a way of varying the theme (variation).

Summary of Step 2

If you have followed along and carried out the preceding activities, you will have discovered activities with objects or toys that will be used as the main theme of a joint activity. See if you agree with most of the statements in the following checklist. If so, you are now armed with important skills for taking turns and teaching during joint activities—knowledge you will use in **Step 3**. If not, start experimenting during play and caregiving routines until you have found some activities that work for each statement.

Activity Checklist: Am I Setting Up a Joint Activity with My Child?

____ My child is playing with toys or objects that other children his or her age would be using.

____ The objects or toys have multiple pieces that can be shared during play.

____ Different actions can be performed with the object or toy, to prevent my child from doing the same thing repeatedly.

____ Any mechanical toy or object with an on–off switch has been removed and hidden, or the batteries removed.

____ I remember to situate my child in front of me and sitting or standing comfortably—sitting on the floor, sitting in a chair that fits, or standing at a table that is a good height for playing.

____ I remember the rules for how to follow my child's interests, join in, and imitate or elaborate on my child's action in play.

____ I am conscious of the four parts—set up, theme, variation, and closing—as we go through them.

Kylie's parents thought about the different objects that Kylie enjoyed that also would be good for developing joint activities and turn-taking skills. They decided to experiment with only those toys involving multiple pieces. They rearranged Kylie's toys, with the multipiece objects or toys being in sight and other toys moved to closets or placed in storage (for the time being). The result was a play area containing plastic blocks, animal puzzles, markers and stickers, dress-up items (necklaces, purse, hats, bracelets, sunglasses), play dough, farm animals, and toy drums. Kylie's parents decided to include Kylie's favorite books as well as some new ones, because they wanted to encourage and share this interest with her. They figured that they could take turns turning the pages of a book with Kylie. They placed each toy in a clear plastic shoe container, so that all pieces could be kept together but would still be visible to Kylie when she and a parent were deciding which one to use for play. That way they would encourage Kylie to ask for help getting things out of their containers, and would also prevent Kylie from becoming disorganized by having too many toys available at once. They found that doing so helped organize Kylie's play from the start, because parents and child were able to select together which shoe container to take to the table, couch, or floor. Similarly, when it was time to clean up the play, the shoe container was in close proximity for Kylie's parents to teach her how to put away all items and place the container back on the shelf before selecting the next shoe container.

What about Rascheed? *After reviewing the activity checklist for Step 2, Rascheed's parents decided to get rid of his electronic toys. Not only was it extremely difficult to get their son to look at his parents while he was fixated on the toys' sounds and lights, but the more time he spent with these toys, the more he engaged in arm flapping and body rocking. Rascheed's parents understood, however, that their son might need encouragement and help to develop interest in nonelectronic toys. Before starting on joint activities, they set out different objects and toys to find out what he might like. They watched Rascheed play with a ball ramp toy (placing a ball at the top and watching it roll down the tunnel), push pegs through their holes, and touch the pages of books that had textures on them. His parents were thrilled that Rascheed paid attention to and seemed to enjoy a few nonelectronic toys. Also, his selection of toys involved multiple pieces (balls, pegs, pages) that could be touched, handed over, taken turns with, and imitated during play. Rascheed's parents now felt that they had an initial blueprint for starting joint activities with their son, and revisited the Step 2 activity checklist questions with these new routines in mind.*

Step 3. Set the Theme

Rationale. You need to create a theme inside the play—something that you and your child can each take turns doing to turn the activity into a shared interaction—so that the activity does in fact become a joint activity and turn taking can occur. If your child sets the theme (for example, picking up a rolling pin to roll play dough, rolling the car back and forth, or starting to stack the blocks), follow your child's lead and take a turn doing the same thing. When it's your turn, you could simply imitate what the child is doing using other pieces of the material. For example, your turn could be adding another block to the tower, using a second rolling object on a piece of play dough, or taking another ball and inserting it into the tube after your child has done so.

What If Your Child Doesn't Take the First Turn?

If your child doesn't take the first turn, or if you want to demonstrate a new toy, you can show the child what to do and then give the materials to your child, or you can demonstrate and then give your child his own materials just like yours and help your child copy what you just did. For example, to play with play dough, you might make a shape out of the dough with a cookie cutter and then label the shape by saying, "It's a star." In your first turn, you have set a theme: you've shown your child how to use a cutter to make a shape and also provided a new word to build your child's vocabulary. Or if your child likes bubbles, you might puff your cheeks and blow air out of your mouth in your turn with the bubbles, so that your child looks at you and you have a chance to demonstrate the gesture. You could then say the word "blow" after doing this to name the action, and then label "bubbles" when you've blown some. Eventually you will find a joint activity in which the two of you can take turns.

 Activity: *Name Objects and Actions While Engaging in Turn Taking*

Adding words to your play as just described is something that most parents do automatically. It's good to add some words, name objects, add sound effects, and label the actions. But for a child with ASD, it's particularly important to keep your language simple—almost as simple as your child's, as described in more detail in Chapter 13. If your child is not talking yet, then keep your language short and direct. For example, if the activity involves play dough, you can label objects and actions like "dough," "open," "roll," "push," "poke," "cut," and the names of the cookie cutters (e.g., "square," "circle," "tree," "plane"). Appropriate two-word action and label phrases might include "Open dough," "Cut dough," "Push square," "Take out," "Put in," "Blue dough," "Top on," and so forth.

> #### Helpful Tip
>
> To learn about turn taking, your child needs to be watching you take your turn. If he doesn't seem to be paying attention, shift your position if you're not already face to face. If possible, position materials in front of your face, so that your child looks at your face as well as the materials. Do not be afraid to take a toy quickly, say "My turn," take a turn, and then give the toy back. That usually brings attention! Your child may fuss at first because he doesn't know the routine, but if you take short turns and always give the object back right away, your child will become accustomed to the turn-taking routine.

Here are some ideas for words to go with joint activities:

- During toy play, as your child is taking her turn, think of what the object or material is called, and name it out loud when your child is holding, touching, or reaching for it. Do the same for simple actions that you and your child do with the object—"put in," "take out," "shake," "roll," "bang," "open," "close," "scribble," "clap," "hop," "up," "down," and so on. Repeat the word when it is your turn to use the object.

- Do the same during social games without objects. What actions, gestures, and body movements happen during songs and physical games? Start giving names to all of these opportunities.

Summary of Step 3

The theme might feel a little repetitive in these first few turns, but that's necessary so your child can learn what will happen next and also learn to wait for your turn. But it should also be interesting and fun, and that means your child gets her turns quickly. Once you and your child have gotten the hang of this, it should feel balanced, with roughly equal numbers of turns. *In play, partners are equal.* See if you agree with most of the statements in the following checklist. If so, you are now armed with important skills for taking turns and teaching inside joint activities—knowledge you will use in **Step 4**. If not, start experimenting during play and caregiving routines until you have found some methods that work for each statement.

Activity Checklist: What Is the Joint Activity Theme?

_____ I have found objects or games that provide opportunities for turn taking with my child in play.

_____ I follow my child's lead and imitate his or her action when taking my turn.

_____ I have my child's attention when taking my turn.

_____ I use simple language to name the objects and actions during play.

_____ My child and I take turns, acting as equal partners, to create a theme when playing together.

What about Kylie? *For Kylie's parents, the biggest challenge was how to take turns without upsetting Kylie. Her parents continued practicing the setup with Kylie—helping her take down the shoe container she wanted to play with, and setting up the materials at her table or on the floor. Kylie had become accustomed to this routine and understood that her parents were there to help and support her interest—to play and have fun! Once the materials were set up, though, Kylie's parents weren't sure* *how to continue their involvement or take their next turn in the activity. They desperately wanted to play with and show her things they thought she might enjoy, but they didn't want their turns to upset her.*

So they reviewed Chapter 4 and paid particular attention to the strategies of following their child's lead and using imitation for becoming more involved play partners. Having the toys already organized in the shoe containers and having multiple pieces made it easier to take the next object out and do exactly what Kylie had done with the prior piece: put in the next puzzle item, stack the next block, bang the drum, or scribble on the paper with the marker. They continued naming the objects and Kylie's and their actions: "Cow, put in," "Block, on," "Bang, bang, bang," or "Marker. Here's paper. Open marker. Scribble, scribble, scribble." They also started paying attention to the pace and how rewarding the play was to Kylie, because they wanted to make sure that Kylie would pay attention to their turns without finding it a negative experience. They decided their turns needed to be fun, fast, and focused, so they made quick motions with their turn—putting one piece in the puzzle, placing one block onto the tower, hitting the drum once, or scribbling once on the paper. They also started experimenting with new actions, gestures, and sound effects to add to their turns, such as making animal noises when placing pieces into the puzzle, having the block "blast off" from the ground and land on the tower, or drawing stars and hearts (Kylie's favorites) on paper.

Kylie soon started paying more attention to her parents' turns, and then smiling and laughing at the sounds or effects added to the play, and finally imitating their actions in her turn. She liked their play better. Sometimes she still wanted to play with toys her way and didn't gravitate toward their ideas right away, but that didn't concern her parents anymore. If things started to deteriorate, they felt confident with their "repair plan" and applied the same strategies of helping, imitating, and narrating play before gradually taking more deliberate but fun turns in the activity. The outcome was a repertoire of common themes or play actions that both parents and daughter could construct and enjoy together.

Step 4. Elaborate the Joint Activity—Add the Variations

Rationale. When we play, we pick an idea or theme and repeat it during play, but we don't remain stuck or limited to repeating the same theme over and over again in the same way. The natural tendency in play is to start a play theme and after a little while begin elaborating creatively on the theme, to add interest and enjoyment. This is the basis of creative play. One minute children might be playing house, and the next they're action heroes flying around the room to save the day. Or an activity that started off as squeezing play dough through fingers can turn into making animals and then making those animals run, hop, and crawl across the table. Children's play typically evolves and varies as it goes along, and we want children with ASD to be able to participate in creative play with their peers, as well as to initiate and contribute their own ideas during play. That's how they learn about different concepts: make-believe, role play, ways to carry out conventional or customary actions with everyday objects. Adding materials, ideas, or actions to the initial theme is called *variation* or *elaboration*. It highlights different aspects of an activity so that a child learns different concepts, including that objects can be used in many different ways (flexible play); it helps develop your child's creativity and imagination; and it also prevents boredom so the learning can continue.

Activity: *Try Different Ways of Varying or Elaborating on the Theme*

There is no right way to vary or elaborate on a play theme. The only "wrong" way, in fact, is if you start directing the play, expecting the child to imitate every new move you introduce. Be sure that the theme is really well established first (you have repeated it several times), and that you are following your child as much as you are asking your child to follow you. If variations are hard to think of, just do something different with the same materials while your child is looking, and if she doesn't copy you or try something else, then help her do what you just did. Praise your child for trying. Then let your child do whatever she wants to do with the materials.

Here are some ideas for varying the theme:

- Add new materials. After taking turns with a toy or object, begin to add more pieces to the play activities, and show your child how to add them to the theme. For example, if the theme is scribbling on paper with a marker, add a marker of a different color; add some stickers that you can peel off, put on the paper, and color over; or add chalk and show your child how chalk can also be used to make marks.

- Vary the actions. After taking turns performing an action, change the action slightly. For example, if the theme is stacking blocks and you have established the theme of taking turns putting a block on the stack, begin lining them up rather than stacking them. And then maybe drive little cars over the lined-up blocks as if they were a road.

- Add more steps to the action you are performing. For example, if the theme is putting pieces in a puzzle, and you and your child have been taking turns taking each piece out of a container and putting it in, then the variation might be taking all the pieces out of the puzzle, spreading them around on the table, and then showing them to each other and naming the pictures before each one goes in. Or a different variation, for a child who can make simple requests and name the pictures, could be requesting a certain piece from the other person.

Summary of Step 4

If you have followed along and carried out the preceding activities, you will have developed different strategies for varying or elaborating the joint activity. See if you agree with most of the statements in the following checklist. If so, you are now armed with important skills for taking turns and teaching inside joint activities—knowledge you will use in **Step 5**. If not, start experimenting during play and caregiving routines until you have found some methods that work for each statement.

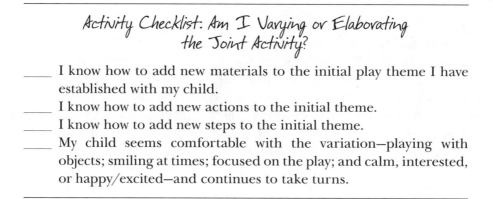

Activity Checklist: Am I Varying or Elaborating the Joint Activity?

_____ I know how to add new materials to the initial play theme I have established with my child.

_____ I know how to add new actions to the initial theme.

_____ I know how to add new steps to the initial theme.

_____ My child seems comfortable with the variation—playing with objects; smiling at times; focused on the play; and calm, interested, or happy/excited—and continues to take turns.

What about Rascheed? *In place of the discarded electronic toys, Rascheed's parents set out a variety of other toys to see what he might enjoy, which turned out to be a ball ramp toy, a peg toy, and a book that provided textures to touch. These toys were used to set up joint activities with Rascheed. Rascheed chose which one to play with each time, and his mother imitated his actions to establish turn taking and initiate the first theme. With the ball or peg toys, turns involved each partner's pushing through or placing the object in the hole, whereas books involved Rascheed's holding them and turning pages, and Jocelyn's touching the textures and pointing to pictures after each page was turned. She also made sure to name each object or picture and action happening in the play: "Push ball," "Peg in," "More ball," "Open book," "Turn," "There's a mouse," "That's soft," and so forth.*

Jocelyn then thought that expanding on the play theme might increase her son's interest and time spent in the activity. She decided to start with adding materials to the activities, so as not to disrupt or change the actions Rascheed had become accustomed to and enjoyed. For the ball ramp toy, during her turn, Jocelyn showed Rascheed how to hit the ball with the hammer to make it go down the ramp. She repeated the action with the new item during her turns while Rascheed continued using his hand to push the ball in, but she exaggerated the motion with sound effects and alternated between hitting the ball slow–fast and light–hard with the hammer. After a few turns of modeling the hammer, she then handed it to Rascheed and quickly helped him hold it to hit the ball. She alternated between having him use the hammer and letting him use his hands, so he wasn't turned off by the new theme's seeming too hard. She also offered choices at times between "ball" versus "hammer" and "hit" (with hammer) versus "push" (with hands), so Rascheed felt that the interaction and the turn taking were balanced. She continued naming each object and action in the activity, to help Rascheed understand and begin to imitate single words related to the things he wanted to do.

Once adding materials (such as the hammer) proved successful, Jocelyn decided to try introducing other new actions. First she started showing him other actions to do with pegs. For instance, instead of hammering them, she showed him how to stack them into a tower with the connectors on each end and then, once the tower was a reasonable size, how to roll the tower across the table. Rascheed was not expecting this change, but he watched intently as the multicolored tower rolled from his mother's side of the table over to him. Jocelyn then said "roll" and helped him push it back over to her. She added another peg to the tower and rolled it again, helping Rascheed now do the same. After a few back-and-forth rounds, Rascheed began rolling the tower by himself with smiles and delight, until the tower became too long to roll and fell apart into pieces. But that didn't worry Jocelyn, because now she had another action to name—"Uh-oh, pegs fell off"—and an opportunity to build the joint activity with several themes all over again!

Step 5. Close the Joint Activity and Transition to the Next

Rationale. After you have played for a while, one of three things is bound to happen. Either your child's interest wanes, or your interest wanes, or you cannot think of anything else to do and the play has gotten really repetitive. When there's nothing more to teach, or you or your child loses interest, it's time to put the toy away and transition to something else. This is the closing. In an ideal closing, one of the two partners makes a move to end, and you keep operating as partners: Follow your child's lead, but offer guidance through the closing.

♟ Activity: *Maintain the Balanced Partnership While You Close and Transition*

Here are some ideas for closing the joint activity and moving on:

- If you see signs that the activity has lost its teaching potential, suggest something like "Are you all done? Should we finish?" and get out the container that holds the pieces, putting a piece in and encouraging your child to do the same. The two of you will put the pieces away together, close the container together, put it back where it goes together, and then make a transition to a new activity.

● Or your child may signal you that he's finished. If your child refuses to play with the materials any longer, pushes them away, starts to move away, starts being very repetitive in a way that makes it hard to take turns, or shows loss of interest by losing energy, suggest that it's time to be all done and help the cleanup begin. Some children, after they learn the routine, may say "All done" on their own or begin to put materials away and lead you through the process of closing.

● If the activity becomes really repetitive, but your child wants to continue, offer a new activity that will be very attractive to the child so that she stays motivated to play with you. Present the new toy to your child while she is still playing repetitively with the first one. Offer it to her, operate it, and make it look really great. See if your child will reach for it—if so, do a trade, giving her the new toy and taking away the old one (get it out of sight fast). Chances are that this will work well, and you will then be at the initiation phase of a new joint activity. If it doesn't work well and your child protests, go ahead and give a piece or two back (but a minimal amount), and then try again in a few minutes with a different toy. Eventually your child will get bored.

● When you transition to another activity, how do you decide whether to do a sensory social routine or a joint activity with objects? We recommend going back and forth between sensory social routines and object-focused joint activity routines to keep things lively and varied. Sensory social routines are best at times when you want to optimize your child's arousal and motivation for learning. Some children have a preference for one or the other. For example, for a child who prefers object-oriented joint activity routines, you may have to make a concerted effort to add sensory social routines; for a child who does not enjoy objects, you'll have to build up object-focused joint activity routines more gradually. Over time, and as your child's play gets more mature and sophisticated, you will find that you will naturally start incorporating more and more social exchanges into object-focused joint activity routines. The two kinds of routines will naturally become more similar over time. Think about preschool children playing dress-up or action figures. There are as many social elements to their play as there are object-focused actions. However, all the way through preschool and into kindergarten, school programs provide both kinds of activities. Free play often involves more actions on objects, and circle time generally involves songs, finger plays, and other sensory social routines. Book activities and pretend play often blend both. Making sure that you are using the same kinds of play routines other children your child's age are using, in both your sensory social and your object-focused joint activity routines, prepares your child for group learning experiences.

Summary of Step 5

If you have followed along and carried out the preceding activities, you will have developed all of the stages or steps of a joint activity and now have several routines that you and your child can do daily and share with one another. See if you agree with most of the statements in the following checklist. If so, you are now armed with important skills for taking turns and teaching inside joint activities. If not, start experimenting during play and caregiving routines until you have found some methods that work for each statement.

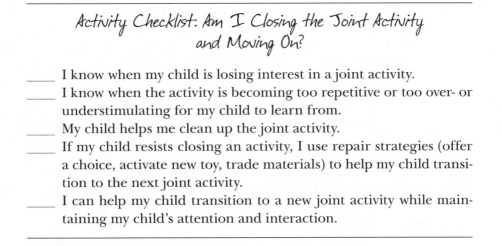

Activity Checklist: Am I Closing the Joint Activity and Moving On?

_____ I know when my child is losing interest in a joint activity.

_____ I know when the activity is becoming too repetitive or too over- or understimulating for my child to learn from.

_____ My child helps me clean up the joint activity.

_____ If my child resists closing an activity, I use repair strategies (offer a choice, activate new toy, trade materials) to help my child transition to the next joint activity.

_____ I can help my child transition to a new joint activity while maintaining my child's attention and interaction.

What about Kylie? *Kylie's parents were concerned about her lack of interest in sensory social routines. Without objects, she just didn't seem to care. But they had seen how much Kylie enjoyed being tickled with objects, and recently she loved it when Dad used an animal puzzle piece and made the animal sound before placing it in the puzzle. They knew from reading Chapter 5 that props can be used to support children's attention to people's faces and bodies during these routines, so Mom began taking turns with Kylie hitting her toy drum with a stick or hands. After a few rounds of this exchange, Mom covered her face with the drum and started a game of peekaboo. She did this a few times, exaggerating the "boo" and even tickling Kylie after appearing from behind the drum. Next Mom placed the drum in front of Kylie's face and said "boo" for her as she pulled the drum away and tickled her daughter. Kylie liked this game for a few minutes, but then started backing away as if to say she was done. Mom responded by acknowledging that Kylie was "all done with peekaboo" and took out a party horn to blow. Kylie had not seen this toy before and quickly approached Mom to take the horn. Kylie's mom blew it a few times; each time, she first sang, "If you're happy and you know it, blow your horn," followed by the "toot-toot" of the horn. Then she held the horn for Kylie to blow, and each time Kylie* *exhaled air, Mom would blow the horn and sing a verse of the song. She wasn't sure Kylie really liked the song, but it didn't matter so much now, because at least there were two sensory social routines that Mom could do in between more object-related games. Mom also realized the importance of practicing these more often throughout the day, so that Kylie could become more familiar with the routines and over time enjoy them more.*

Step 6. Create Joint Activities during Other Daily Routines, to Foster Multiple Areas of Development

Rationale. All kinds of daily caregiving routines have a joint activity structure. For example, mealtimes have an initiation (getting your child into his chair, putting on a bib, wiping off hands), a theme (putting food out so your child begins to eat), one or more variations (you eventually sit down too, usually near your child; interact with your child; eat something yourself, and perhaps share some of your food with your child; respond to your child's requests and refusals; offer a cup and something different to eat), and a closing (asking, "Are you all done?"; wiping off hands and face; untying the bib; taking off the tray; getting the child down).

In Chapter 5 we have discussed the importance of finding ways to include as much time as you can for brief social interactions with your child during your everyday caregiving routines. Thinking about each daily routine as an opportunity for a joint activity may help you think of new ways to carry out these interactions. It is sometimes difficult to set aside enough time to sit down and play with your child, so figuring out how to engage in joint activities during the daily care routines that make up your day is a way of ensuring that your child gets plenty of practice and learning opportunities. We have just reviewed the four phases of a mealtime that fit within each of the four steps for carrying out a joint activity. Take a minute and think through bath time. See if you can think of how the four steps (initiating/setting up a joint activity, establishing a theme, elaborating on/varying the theme, and closing the activity/moving on) would fit there. After you think it through, read on and see how yours is similar to, and different from, our "script":

Initiation/setup: Going to the bathroom, turning on the water, taking off clothes

Theme: Getting into the water, soaping up, and rinsing off

Variation/elaboration: Talking about body parts as you wash them; playing with the suds and bubbles; playing with the bath toys; pouring and dumping water; splashing, kicking, and blowing bubbles; and many more

Closing transition: Getting out, drying off, and putting on PJs

Now how do you create the kind of interaction we have described earlier, so your child is really participating and taking turns in the activity? Your child could participate in the initiation by walking into the bathroom with you (instead of being carried), by helping turn on the water, or by putting her hands under the water and feeling it; by throwing bath toys into the water; by helping take her clothes off, even if it just means pulling her shirt over her head or socks off her toes and putting the clothes in the hamper; and by responding with outstretched hands and maybe some words to your offer to be picked up and put in the water (rather than picking up your child from behind and placing her in the water).

How can your child participate in the theme phase? By taking a turn washing her belly, chest, arms, and legs with the washcloth; by handing you the soap; by helping rub the shampoo into her hair; by holding the cup while you fill it with water; by pouring water on her soapy chest or belly. These are all opportunities for turn taking, with accompanying language and modeling.

The variation phase is probably the easiest to think through, because it is the playtime that goes with bath time. It is an excellent time for playing together in this back-and-forth way. Instead of putting soap on the child's belly, put it on her head. While playing with the rubber ducky, place soap on top of the ducky ("Soap on ducky!").

The closing can involve your child in putting the bath toys in a container; putting the soap in the soap dish; sitting down for drying; offering hands and feet when you request them for drying; helping to pat wet hair with a towel; rubbing lotion on belly and legs; helping comb through hair; and so forth. All the activities you typically do can also include your child and become very rich in language and social learning experiences.

Does this take more time? Absolutely—it's taking all your typical activities and turning them into back-and-forth play and teaching opportunities that your child can absorb. It's much easier to do these caregiving routines without much of a structure; after all, we often just want to get the bath finished! It is easy and fast to change, dress, or feed your child while a video is on and your child is watching. However, when you add the four steps of a joint activity and the turn-taking structure into your daily routines with your child, you're providing a number of important learning elements for your child. You are helping your child learn what is coming, how the whole activity goes, when it will begin, and when it will end. This makes it more predictable for your child and gives your child ways to participate instead of being a passive receiver of your care. You're helping your child learn the meaning of words, of gestures, and the structure of daily life. You're helping your child learn to imitate, to watch and do, to pay attention to other people, and to respond when someone addresses her.

Almost every activity you do with your child can become a joint activity routine: brushing teeth, having your child help with a cooking project, dressing and undressing, going for a walk, bedtime routines, and outings. When a child's daily life includes all these learning opportunities in ongoing interactions with you and other caregivers, your child is getting intervention all day long. You are also likely to find this more fun, because you will be finding your child's smile throughout these exchanges, and nothing is more satisfying to a parent than a happy, enthusiastic child! The following activity will give you tools for identifying potential joint activity steps inside your daily play and caregiving activities with your child.

Activity: *Figure Out a Joint Activity Structure for Your Daily Activities*

Spend a few minutes over the next few days observing how you and your child do the six types of activities discussed in Chapter 4:

1. Toy or other object play
2. Social play
3. Meals
4. Caregiving (bathing/dressing/changing/bedtime)
5. Book activities
6. Household chores

Here are some suggestions for thinking about your daily routines in terms of joint activities:

- For each of the six types of activities just listed, think about how much you use the four-part joint activity structure within them. Which of these include a setup, theme, variation, and closing/transition to the next activity? Which ones lack this structure and might benefit from it? As you identify activities that would benefit from more of a joint activity structure, use the form on page 136 to think through and plan out how you could build a joint activity structure around it. (Make extra copies of the form if you need more space.) Start by making a list of potential themes—the actions you could do in each step that your child would enjoy. If you're not sure how your child might respond, don't worry. You can always try it and make changes based on what worked and didn't work. After you have identified the theme, identify a variation for that theme. Then think about the closing. How can you and your child together close up the activity so your child is participating in the closing? Finally, think about the setup the same way. How can you and your child together begin the activity so your child is expecting what is coming next and is ready to participate?

- Next, try to answer these questions from your observations during this step. For each of the six activities:

    - How can my child and I set up the joint activity?
    - What is the theme of the joint activity? How do we take turns with the theme?

- How can I vary or expand the joint activity? How will we take turns in the variation?
- How can my child and I end and transition to the next joint activity together?

Now here are some specific ideas for structuring your daily routines as joint activities:

- Book activities:

  → **Setup:** Choose a book from a choice of two, and then get positioned face to face.

  → **Theme:** (Child's turn) Child opens book and looks at picture, which you point to and label. (Your turn) You point out next picture and label. Repeat a few times.

  → **Variation:** You add something different—perform an action in an action book, or add sound effects, or count the ducklings, or add a related song. Variations also include going farther in the book, adding more pages, having your child point, asking questions. Don't struggle to think of variations unless the book activity seems to be getting too repetitive.

  → **Closing/transition:** Your child helps put the book back where it belongs, and goes to choose another toy.

- Diapering:

  → **Setup:** Hand your child the diaper (this tells your child what is coming next), and walk together, hand in hand, to the diapering area. Get your child to extend hands for the pickup.

  → **Theme:** Have your child hand you the diaper, the wipe, and so on.

  → **Variation:** Play a social game while your child is still lying down after the clean diaper is on (pattycake, chase/"I'm gonna get you," bumblebee, etc.).

  → **Closing/transition:** Your child sits up, put hands up to be lifted off, throws the dirty diaper in the trash, and leaves the area.

- Meals:

  → **Setup:** Your child puts hands up to be lifted into high chair, helps put bib on, chooses drink or food first.

  → **Theme:** First your child and then you begin to eat or drink.

  → **Variation:** New food, new choices, giving you bites, imitation games, using spoon or fork, trying new foods, pretending to give a doll or stuffed animal a bite.

→ **Closing/transition:** Have your child hand you the dish, the cup, the spoon; help wipe hands and face; help wipe tray; reach for the pickup to get down.

● Outdoors:

→ **Setup:** Get shoes and socks; have child sit down near door; put on jacket, shoes, and socks while child helps with each. Open door, close door.

→ **Theme:** Whatever activity your child chooses. Turn taking can involve signaling to you for pushes on the swing (swing the child from the front rather than the back so you can interact, touch feet, etc.), throwing the ball back and forth, digging together in the sand, catching your child at the bottom of the slide, or the like.

→ **Variation:** A second activity.

→ **Closing/transition:** Put away the balls, shovel, or other equipment. Take hands to walk inside. Take off shoes, socks, jacket, and put away. Wash hands and get drink of water.

● Dressing:

→ **Setup:** Get clothes out and put on floor, bed, or wherever you dress.

→ **Theme:** Hand child shirt and help child put shirt on head; wait for child to pull shirt over head; and so on.

→ **Variation:** Each additional piece of clothing.

→ **Closing/transition:** Finish with a song, applause, closing drawers or closet doors, looking in the mirror and labeling clothes, or other ritual.

Summary of Step 6

If you have followed along and carried out the activities above, you now have ideas or "blueprints" for what kinds of joint activity routines you can embed in all your daily activities. You are now thinking about these activities more as child participation opportunities. These activities will serve as the framework for taking turns and teaching various skills to your child. See if you agree with most of the statements in the following checklist. If so, you are now armed with plans for using the joint activity structure to engage your child in many more back-and-forth learning opportunities throughout your daily activities. If not, start experimenting with the joint activity structure during play and caregiving routines until you have found some methods that work for each.

Activity Checklist: What Kinds of Joint Activities Can I Do with My Child?

_____ I know how to set up a number of games with toys or other objects my child likes to play with, or social games without toys.

_____ I know how to carry out the theme or main action of the game that will make my child smile.

_____ I have ideas for how to vary these activities or add new materials or play actions that I think my child will like.

_____ I have ideas for how my child will help me end the activity and choose the next one.

_____ I have ideas for how to use the four-part joint activity structure during my child's mealtimes.

_____ I have plans for how to use the four-part joint activity structure for outdoor play.

_____ I have tried the four-part joint activity structure for book activities.

_____ I am using the four-part activity structure inside bath times and other caregiving activities.

Chapter Summary

This chapter has focused on how to develop a back-and-forth "dance" with your child during four-part joint activities with toys, social games, and daily caregiving routines. Developing this turn-taking way of interacting with your child and devising these joint activities to frame play and daily caretaking routines involves increased learning opportunities for your child, increased language exposure, increased social interactions, and the opportunity to participate and learn the ins and outs of daily life. Now it's your turn—have fun!

Four-Phase Joint Activity Record

Example	Setup	Theme	Variation	Closing/ transition
Toy or other object play Trains	Choose which trains to use and where to sit.	Take turns laying down the track, connecting cars, and pushing trains around the track.	Trains can crash, go up or down bridges, go through tunnels, circle fast or slowly around track. Or add people or animals to ride in or on top of trains.	Put trains and track into container and choose next activity.
Toy or other object play				
Social play				
Meals				
Caregiving (bathing/ dressing/ changing/ bedtime)				
Book activities				
Household chores				

Refrigerator List

Goal: To teach your child the back-and-forth structure of joint activities.

Steps:

✓ Position yourself and the important materials between you and your child.

✓ Stay in the spotlight! Make sure your child is watching your turns.

✓ Narrate; label; and put in simple words, songs, and sound effects.

✓ Frame play and caregiving activities with the four-part joint activity structure:
  - initiation/setup
  - theme
  - variations
  - closing/transition

✓ Maintain a turn-taking, back-and-forth style through each of the four parts of your joint activities.

7

Talking Bodies

The Importance of Nonverbal Communication

> **Chapter goal:** To provide you with ways to help your child
> (1) learn to express desires, feelings, and interests by using
> body language, and (2) learn to understand your body language.
> Nonverbal communication is a foundation for speech and language.

Why Nonverbal Communication (Body Language) Is So Important

Although most of us think of speech when we think about children's communication, there is much more to communicating than speaking. Long before their speech develops, most babies and toddlers become very skilled at getting their messages across by using their eyes, facial expressions, hand gestures, body postures, and sounds. They also learn to understand their parents' body language very well. Bodies talk! Recognizing and using nonverbal communication teaches them that one mind can choose to send thoughts and feelings to another—through eye contact, actions/gestures, and sounds—and that the other mind can interpret these messages that travel from the body, through the air, into the eyes, and into the mind of the partner. This is what communication is all about.

Through body language, your child will come to understand that he can interpret your thoughts, feelings, desires, and interests, and that you can interpret his. This is why nonverbal communication is so important: It allows your child a new way of understanding other people and himself as people with inner lives, with mental states that can be shared. In other words, you can read each other's cues, which in a sense means reading minds! This is how we interact with each other—by sharing what is going on in our minds and hearts.

And it's not just that nonverbal communication allows a child who doesn't speak a way to express himself. Nonverbal communication, most language researchers believe, provides a crucial foundation for speech development. Once a child understands that communication exists, speech and gestures take on meaning. Speech becomes an additional communication system, built on our first communication system, which we call ***talking bodies***.

What's Happening in Autism?

Autism interferes with learning about others' minds. Young children with autism have lots of difficulty learning that messages are sent from one person to another, from the mind, through the body, and into the eyes, ears, and mind of the other. This process of choosing to send messages and "reading" others' messages may not seem to exist for them. Many young children with autism seem unaware that communication occurs between two people; they do not recognize the importance of gaze, gestures, speech sounds, and facial expressions. A child who doesn't know that there is meaning in those signals will not pay attention or look for meaning. Some children move their parents around and push their hands toward things to try to send messages. Some young children with autism do not use any clear signals at all to communicate their needs or wants. Their parents have to decide when it is time for the child to eat, to be changed, to go to bed, without many cues from their child. Other children may fuss or demonstrate distress, but they don't communicate what their unhappiness is all about, so that their parents have to work very hard to figure out what their child needs.

Why Is It a Problem?

When a child doesn't communicate at all, or communicates distress but not the cause of it, her parents may get so accustomed to making decisions for her that their child no longer has any unmet needs. Life is easy! Everything is being managed by someone else! Why would a child whose every need is met be motivated to start communicating?

These autism-caused barriers to nonverbal communication can severely delay all communication development, and these barriers to communication can remain in place for many years—holding up speech and language development, preventing social exchanges based on shared meaning with parents and others, and severely limiting children's access to learning. Before early intervention was available to most children, it was not uncommon for us to see some children as old as age 8 or 10 who were still completely unaware of communication. They were without speech, gesture, or alternative communication, which meant that they were also without social exchanges or interactions with peers and siblings.

Juliana's parents don't know what to do about their 2½-year-old's mealtimes. Instead of sitting in her high chair at mealtimes, their little girl wants to have access to her cereal, sandwich, and fruit bars while she is moving about the house, cup in hand. To accommodate her—since she screams, throws herself back, and will not sit when they try to put her in the high chair—her parents keep a little stash of food (cereal bowl, crackers, bits of breakfast bars) on a low shelf in the kitchen where she can always reach them. But this means that crumbs and sticky little fingerprints end up everywhere.

When Juliana wants something special, she pulls her mother by the hand to the kitchen and stands in front of the pantry or the refrigerator. However, when her mother opens the pantry, Juliana has no way to communicate what she wants, since she has not yet learned to point or speak. Her mother has to hold up one item at a time and offer it, and Juliana cries and gets upset each time her mother offers her something she doesn't want. Since Juliana has no clear gestures, her mother might have to offer 10 different choices to find something she will eat, and Juliana often takes only two bites and then rejects the food and begins the process all over again. This goes on many times a day and is an ongoing source of stress for both Juliana and her mother. Juliana's aunt criticizes her mother for "spoiling her," but Juliana is on the slender side for her age, and her mother is really worried about her nutrition. She has no idea how to solve this problem. She wishes that Juliana could communicate what she wants by pointing or labeling.

▶▶▶▶ What You Can Do to Increase Your Child's Nonverbal Communication

Developing nonverbal communication—talking bodies—builds a road to speech and language and lays down a two-way communication road to other people. Here are five specific steps you can take to help your young child with autism develop a talking body and take more responsibility for communicating his needs, interests, and feelings—that is, for being a more active communicator:

Step 1. Do less so your child does more.

Step 2. Wait a little.

Step 3. Create lots of practice opportunities.

Step 4. Persist.

Step 5. Position yourself.

In the following pages, we describe how to carry out each of these steps, give you some ideas for activities to try, and suggest what you can do to solve problems that may come up.

Step 1. Do Less So Your Child Does More

Rationale. Young children with autism, like all young children, need to learn to use gestures, eye contact, expressions, and sounds to make choices, to indicate what they want, to share their feelings, and to reject things they don't want. Doing less to anticipate a child's needs—giving choices among objects, rather than giving your child free access to everything; offering your child more than one choice; or offering your child things you know she does not want—encourages her to communicate.

♟ Activity: *Figure Out How to Encourage Your Child to Communicate More Throughout the Day*

Spend time over the next few days observing your child during the six types of activities discussed in Chapter 4:

1. Toy or other object play
2. Social play
3. Meals
4. Caregiving (bathing/dressing/changing/bedtime)
5. Book activities
6. Household chores

Here are some ideas for encouraging your child to do more to communicate:

● In each of the six activities just listed, think about the theme of the activity and how you can help your child do more during the activity. Can you break up his cracker into several pieces for your child to request, or place only a few cookies in his bowl before he has to ask for more? Can you offer more choices during the activity to increase your child's participation? What about the setup? Do you think your child can be more involved in helping you open up containers, take materials out, choose which items to use? Remember the four-step joint activity sequence of setup, theme, variation, and closing/transition that you have learned in Chapter 6.

> *"Often parents feel that without verbal language, or with this diagnosis of autism, their children are incapable of doing things. They think they are helping them by overdoing things for their children, but they are decreasing independence and hindering the learning process unintentionally."*

● Next, for each one of these four phases, make a list of what actions you could do that will help your child participate more in the activity. (We have provided a form for you to use to keep your list right in this book if you want to. It's near the end of this chapter.) If you're not sure how your child might respond, try it and make changes based on what worked and didn't work.

Step 2. Wait a Little

Rationale. One way of doing less is by waiting for a cue from your child before you hand over what she wants. Start to wait for your child to communicate with you about what she wants. You will build up your child's repertoire of communicative behaviors—gaze, hand gestures, sounds—and your child's awareness that each of these ways of communicating sends a message and gets her what she wants.

 ### Activity: *Wait, but Actively Watch for Your Child's Cue*

When your child clearly wants something—to be picked up, to be given a drink, to get a bath toy, to reach a favorite object that you have retrieved from under the couch—hold the desired object up in front of your body and wait. Wait for a small gesture, wait for brief eye contact, wait for a vocalization. Wait for your child to do something to communicate what he wants. Look for eye contact, an outstretched hand, or a vocalization—some sound or gesture that is your child's expression of his desires or feelings. When you see that gesture or hear that sound, quickly give your child what he is requesting with that single communication.

 Helpful Tip
Although most young children tend to use their voices, hands, and eyes all together to cue their parents, children with autism tend to use these separately. Eventually your child will learn how to combine gesture, gaze, and voice to communicate wants, needs, feelings, and interests to you. In Chapter 13, we'll discuss how to help your child combine these behaviors in communications.

 ### Activity: *Problem-Solve to Minimize Your Child's Frustration*

Here are some ideas for problem solving as you wait and watch:

● **What if your child uses crying and screaming as the communication, like Juliana?** Waiting will only result in more crying. If your child uses crying to communicate, then you will have to start to offer the choice *before* your child has the idea, before the crying begins. If your child is approaching you to be picked up, notice that the approach is coming before your child fusses to be picked up, bend down, and extend your hands toward your child's hands. As your child extends his hands to you (there is the gesture), follow with a pickup.

> **What about Juliana?** *Juliana's parents started initiating the trip to the pantry. While Juliana was doing something else, they would line up three or four favorite foods from the pantry along the edge of the counter. They would then find Juliana, take her by the hand, and say something like "Let's get some food." They would then walk to the kitchen, bend down beside Juliana, and point to the objects: "What do you want?" As Juliana reached for one of the items, her parents would take it down, hold it in front of her, and offer it partway, so that she had to reach again toward them. As soon as Juliana reached, they would give her the food, because Juliana had communicated with the reach.*

- **What if your child just stands there and doesn't do anything?** Get down a favorite item, squat down so you are face to face with your child, and offer the object partway to your child: "Do you want bunny [or other favorite toy]?" As she reaches to take it, say "Yes, you want bunny," and give it to her. Your child has communicated with a gesture—the reach!

Step 3. Create Lots of Practice Opportunities

Rationale. For your child to learn how to use his body to communicate, he will need lots and lots of practice. You can create many opportunities every hour that you are with your child, by not ignoring his needs but finding ways to hold back a little from giving things to your child without requiring him to communicate. The idea here is to create communication temptations.

♟ Activity: *Creatively Hold Back before Giving Things to Your Child*

Here are some ideas for creating communication temptations:

- Before you pick up your child, offer your arms—but wait to pick your child up until she looks at you or raises her arms in response to you. The look can be fleeting at first.

- When your child needs a drink of water, put some water in his cup, bend down so you are face to face, and hold the cup in front of you—but wait to hand it over until your child looks, vocalizes, or reaches.

- Create situations in which your child needs your help. Sometimes children have access to everything they need without needing to communicate to anyone for help. If this is true for your child, you can begin to keep your child's favorite toys, cup, snacks, or other special objects visible but out of reach (on a shelf or in a closed clear container), so that your child has to request your help to get what she wants. What would this look like? Your child may reach to the shelf, may bring you the container, or may stand there and fuss. You can say, "What do you want?" If your child reaches or points for the object, gestures to be picked up, vocalizes in a way that is not crying or fussing, or looks at you for help, say, "You want the [object]" as you get it. Then say, "Here's the [object]."

- If your child stands there but doesn't make any communicative action, help your child make a clear request with his body. You can pick up the desired object and move it closer to elicit a reach ("Want [object]?"), offer your arms to elicit an arms-up gesture to be picked up ("Want up?"), or position yourself at your child's level and right in front ("What do you need?") to elicit a brief look or a sound of some type. Pick up the child right away or get the object if your child gives you eye contact or makes some type of sound other than fussing in response to your question.

- If your child is fussing about wanting an object and is headed toward a bigger upset, offer your arms for pickup, pick her up after she extends her arms, lift her toward the object, and watch for a reach. If there is no reach and no gesture, pick up the object with your free hand, but keep it out of your child's reach; then wait until the look, reach, or vocalization occurs before giving it to her. Or, while your child is still on the floor, pick the object up off the shelf and move it slightly closer to her to elicit a reach before you give it. Because you give her the object right after the gesture, sound, or eye contact, she will learn that it was one of these nonverbal cues that resulted in your handing her the toy.

- When you give your child something, it might still be in the closed container. Then your child will need to give it back to get your help to open it. If he doesn't readily give it back, extend your hands and say, "Need help?" He will likely hand it to you, but if he doesn't, help him put it in your open hand. Then open it and give it back right away, saying something like "Here's the [object]!"

- Instead of getting the one cereal box from the shelf that you know your child wants, get two, including one your child doesn't like. Hold the two cereal boxes in front of your child to elicit a reach or touch to the one she wants. Or give the child the one she doesn't want, and when she begins to protest or refuse to take it, say, "Janie says no" (with a vigorous head shake) while you offer your open hand to take back the unwanted cereal. Then immediately offer her preferred cereal box to her, and when she reaches to it, say, "Janie says yes, Cheerios!" while you nod your head yes and start to pour the cereal. Now Janie has communicated two feelings nonverbally—protest and desire.

● Instead of picking up your child repeatedly to swing, tickle, or hug him, do the action once and then put your child down. Then look expectantly at your child and wait a second to see if your child comes back for more ("Want more swing?"). If so, there is some body language! Do it again right away ("Yes, Ethan wants swing!"). If your child looks at you but doesn't act, respond right away and swing. If your child stands there but doesn't communicate in any way, reach down and offer your arms and wait for the child to reach back. If he does, proceed to swing. If your child does not respond to the offer and is still there waiting, go ahead and deliver the swing or other action again ("Swing!"). Do it a couple of times and then stop again, offer your hands again, and wait, just like you did before. See if your child will reach for your hands, look in your eyes, or make a sound communicating that he wants you to repeat the game.

● Instead of blowing bubbles, a balloon, a windmill, or a noisemaker repeatedly, do it once or twice so your child gets interested. Then get ready to do it the third time, but wait! Stand there with the bubble wand or other toy posed at your mouth, and look right at your child's eyes. Ask "Blow?" and make a little blow, but don't blow the toy. Your child may look right at your eyes, may try to blow, may reach out, smile, or make a sound. If your child does any of these, blow! Do this repeatedly, waiting for a communication before many of the blows. But give a couple of "freebies" too, so that this is easy rather than hard, and your child gets plenty of effects to keep her motivated.

● Mealtimes and snack times at the table are great times to practice. Before you put the food on your child's high chair tray, hold it in front of you and in front of your child, offering it but waiting for your toddler to communicate somehow that he wants it. Give five Cheerios on the high chair tray instead of filling it, so that your child has to request more again and again. Pour a little bit of milk or juice into his cup rather than filling it, so that he has to request more and more. Don't set out cups of water or snack items for your child to help himself to. Offer all these as choices so that your child needs to request them.

Later in the chapter, we discuss how, over time, you will begin to ask for more elaborate communications—such as using a point instead of just a reach, or using both gesture and a vocalization at the same time. For now, the goal is to help your child develop a talking body by learning to use simple nonverbal communications like eye contact, sounds, reaches, directed smiles, and other body gestures.

"We used these techniques at mealtime, but it was always tricky to decide exactly how hard to push my son to respond, [since] he was underweight and we didn't want to reduce his nutritional intake. One helpful suggestion was that we should always provide food or drink on request, but could give a less favored item if he didn't give any indication of a want or preference. That helped us be consistent, rather than worrying that he would lose weight due to our efforts. You could also use this technique for snacks or desserts instead of mealtime."

Helpful Tip

Consider behaviors your child might use when wanting something to happen:

- Wanting your attention: raising arms; looking up at you; making a sound; touching or tapping you; holding up an object to show you
- Wanting something out of reach: pointing to or asking for the object; giving a closed container for you to open; nodding for you to retrieve the object; showing where the object goes; looking at the object and reaching
- Refusing or being "all done" with something: giving an object to you; putting an object on the table or in the container; shaking head; verbalizing "no" or "all done"; throwing the item away (if appropriate), leaving

Here are more ideas:

- Instead of plopping all the bath toys into the tub, offer one or two while naming each, and wait for your child to communicate the request before you hand it to him.

- Instead of having your child's toys all out and available, organize some of them in clear shoeboxes (with snug lids) on a shelf, and have your child choose a box. Once she gets the closed box, wait for a nonverbal communication that your child needs help to open it. Offer your hand and ask if she needs help.

- Instead of dumping out the pieces of a puzzle all at once, keep the pieces and offer them to your child one at a time as you name each one, or as a choice between two ("Bear or horse?"). Elicit a reach, gaze, or another nonverbal communication for most of them. Name it as your child gets it: "Bear! You wanted bear!" Give a few here and there as freebies when your child looks at them ("Here's pig!") to keep motivation high. Do this when playing with any toys that have multiple pieces.

● When changing your child's diaper, give her the diaper to hold and then ask for it when it's time to put it on (hold out your hand and say, "Give me diaper!"). If she doesn't give it to you, then take it: "Give me diaper. Thank you. Here's diaper." When putting your child's shoes on to go outside, tell your child to sit down on the floor or couch in front of you. Put her shoes and socks between the two of you, and have her hand you each shoe and sock one at a time (help as needed) to put on as you ask for them ("Give me sock," "Give me shoe"). Narrate as you put each item on, as described in Chapter 4. With dressing, have your child hand you each piece of clothing when you ask for it. Help as needed, and narrate as you go.

● When bathing, ask your child for each hand and each foot. Ask for the shampoo and washcloth. Offer each toy before you give it. For each, name objects as you go, offering choices or help as needed. Doing all these caregiving activities in this way gets your child actively engaged in the activities and gets your child attending and responding to you, rather than being a passive participant in the process.

We have described many ways you can help your child develop a talking body and use her body to communicate, but how should you respond when she does it? With your body *and* your voice. Follow through on your child's communication—do the action or give the object requested, and narrate! Add some words to describe what the child wanted, or what he or she was doing, or what was happening:

> *"My son wasn't willing to help with dressing or shampooing at first, but using narration while guiding him helped us reach the point where he would participate."*

- "You want cereal."
- "More juice."
- "Get the bubbles."
- "Bang bang" (when banging toys).
- "No milk" (when your child refuses).
- "Blow balloon."
- "Up."
- "More swing."
- "Pour water."

In Chapter 13 we discuss in much more detail how to choose your language.

The ideas listed for this step show how many times an hour you can set up an opportunity for your child to communicate with you by using body language. You might find that your toddler can communicate with you as often as 60 times in an hour of play or caregiving activities—once a minute—if you really slow down and stop handing things over and doing things *to* your child, and instead *involve* your child in the activity and draw out nonverbal communication *from* your child.

♟ Activity: *Choose Certain Gestures to Teach*

We have been discussing at length how and when you can encourage your child's gestural communication. But which specific gestures are good choices to teach first? In choosing gestures, you will want to consider two issues: (1) what gestures you can easily prompt, shape, and elicit from your child during the teaching/learning phase and (2) what messages the gesture needs to convey.

There are three main types of messages that very young children tend to deliver in the preverbal communication period: desires for social interaction, efforts to control other people's behavior (called "behavior regulation"), and efforts to share attention with other people about interesting objects and events—joint attention. We will hold off discussing joint attention until Chapter 10 and focus now on gestures you can help your child learn to convey her desires for social interaction and behavior regulation.

Young children communicate their desire for social interaction with all kinds of body language. They look intently and smile to invite an interaction or to respond to a fun game. They reach to people they want to play with. They make gestures to cue parents to sing favorite songs, to tickle them, to chase them. They reach for more when their parents start and then stop a social game. They use their voices to call, laugh, or chuckle. They come right up to parents to gain their attention and begin an interaction. They clap, wave bye-bye, give high fives, and make gestures for simple games like peekaboo at parents' request.

In Chapter 5, you worked on developing many of these gestures with your child during all kinds of social activities. You very likely have already helped your child develop gestures like looking, smiling, reaching, and carrying out some gestures as ways of beginning a social game with you or continuing these games when you pause. You have also been working on teaching your child the "arms up" gesture when requesting a pickup or hug. Other communications in this group that are often easy to teach young children with ASD are looking and waving during greetings and high five. We will briefly describe how to go about teaching your child each of these.

- To teach your child to look and wave during greetings, begin by developing a very clear routine with your child for "hi" and "bye." When you go into his room for the first time each morning, and every time you return to him from being away—in another room, on an errand, after a nap—say "Hi!" with a big smile and an exaggerated wave as soon as you see him. Then walk right up to your child and repeat the "hi," smile, and give a big wave when you are right in front of him and face to face (you'll have to squat down if your child is standing on the floor). Then take your child's arm at the wrist or below and help your child wave as you say, "Hi, Mommy." Do the same thing whenever you are leaving, "Bye-bye." Say, "Bye-bye!" and wave when you are close to and right in front of your child so you can prompt him, and then, as you walk away, turn back and repeat it just before you walk out. Try to find multiple times each day to repeat these greeting routines when you are approaching or leaving your child. You can also cue other people to use the same greeting routines, and even make stuffed animals do these greeting routines. Always help your child respond, with a wave and with your words, "hi" or "bye-bye." After a few days of this, continue your routine, but try to provide less of a prompt when you cue your child to respond. Instead of taking your child's hand and prompting the full wave, try waiting a few seconds and then prompting more from the elbow than from the wrist. Be very consistent with this, offering many practice opportunities a day. It is quite likely that within a month your child will begin to respond to your greetings with a wave, eye contact, and perhaps even the words.

● High five is another gesture that is a good early choice. To teach it, choose a time when your child is sitting facing you and you are at eye level. Offer your open hand to your child, aimed toward one of her hands, saying, "Give me five," and then with your other hand, take your child's hand and slap it gently against your palm. Follow with a tickle and then practice it again a few times. Practice every day, multiple times, providing less help each day than the day before: Instead of operating your child's hand, drop back to her wrist, and then in the next few days drop farther back, to her lower arm. In a week or two you will likely see her responding to your offer of your open hand and your verbal request for "high five" by placing her hand on yours. Once she places her hand on yours without any help, start to practice the gentle slap that goes with high five by playing a kind of two-handed pattycake. This will very likely evolve into a full high five in the next few weeks.

Young child's behavior regulation communications generally have two meanings: requests ("Do this for me") and protests ("I don't want that; no"). You have been focusing on developing clear requests for desired objects and interactions through communicative reaching for several chapters now. A second important request that young children need to communicate is to ask for help.

● You can teach your child to hand you things and look at you to request help. We have already discussed the use of baggies, plastic containers, and other barriers you can place around desired objects, so that your child needs to hand them to you, and look, to request help in opening them. Other objects that easily support requests for help are windup toys, flashlights with difficult switches, bubbles with tight lids, juice boxes and food containers that need to be opened, and so forth.

In all of these situations, you can offer your child the closed, familiar container, which your child will take but will be unable to open. You then offer your open hand (the "give me" gesture), while you ask, "Help?/Need help? Sure, I'll help you!" Help your child give it to you and then open it fast and give the object back right away (this is the reinforcer for his gesture). Practice this often, with many materials. As your child becomes skilled at putting the object in your open hand, close your hand so your child has to do more to get your help, by putting it against your closed hand. The next step is to have your hand available but on your lap, so your child has to do more to put the object in your hand. As the last step, hold something else in your hands so your child has to do a full approach and offer to you to request your help. Every time your child makes a help request you say, "Help?/Need help? Sure, I'll help you!" (or the like) and give help right away. Over the course of this procedure, your child may very well begin to imitate your word "help" while she gives you the object with which she needs help.

● All children need to have some way to communicate "no." Providing a gesture for "no" may replace crying, throwing, or other unwanted behavior that your child currently uses. Teaching children to shake their head "no" is a rather difficult task until they have mastered facial and gestural imitations. The first protest gesture that most toddlers use is to push unwanted things away. You can easily teach this to your child once your child has a clear requesting gesture for desired objects. Pushing away for "no" is easiest to teach during a meal. The meal should be made up of at least one finger food your child likes a lot and one that she does not like (raw carrots, celery sticks, or green pepper slices work well). Begin by offering your child several bites, one at a time, of a preferred food, like a cracker. ("Want cracker? Yes, you want cracker.") Wait each time for the reach request before you hand it over. Then, after three or four bites, offer the unwanted food instead of the cracker, in the same way you offered the desired food ("Want carrot?"), moving it toward your child. If your child takes it, wait until she starts to put it down or get rid of it. Then take it back, saying, "No, you don't want carrot. You want cracker." And freely give a cracker ("Here's your cracker"). After a few more bites of the preferred food, offer the carrot again. After enough repetitions of this routine, your child will start to push away the carrot before it gets too close—that is the behavior you are trying to teach. As soon as she starts to push it away, pull it back while saying, "No, you don't want carrot; you want cracker," and then freely give the desired food.

Once your child begins to push away unwanted food at mealtimes, you can practice this in toy play as well, occasionally offering an unwanted object (a tissue, an empty small box, etc.) when you are handing toys over one at a time—as you might during a puzzle routine, building block towers, or putting shapes in a shaper sorter—at your child's reaching request. Teach your child to protest by pushing things away and giving things back to you, always using the "no" script.

The gestures just described are the first ones that we teach in our intervention work, and they provide a very strong initial foundation for communication.

Step 4. Persist

Rationale. With all of these new routines, your child will likely not understand at first what you want, and may fuss or resist because you have changed the way you are doing things. You will help things go smoothly by making it easy for your child to communicate and get what she wants. But persist so that learning occurs.

Activity: *Keep It Very Easy for Your Child*

Here are some ideas for keeping these new routines easy for your child:

- Look for communications (gaze, reach, sounds) you know your child can easily produce.

- Help your child do what you want him to do (reach, point, raise arms).

- Hand over the desired object or activity really fast after your child communicates, so your child quickly learns that this communication—no matter how small—is powerful. It has big effects and brings rewards.

- Be sure that each of these new routines is leading up to something your child wants, so there is a reward at the end. High chair choices mean food! Pointing to toys on the shelf gets toys! Maybe handing over a diaper at the changing table is followed by a favorite tickle game or by a moving mobile or music to see and hear, or by a favorite toy to hold for a few minutes while the diaper is changed. Get a hands-up at the end of diapering before you lift your child down from the table or up from the floor.

- Once you have had a success, keep repeating the new routines. You are likely to see your child learn your new way pretty quickly, and your child will begin to anticipate the routine, your expectations, and your cues. Over time, you will see your child use more and more nonverbal communications in your routines.

Step 5. Position Yourself

Rationale. When people communicate, they face each other. Especially for fostering eye contact, you must be facing your child, and your face should not be too far away from the child's face. Communicating with your child face to face also makes it much easier for your child to get the idea of directing her eyes, voice, and gestures to you, not just out into space somewhere.

♟ Activity: *Find Ways to Position Yourself Face to Face with Your Child and Put the Desired Objects between You*

All the ways we have suggested in Chapter 4 for positioning yourself to promote your child's attention to you can be used here. Even for a book activity, try to position yourself in front of your child on the couch, on a bed, or on the floor (with the child in a bean bag chair or sitting with his back against a chair or couch) so that you are an active and communicating partner in the activity, not a faceless book-reading machine. When you are in front of your child with books, and draw your child's attention to pictures with your pointing, words, and sound effects, your child has much more experience of you as the *partner* in the book activity, rather than being a voice from behind and a hand on the book. Your child sees you form the words and sees you gesture, and begins to understand reading as a social rather than a visual activity.

Summary of Steps 1 through 5

If you have followed along and carried out the preceding activities, you will have found a number of ways to increase your child's nonverbal communication—use of gestures, gaze, and expressions—to communicate his wants, feelings, and thoughts. You will find yourself doing more *with* your child, and less *to or for* your child. As a result, you are probably beginning to see your child use much more body language to communicate spontaneously. See if you agree with most of the statements in the following checklist. If so, you are now armed with important skills for helping your child develop nonverbal communication—knowledge that will also help your child develop speech and language. If not, try to experiment with the preceding activities until you have experienced some success with each of the statements in the checklist.

Activity Checklist: Am I Doing Less So My Child Is Doing More?

_____ I know how to wait for my child to communicate; I do this many times a day.

_____ I have found many opportunities during the day for my child to communicate.

_____ I have made communication opportunities for my child during many different play and caregiving routines, and we do these most days.

_____ Once I expect my child to communicate, I know how to persist and to help my child so we usually have success.

_____ I routinely position myself in front of my child, and close to eye level, so it is easy for my child to direct communications to me.

_____ My child is learning how to use his or her body to communicate in many more situations at home then he or she used to.

⫸➡ What You Can Do to Increase Your Child's Understanding of Others' Nonverbal Communication

Children with autism are often remarkably unaware of the meaning of other people's nonverbal communications. It is not unusual to see a young child with ASD who does not understand the "give me" gesture of an open hand or the meaning of a point. Your child may not understand the significance of an angry or sad facial expression on another person. Sometimes people interpret the child's lack of interest or response to others' expressions as a lack of cooperation, but many children with ASD just do not understand what is being asked. We need to teach young children with autism to pay attention to people and what they are doing and help them understand what others' body language means. Children without communication problems seem to learn this effortlessly. For children with autism, however, we need to throw a spotlight onto other people's body language so it really stands out for them. How can you do that?

Here are three steps you can take:

Step 1. Exaggerate your gestures.

Step 2. Add predictable steps.

Step 3. Provide needed help.

Step 1. Exaggerate Your Gestures

When you are playing with toys with your child, highlight your own gestures in your toy routines, along with your speech. Ask your child to give you pieces, to pick up pieces, or to put them in, by extending your hand for the pieces or pointing to where they go while you speak. Use your hands and body as well as your words to convey this, and then help your child follow through. Use hand and body gestures that are relatively easy for your child to imitate, such as reaches, points, open hands, and pushing away—gestures that can easily be incorporated into your joint activity and sensory social routines.

- Object-based gestures: showing, pointing, giving, putting in/taking out, turning, pushing, crashing, rolling, banging
- Sensory social gestures: showing, pointing, clapping, patting, jumping, creepy fingers, tickling, stomping

Have your child help to set up or clean up an activity or to take the next turn, using your body to communicate this by showing her how, by handing pieces, pointing, using hand gestures. Ham it up! Help your child follow through; be sure your child achieves her goal as soon as she follows through; and give your child lots of praise for following through. All of your routines are vehicles for body language.

Here are some ideas:

- When dressing, show and label each piece of clothing before you put it on. When you involve your child in helping or giving, use big gestures like holding your hand out for your child to give.

- When diapering, show the diaper and name it before you give it to your child to hold. When you ask for it back, use a big gesture to get it, and a give the child big "thank you" afterward.

- At mealtimes, give your child a few bits of food on the high chair tray, and then point to one for him to eat: "This one—get this one!" Help your child follow your point to get it. If he doesn't, then next time, give just one and point to that one before your child gets it. That way, your child *has* to be following your point.

- At bath time, ask for a hand or foot to wash by pointing, asking, and holding your hand out. Ask for the bath toys at the end, and point to them to be put away, one at a time.

- During sensory social games, exaggerate the gestures for chase, tickle, swing, spin, "Itsy-Bitsy Spider," and other songs and finger plays. Get down on eye level, face your child, make a big excited smile, position your hands dramatically, and then start the game with big energy. Help your child anticipate what is going to happen from your face and body posture, and build her excitement and anticipation.

Step 2. Add Predictable Steps

It will help your child a great deal to understand your gestures in routines if you add routine steps and sequences to the play and care routines, and then use a gesture or other nonverbal action to cue your child to take the next step. Carry out your activities or games in predictable steps, repeating the routine in step-like fashion a few times in a row, so that your child understands the steps of the routine and can anticipate what is next. Then the next time you repeat the sequence, pause at one of the steps, use an exaggerated gesture, and wait for a response.

> *Lindee has built a very predictable routine around bubbles for her 18-month-old son, Anthony. The bubbles sit on a bookshelf above Anthony's reach, along with other favorite toys.*
>
> ***Setup:** First (Step 1), Lindee says, "Want to play?" while she offers her hand. He takes it, and they walk together over to the bookshelf. Step 2: Then she turns to face him, and she waits for him to extend his arms and look at her for a pickup. If he does this, she says, "You want up," and picks him up. If he doesn't, she extends her arms and says, "Want up?" Then she waits for his arms and eyes before she lifts. Step 3: She lifts him toward the shelf, and he reaches towards the bubbles. Step 4: With her free hand she picks up the bubbles, saying, "You want bubbles! Here are the bubbles," and hands them to him. She then puts him down. Step 5: He tries to open the bubbles but cannot, and she extends her hand: "Need help?" He looks at her and puts the bubbles in her hand. Step 6: "Open. Open bubbles," she says as she opens them. She pulls out the wand and positions herself to blow.*
>
> ***Theme:** Lindee looks right at Anthony's eyes, says, "Blow bubbles?", and makes a little blowing gesture with her mouth. Step 7: Anthony looks directly at her, smiles, and blows. She immediately blows a stream of bubbles for him. He smiles, reaches for the bubbles, and bats them.*
>
> ***Variation:** Step 8: Lindee catches a big bubble with the wand, holds it out to Anthony, and says "Pop?" He points his finger and pops the bubble as she says "pop." Step 9: She extends her finger and pops another as he watches, which he then imitates, poking while she says "pop." Step 10: The bubbles are all done, and Anthony looks around, sees the bubble container right there, and picks it up. He hands it to Lindee with eye contact, and the process begins again.*

Look at this episode. It takes 2–3 minutes, and inside this routine are 10 different communicative steps. Anthony produces one or more nonverbal communications inside each step, several each minute. For a child who 3 weeks ago produced absolutely no communicative gestures, this is a huge transformation. And the set routine that Lindee uses to do this simple game helps Anthony anticipate each next action and cue her for it. He is now an active communicative partner, fully engaged and co-constructing each step of this simple routine. If a simple bubble routine can foster so many communications, imagine how much can be done with a more elaborate routine like a meal or a puzzle.

Here are some examples of talking body signals you could use throughout your interactive routines during the six target activities (toy or other object play, social play, meals, caregiving, book activities, and household chores):

- Use a hand or body movement to "ask" whether your child would like to continue a song or game.

- Use eye contact and an expectant look to "ask" whether your child would like to receive or take an object, cup, or food item.

- Use a sound effect to cue the child that you are about to create an action with an object.

- Smile or laugh and wiggle your fingers to indicate that you are about to tickle your child.

- Extend your hand to indicate that you are about to play a physical game.

- Mimic the blow gesture to indicate that you are going to blow bubbles or blow up a balloon.

The example with Lindee and Anthony illustrates one of the reasons we place such importance on using the structure of joint activities for play and for care routines. It is much easier for your child to understand what you are indicating and saying if she already knows what will happen next. So, as much as you can in all your daily child routines, think about a consistent setup, theme, variation, and closing. This is every bit as important for bathing, diapering, dressing, meals, and so forth as it is for object and social play. If you need a reminder, go back to Chapter 6 and review the section on joint activity routines.

Step 3. Provide Needed Help

An effective way to teach your child to "ask" for help, by giving materials to you or by looking at you for help, is to use something that is a little too difficult for your child to do alone. While you are providing the help your child needs, you will also be using different gestures to help your child learn to understand nonverbal communication.

Here are some possibilities:

- For a child who likes puzzles, you could use a puzzle that's a little too difficult for your child to complete alone. As you and your child are completing the puzzle together, *point* to the holes for each of the pieces, while saying "It goes here! Here!" When your child follows your point, then the pieces go in. Voilà—there is the reward for noticing and following your point!

- You might put the puzzle pieces for a favorite puzzle in a plastic container or bag that your child cannot open himself. Give him the puzzle and container of pieces, and wait for him to need your help. When your child realizes he can't open it by himself, ask if he needs help, *using an open hand to request it* along with words. Then, when he puts it in your hand, open it and give it right back. His reward for responding to your open hand and making the request is getting access to the pieces.

● You might start a windup toy that your child loves to watch. Don't wind it up too much! When it runs out, wait to see what your child does. She may look at you or give it to you. If so, say, "You want more?" as you wind it up and do it again. If not, ask your child to give it to you by using an *outstretched hand* and words. Then, as soon as your child gives it to you (even if you need to help), wind it up fast and get it going again.

In addition to these activities in which you are providing help, sensory social routines can be used to teach children the meaning of nonverbal communication. When you are playing games like chase/"I'm gonna get you," airplane, "Ring-around-the-Rosy," pattycake, or peekaboo, *highlight your expressions, gestures, and body movements*, so that your child learns the relationships between your movements and the game. Your movements and words will "label" the game for your child. Playing games and performing caregiving activities in a kind of ritualized way—the joint activity structure—with toys, with sensory social routines, with diapering/dressing/bathing/bedtime routines, and with mealtime routines will help your child learn to associate your gestures, facial expressions, and words with the routines. You are teaching your child how to read and interpret the meaning of your face, gestures, body movements, and words.

> ### 🖐 *Helpful Tip*
>
> Just as with increasing your child's nonverbal communication to you, increasing your child's understanding of your nonverbal communication requires that you create lots of practice opportunities, persist, and position yourself to get your child's attention.
>
> Tape notes or reminders to yourself in the areas where you provide your child's care and play—over the changing table, over the bathtub, on the kitchen table, by the child's bed, on the wall by the play areas—to remind you to set up routines and gestures.

⋙➡ Planning Activities to Increase Nonverbal Communication

It might help you get into the swing of incorporating all the preceding steps into your daily routines if you use the two forms discussed in this section to plan. First, think of an object-focused joint activity and a sensory social routine that your child really enjoys doing with you. Imagine going through the steps and sequences of that routine. What gesture could your child use to request these preferred actions, movements, or consequences from you? Look at the two examples in the form on pages 160–161, and then try filling out a few more activities to practice with your child this week. Make extra copies of the form to record information about additional activities besides those listed on the left, if you like.

For some parents, it is helpful to dissect the day into the six types of play and caregiving activities or routines that occur throughout the day, and then to break down the joint activity steps that each routine involves. When you do this, you have a framework for thinking through the different gestures, actions, facial expressions, and words that go with those steps. The form on pages 162–163 provides you with some examples that other parents have developed. Try one or more of these out, varying the steps to fit your own home and materials. Be sure to narrate each step, provide clear gesture cues, and cue your child to take some active role with every step. Next, try writing out a "script" for yourself for an activity in one of the form's blank rows. Then try out the script during the activity, and see if it helps you break down the activity into simple steps that each contain a simple narration and a nonverbal communication for you and for your child (see the case example of Lindee, Anthony, and the bubbles, above). You may be surprised by how quickly your child begins to participate in each step and how much more your child begins to communicate with his or her body.

If you have followed along and carried out the preceding activities, you will have found a number of ways to increase your child's awareness and understanding of your nonverbal communication—your use of gestures, gaze, and expressions. You will see your child's understanding in the gestures, sounds, and looks he uses to respond to you. See if you agree with most of the statements in the following checklist. If so, you are now armed with important skills for helping your child learn to understand nonverbal communication—knowledge that will also help your child learn to understand and develop speech and language. If you do not feel successful yet, try to experiment with the preceding activities until you have experienced some success with each of the statements in the checklist.

Activity Checklist: Am I Helping My Child Learn to Read My Body Language?

_____ I have found many opportunities during the day to highlight my body language for my child.

_____ I have created gestural communication opportunities with my child during many different play and caregiving routines, and we do these most days.

_____ When my child uses a nonverbal cue (no matter how small), I try to

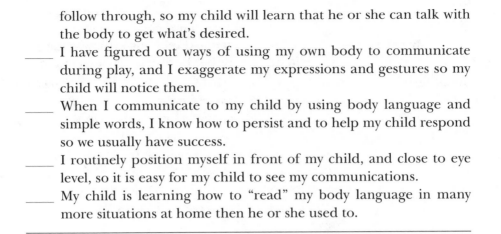

follow through, so my child will learn that he or she can talk with the body to get what's desired.

_____ I have figured out ways of using my own body to communicate during play, and I exaggerate my expressions and gestures so my child will notice them.

_____ When I communicate to my child by using body language and simple words, I know how to persist and to help my child respond so we usually have success.

_____ I routinely position myself in front of my child, and close to eye level, so it is easy for my child to see my communications.

_____ My child is learning how to "read" my body language in many more situations at home then he or she used to.

What if your child doesn't start signaling you in desirable ways? *Bethany's mother came into a parent coaching session with this concern: "The only messages Bethany communicates to me when I try to wait for a signal are crying and screaming. She tries to grab an object as soon as it is visible, so I can't figure out how to hold it back so she can provide me with a gesture. What should I do?"*

The therapist knew Bethany well enough to know that she did not like change. The therapist suggested that, rather than holding objects back, the mother try giving her daughter items in containers, plastic zipper bags, or jars that she can hold on to but cannot open. This way Bethany could have some control over the object, but would still have to signal that she needed help. To help Bethany request help with a gesture rather than by crying, her mother needed to have her hands right in front of Bethany's so she could quickly ask her if she needed help, and then open it quickly for Bethany and give the bag right back to her before Bethany would have a chance to start crying.

A second strategy the mother began to use was to use lots of baggies—just two or three crackers in each (for snacks), one toy in each (for toy play with little objects), one color in each (for crayons)—in activities when there were lots of chances to practice. Having this happen frequently also helped Bethany get used to the new demand and get over crying. This took some time, but her mother knew from experience that Bethany did best at learning new things when they were repeated frequently. Practice over time developed the skill into an automatic, independent behavior. And there was little frustration, since Bethany reached her goal quickly and easily—getting the item out of the container/baggie when she handed it to her mother.

The mother also tried a suggestion we have discussed above: She offered Bethany something she liked before she started to fuss. She held out a preferred toy, as well as a nonpreferred toy, slightly out of reach. When Bethany reached for the preferred toy, her mom quickly gave it to her, so she could learn that she could reach for things instead of only fussing when she wanted something.

Planning Activities to Encourage Nonverbal Communication

Activity	My child likes to:	I can join by:	My child can request with his or her body by:	The body language I am waiting to respond to is:
Toy or other object play Trains	Roll the trains back and forth	Handing trains for him to roll Handing tracks for him to connect and roll the trains back and forth on Rolling another train back and forth	Handing me the box of trains he cannot open Pointing to which train he would like to have Telling me which color train he would like to have Giving me a track that he cannot connect on his own Pointing to or telling me where to lay a track down Giving me a train when he wants mine	Giving me a train or track Pointing to a train or track Saying a word while looking at me
	Hear the "choo-choo sound"	Making "choo-choo" sound while rolling train back and forth or crashing my train into his	Making a "choo-choo" sound, looking at me, doing both, or crashing or moving his train near mine	Making a sound with or without looking at me Copying me with his train
Social play Tickle	Have her legs and tummy tickled	Tickling her legs and tummy	Scooting her body closer to my hands to be tickled Saying "tickle" or the name of a body part to tickle Showing me her tummy Raising her legs Looking at me Looking and laughing/smiling at me	Body movement directed toward me Saying a word while looking at me Looking at me Looking and laughing/smiling at me

(cont.)

From *An Early Start for Your Child with Autism*. Copyright 2012 by The Guilford Press.

Activity	My child likes to:	I can join by:	My child can request with his or her body by:	The body language I am waiting to respond to is:
Meals				
Caregiving (bathing/ dressing/ changing/ bedtime)				
Book activities				
Household chores				

Breaking Down Activities into Nonverbal Communication Steps

Daily routine	Steps	Talking body options
Caregiving (bathing/ dressing/ changing/ bedtime) Getting dressed	1. Getting clothes ready to put on 2. Putting on shirt 3. Putting on pants 4. Fastening buttons or zippers 5. Putting on socks and shoes	1. Handing clothes to caregiver to be put on, one by one, on request 2. Pulling shirt down over head, raising each arm for shirt, pulling down over belly 3. Standing up on instruction, lifting each leg for pants, helping pull over leg, helping pull up over hips 4. Pointing to buttons or zippers or pulling them through when they are almost finished 5. Sitting down on instruction, handing over each piece, and raising foot for each sock/shoe to be put on, helping pull sock up or push shoe on, standing up on instruction at end
Household chores Cleaning up dirty clothes	1. Picking up clothes 2. Opening hamper 3. Throwing clothes into hamper 4. Closing hamper	1. Picking up requested dirty clothes from floor and carrying to hamper or handing to caregiver 2. Vocalizing for hamper to be opened 3. Vocalizing or pointing to which item to be thrown into hamper from choice of two 4. Following gestural or verbal instruction to close hamper
Toy or other object play		

(cont.)

Breaking Down Activities into Nonverbal Communication Steps (cont.)

Daily routine	Steps	Talking body options
Social play		
Meals		
Outdoor play		
Book activities		

How do you build on success? *For Robert, who learned how to gesture to get items from a bag very quickly, his dad "upped the ante" and used the same format to teach additional gestures. Robert's father added a second expectation: When he opened the bag upon Robert's physical request, he held up the two objects inside and offered them to Robert, who needed to point to the one he wanted. Robert reached for the desired object, and his dad said, "Point," while modeling a point and then shaping Robert's hand to a point as he touched the object. As soon as Robert touched the object with his point, his father gave it to him.*

Chapter Summary

Our first way of communicating is with our bodies and facial expressions. Long before speech emerges, most young children learn that people use body signals to send messages back and forth. They become quite skilled at communicating many kinds of messages nonverbally, before they can say their first words. Speech develops later, out of an elaborate nonverbal communication system. As you help your child with autism learn to use his or her body, eyes, and voice to send and understand simple communications, you will gradually continue to add expectations and opportunities for gestural communication, starting with easy or familiar gestures for your child to use and slowly teaching some new ones. You are teaching your child a critical life lesson about how we communicate and interact with one another, which is not by grabbing, screaming, crying, or manipulating bodies until a need is met. Instead, we send messages to others about what we want, feel, and want to share, and we attend to their messages as well. Our messages are about the thoughts, feelings, desires, and needs that motivate us to approach, engage, and converse with others, and we do this through our facial expressions, gestures, postures, eye contact, and finally words. Your child's spoken language will develop out of this framework.

Refrigerator List

Goal: To provide you with ways to help your young child with autism learn to express desires, feelings, and interests using body language and to understand your body language

Steps:

✓ **Do less so your child will do more!**

✓ **Pause and wait—for a gesture, eye contact, or a vocalization.**

✓ **Add gestures to steps of joint activities during play and caregiving routines.**

✓ **Exaggerate facial expressions and gestures during play and caregiving.**

✓ **Divide up materials to practice "give me" gestures during play.**

✓ **Build in barriers so your child needs help.**

✓ **Point to objects and pictures, and wait for your child to follow.**

✓ **Put simple words to your child's body language and to yours!**

✓ **Build steps for communication exchanges into key activities—social and toy/object play, meals, caregiving (bathing/dressing/changing/bedtime), and household chores.**

8

"Do What I Do!"

Helping Your Child Learn by Imitating

Chapter goal: To encourage you to imitate your child's sounds, gestures, facial expressions, actions, and words, and to teach your child to imitate yours. Children learn by watching others and doing what they do.

Why Imitation Is So Important

Most young children are natural mimics. They copy what they see their parents do; they copy the sounds and the gestures their parents make and the words they say; they even copy how their parents walk and dress. They often favor imitating other children—especially their brothers and sisters, as well as kids who are the same age or a little older and whom they admire.

Imitation is a powerful learning tool for all of us. Our brains are set up to remember and learn from watching other people, and children remember what they see others do for a long time, even without practicing it. This means that children can imitate an action immediately after seeing someone else perform it, as in the often spontaneous games that even the youngest children play with siblings, friends, and parents. But they can also imitate it later, because they remember what they have observed.

This special capacity comes to us in part through brain cells called *mirror neurons*, which link actions that we see others do to our own action patterns. With the help of mirror neurons, in a way we actually experience what we see others do: Mirror neurons fire in the brain both when we perform an action and when we see it performed. This means that, at least to a degree, a new action becomes a part of an observer's skill set before the observer actually imitates it. This is how we learn by watching and remembering. But we also learn by doing. So the seedling of a skill that resides in the child's brain because the child has watched and remembered that skill in action becomes more fully learned once the child starts putting it into action herself.

Children's neural capacity for imitation lets parents, siblings, grandparents, and others pass learning on to children without even trying or thinking about it. Skills of all kinds get passed from person to person, across generations, in an effortless fashion that allows each generation to start where the last one left off instead of starting over. Many people believe that imitation and language together are what have created the amazingly complex, rich cultures that people all over the globe have developed over thousands of years.

Imitation is an especially powerful tool for learning how to interact socially with others. This is because social behavior involves many complex and subtle rules, many of which we haven't consciously thought about. For example, when we are interacting with others, we naturally know how far or close we should stand apart from the other person; we unconsciously imitate the other person's facial expressions and gestures; and we time our responses so that the conversation has a natural ebb and flow. No one actually taught us to do this. We learned all of these social behaviors through imitation rather than through explicit instruction.

Children's almost automatic imitation of other people affects them in countless ways. When children (and adults) see another person's expression and emotions, their mirror neurons fire, allowing them to feel the other person's emotion. When they imitate another person's facial expression, they actually come to feel that emotion as well, allowing them to share the other person's inner feelings. Have you ever watched people's faces when they are watching an emotional movie? You can see the emotions of the actors played out on the faces of the people watching the movie. This ability to be emotionally connected to others through imitation happens even in toddlers. Children's almost automatic imitation of other people enriches them in countless ways:

- *It fosters empathy, which increases the capacity to learn from others.* When children imitate someone else's facial expression, doing so triggers the same emotion in them that they are observing. This happens even in toddlers, who can be seen to burst into tears themselves when they watch someone they know start to cry. You probably remember times when just seeing someone else in pain or distress has brought on the same feeling in you. You probably felt a wave of sympathy or empathy for that person and a desire to comfort or help. This helps people feel deeply connected to each other, which tends to increase the desire to pay attention to each other, which in turn increases the potential to learn from each other.
- *It helps children learn language.* When babies and toddlers imitate the sounds that they hear around them, using their own "baby talk," they are practicing making the sounds of their own language. Their ability to imitate parents' words allows them both to perceive and to express their native language.
- *It promotes nonverbal communication.* When young children imitate other

people's gestures and postures, they pick up all those extra cues that add meaning to speech—the ones we have talked about in Chapter 7. These nonverbal cues convey emotional meanings and let us express so much more than we can put into words.

- *It teaches them how things work.* When young children imitate others' actions on objects, they learn how things work, what they are, and what they are used for.

- *It helps them learn the social rules for conversations.* In a conversation, two people alternate between the roles of speaker and listener: Person A says something while Person B listens; then Person B responds to Person A's meaning, building on the topic; and so it continues. This kind of conversational structure also underlies imitation games. An adult bangs two blocks together and then pauses while the child reproduces this action, and then the adult does it again, and so forth, with variations added by either partner when the game gets boring. This is exactly what happens during conversations, and this kind of experience may actually help children learn the rules for conversation: Take turns, don't interrupt, stay on topic, keep it interesting for your partner, and so on.

What's Happening in Autism?

As you may have noticed, young children with ASD are much less inclined to imitate words, gestures, and actions than are other children their age. Even though they are very interested in objects and have lots of skills with objects, they tend not to imitate what other people do with objects very often.

There are a number of theories about the problems with imitation in ASD, but no definitive answers yet. Brain imaging studies have shown that although the mirror neuron system in children with autism is less active, it is not "broken"—meaning that, with proper experience, this system can become active and functional. This is one reason it is important to provide early intervention that promotes imitation skills. Possible reasons why children with autism don't naturally imitate others' gestures, facial expressions, and body movement are that they are not paying attention to others' movements or simply aren't motivated to imitate others (rather than being unable to). This is good news, because it means that by getting into your child's attention spotlight and helping to motivate your child to imitate you, you can awaken his mirror neuron system and help this part of his brain develop.

Why Is It a Problem?

If you look back at the list of enrichments that imitation makes possible, it's easy to see how much children who don't imitate others much can miss out on. We think, in fact, that the decreased motivation to imitate may be responsible for a significant part of the delays most young children with ASD show in all areas of development. Imitation is one of the most important skills a young child with autism can learn, because it is such a learning tool by itself and helps children learn so many different types of skills. Children who do not imitate may miss much of the learning that just observing the goings-on in the social environment makes available. Without imitation, kids have to figure everything out anew, rather than learning from others the easiest and most effective ways to do things. For example, imagine how a child would learn a group game like hide and seek or "Red Rover" without using imitation to learn from other children. But even in a structured educational setting, the lack of imitation makes it harder to learn new skills, because children won't necessarily be able to pick up on quick, efficient modeling from teachers or therapists (or parents).

Imitating others also enhances social relationships. You know the saying "Imitation is the sincerest form of flattery"? Imitating a person we admire or enjoy (dressing or styling one's hair a particular way, playing with a certain toy, saying a funny word) creates a moment of sharing or connection between people. It elicits positive feelings in both partners. By extension, imitation is crucial for developing the ability to identify with important others and to share meaning and emotion with them.

⟫⟫⟫ What You Can Do to Teach Imitation to Your Child

Fortunately, it's clear from research that young children with ASD can learn to imitate others well and naturally when their own motivation and attention to imitate are increased. Several studies have shown that early intervention can increase the imitation abilities of children with autism. As with other behaviors (such as making eye contact and using gestures and words), when children with autism start paying attention to others' actions, are shown how to imitate others, and discover that imitating others is rewarding, they become more motivated to do it. In Chapter 4, we have discussed imitating what your child does as a way of joining your child and gaining her attention. In this chapter we are going farther and focusing on how you can teach your child to imitate different skills and behaviors inside your ongoing play and caregiving routines. There are five specific steps you can carry out to increase your child's imitation:

Step 1. Imitating sounds.

Step 2. Imitating actions on objects.

Step 3. Imitating hand gestures and body/facial movements.

Step 4. Imitating and expanding on actions.

Step 5. Putting imitation games into the joint activity frame.

In the following pages, we describe how to carry out each of these steps, give you some ideas for activities to try, and suggest what you can do to solve problems that may come up.

Step 1. Imitating Sounds

Rationale. Children who have not yet learned how to use words to communicate need to build a large repertoire of sounds, to learn how to make a sound intentionally, and to learn how to make specific sounds in order to get something they want (in a goal-directed fashion). Finally, they need to understand the full power of their voices as a way of achieving a variety of goals. Although we deal in depth with developing verbal communication in Chapter 13, here we focus on parents' use of imitation to achieve three things: (1) to help children notice their own vocalizations, (2) to increase the frequency of the sounds they are making, and (3) to increase their intentional production of sounds and specific vocalizations.

♟ Activity: *Increase Your Child's Sounds by Echoing Them*

You may hear your child vocalizing, sometimes in response to something that has happened and sometimes "out of nowhere." Even if you're not sure what a sound means, imitating your child's sounds conveys to the child that you have heard him and that his vocalizations are meaningful and important. You're saying, "I heard you," to your child and assigning importance and meaning to the sound with your actions. Begin by positioning yourself so your child can see your face. Then imitate whatever vowel or consonant sounds or other sound effects your child emits (except for crying, screams, or whining) while playing with his voice. Now wait to see if your child makes the sound again. If he does, you now have the opportunity to imitate him again. With this back-and-forth interchange, you've created an imitation game! If he doesn't make the sound in return, try again, waiting expectantly. Eventually your child will repeat his sounds after your imitation. Developing some vocal imitation games is worth your persistence, since it's a critical step on the road to speech development.

♟ Activity: *Sing Songs and Play Rhyming Word and Finger Games*

Singing songs and highlighting a key word or phrase in each verse helps your child start to hear the pattern and the important parts of the song. You might sing or say that target word or phrase a little louder or even slower, to help your child attend to its meaning. Add gestures and facial expressions to mark the targets. After singing the song verse in its entirety over a few days, so your child begins to recognize it, start to make a little space in the song for your child to join in. Come to the target word or phrase in the song and then wait, looking expectantly at your child, to cue the target. Your child might start to put in the missing word by making a sound. If so, great! When you hear it, continue the song. Or, instead, when you pause, your child might make a small gesture, wiggle her body, give you a quick look, or provide some other cue that shows she wants to participate. If she does this, add the word after your child's cue and continue the song. This skill marks a milestone in speech development, and it is a very important type of activity for fostering verbal imitation. Develop a whole repertoire of songs, chants, and finger plays with your child.

For example, you could sing a song like "The Wheels on the Bus," emphasizing a key phrase: "The wheels on the bus go *round and round, round and round, round and round* (of course with the accompanying hand actions). The wheels on the bus go *round and round*, all through the town." "Round and round" is your target phrase. After singing the song a time or two, this time you would sing, "The wheels on the bus go [pause] . . . " and wait expectantly for your child to make a sound or at least some kind of nonverbal cue. Once he does, quickly and happily continue the song, singing, " . . . *round and round*, all through the town!"

Summary of Step 1

If you have followed along and carried out the preceding activities, you will have developed a new habit—that of imitating your preverbal child's sounds—and you and your child will be making progress in developing some vocal imitation games. These activities serve as a starting place for increasing your child's vocal imitation skills, and we will develop the next steps in a later chapter. For now, see if you agree with most of the statements in the following checklist. If so, you are now armed with important skills for teaching imitation—knowledge you will use in **Step 2**. If not, start experimenting during play and caregiving routines until you have found some methods that work for each statement.

Activity Checklist: Imitating Sounds

_____ I pay attention to my child's sounds.

_____ I imitate my child's sounds back to him or her when I hear them.

_____ I have a repertoire of songs, finger plays, and other language activities that my child enjoys.

_____ I know when to pause and wait in these games for my child to cue me or vocalize to continue the game.

Claire, age 3, has autism and occasionally makes sounds, although these are not directed to her parents. Her parents describe the sounds as more like exhales (e.g., "haa") than like attempts to communicate a word, and they haven't been sure how to respond to them. During one of Claire's favorite activities—making shapes out of play dough—her dad begins to name the cookie cutter shapes and describe the actions as he makes animals out of play dough. He also adds sounds to the animals as he shows them to Claire: "Look, Claire, a doggie," "Doggie says 'woof woof,'" or "Bird goes 'tweet tweet.'" After repeating this theme a few times, Claire's dad pauses as he holds up the next animal and waits for Claire to imitate the sound. She doesn't, but that's okay, and Dad continues the activity anyway. But then, as Claire is looking down at the table and picking up the animal she's just made, she makes the exhaled sound.

Dad remembers what he has read in this chapter and imitates the sound right back. After a few seconds, Claire's dad repeats the sound again, but this time makes it a little deeper. Claire looks up and smiles slightly. Dad repeats the sound, exaggerating it even more. Claire's smile widens. Now Dad asks Claire, "Again?" and when she looks at him intently, he makes the sound again. This time he says to Claire, "You do it," and models the sound again. Claire opens her mouth slightly, but no sound comes out. Dad fills in the sound, and Claire continues to smile. Dad goes back to the play dough activity and holds up the dog, making it say "woof woof" again. As Claire reaches to take the dog from Dad, she makes the exhaled sound. It doesn't matter that she didn't look at Dad while making the sound. Her father imitates her sound, and she repeats it. He imitates it again, and she repeats it again. Vocal turn taking! He is delighted and imitates her sound, and then has the dog go "woof woof," which she loves.

> "We also encouraged my son to speak by using animal noises. It's easy to make the noises fun, and they seem relatively easy to repeat, so playing animal noise games with a farm was a big part of our early attempts to encourage his speech."

Malik is a 26-month-old boy with autism who does not make sounds or speak and seems to drool constantly. His mother says he doesn't seem particularly interested in toys and prefers to suck or chew on them rather than engaging in play. She's not sure where to start in teaching vocal imitation to Malik, given his lack of interest in toys and his very limited speech and communication skills. After reviewing the Step 1 activity checklist, Malik's mother reads about the use of silly mouth games to stimulate motor movement and elicit sounds. She decides to try this, since toys or objects may not work with Malik right away.

She sits Malik in his chair and sits in front of him to ensure good face-to-face positioning. She starts a game by saying "oooaaahhh" while patting her mouth. Malik watches with curiosity, but he does not reach out. She makes the sound again on her own mouth and then pats Malik's mouth. He doesn't make the sound, but he does open his mouth slightly to stick out his tongue. She makes the sound for him as she pats his mouth and then goes back to her mouth, exaggerating the pitch and intensity of sound. She keeps alternating between her mouth and Malik's, pausing when it's Malik's turn to see if he'll imitate the sound.

Although Malik doesn't make the sound, he does continue to stick his tongue out, so Mom decides to vary the game and sticks her tongue out to wiggle back and forth while saying "aaahhhhh." She's added a different action to see how Malik will respond. He continues to stare intently at Mom's face and show interest in the game. He sticks his tongue out again. Mom takes a turn wiggling her tongue, and he repeats it. She adds an "ahh" sound to her tongue movement, and he puts his tongue out again and makes a little noise. She is very excited about this development. She decides to practice these mouth games in other caregiving activities when Malik and she can be face to face, such as diapering and meals. Within a few days, he is reliably imitating her when she sticks out her tongue.

Step 2. Imitating Actions on Objects

Rationale. Imitating your child's actions with objects draws your child's attention to what you are doing, gives you a specific vocabulary of objects and actions for narrating your child's activity, and gives your child the sense of two people doing things together—that is, reciprocally. It takes turn taking to another step: imitating. It should increase the amount of time your child spends on socially coordinated activities, and will most likely increase your child's motivation to imitate your actions. Research by one of us authors (G. D.)[1] found that when parents imitate what their children are doing, children with autism start making more eye contact and smile at their parents more often during the imitative play. The children notice that their parents are imitating them and enjoy this game.

Imitating your child's actions with objects can also increase the flexible, creative, and varied nature of your child's play. Our goal in this step is for children with ASD to pay attention not only to the objects we're holding, but, more importantly, to what we do with them. Teaching them to imitate others gives them ways to learn on their own, and it also allows us to teach new skills through modeling, so we can provide them with new ways to play with objects and expand their repertoire of ideas and actions.

Here are some activities for increasing your child's imitation of actions performed on objects.

♟ Activity: *Use Matching (Identical or Very Similar) Toys, or Multiple Pieces of Toys, to Teach Your Child to Imitate New Actions Quickly and Easily*

For this first activity, you will need some matching sets of objects available during various activities. Make sure that you are right in front of your child, and that your objects are positioned in front of her matching objects. Note that how quickly you move through the sequence of steps involving imitating your child will depend on how your child responds to each of the steps. If he quickly engages, watches you imitate, and begins imitating your actions, you could move

---

[1] Dawson, G., & Galpert, L. Mothers' use of imitative play for facilitating social responsiveness and toy play in young autistic children. *Development and Psychopathology, 2,* 151–162, 1990.

through each of these steps in your first session trying it. However, if your child doesn't watch you or doesn't readily imitate the actions you introduce, spend more time on each step (at least a day, if not longer) until you see the response you want, before moving on to the next step.

Here is the sequence for using matching or multiple-piece toys:

- Begin by imitating your child's actions with your own materials and labeling the objects and actions your child is using. For example, if your child is rolling a car back and forth, you would roll your car back and forth exactly as your child is doing it. When your child stops rolling his car, stop yours too. When he begins again, you begin again too. Your child is likely to start experimenting to see if he can get you to do whatever he is doing. He may smile and may even make eye contact, clearly enjoying the game and the power he has in making you do whatever he does!

- After you have imitated your child's actions precisely for a while, introduce a variation on the action you are performing. For example, you could roll the car more quickly or slowly, or roll the car on your body instead of the floor, and so on. Pause and wait expectantly, and see if she will spontaneously begin to imitate these new variations. All the while, remember to label the actions ("Car is rolling! Car is rolling fast! Car is rolling slowly. Car crashes!").

- After you have gone back and forth a few times, imitating your child by using the action he is doing or a variation on that action, change your action to a different one (of about the same difficulty level), and show your child your new action in a big display. Ideally, you would start by introducing another action that you have already seen your child perform with the object. For example, if you have previously seen your child both roll and bang a car and you have been imitating your child rolling the car, you could start to bang it. Label the action ("Bang-bang!") and repeat it a couple of times. If your child is interested in what you are doing, wait expectantly and see if your child imitates the action you introduced. If not, help (prompt) him to copy you. To prompt him to perform a new action with the toy, gently guide him through the new movement, with your hand over his hand.

- Once your child has made the new action, praise your child enthusiastically and let your child do what she wants to do for a minute with the toy. Imitate your child a few times and then show the new action again. Again make a big display, wait for your child to imitate you, prompt her to do so if needed, praise, and then let your child have control of the materials for a few minutes. This is the basic learning frame for teaching imitation of actions on objects.

♟ Activity: *Use Double Sets of Toys*

Here are some ideas for using double sets of toys to teach imitation:

- Sets of musical instruments—such as two drums and two pairs of sticks, or two sets of maracas—can be used in fun activities with different actions to teach your child to imitate. Follow your child's actions for a few repetitions, and then model something different. Or, you can begin the game by tapping your drum with your sticks or shaking your maracas, and if your child doesn't naturally join in, then help him imitate the action. Take your turn again, making sure to add language, sound effects, or even a song. Then pause and encourage your child to carry out the action. Try to wait a second or two to see if your child will copy you. If he doesn't do it, prompt him to imitate, cheer him, and then after the imitation let your child play as he wishes for a few minutes.

- Another way, useful for introducing a new instrument, is for you to hold on to both sets of items and model for your child how to use the instrument (be sure you are demonstrating an action you know your child can do). Then hand the matching instrument to your child for her to imitate (the reinforcer here is the interesting sound the instrument makes). If she does not try to imitate you quickly, prompt her to do so. If she tries but can't quite do it, help her complete the imitation. Comment enthusiastically (e.g., "You banged it!") and do the action again. Keep taking turns, and when these actions become a little repetitive or dull, switch it up: Bang the drum with your hand instead of the sticks or use the maracas to bang on the floor. Then continue the turn taking to help your child imitate these new actions.

- Toys with multiple pieces (like trains, blocks, balls, or puzzles) can also be used to teach object imitation. You may need to limit the pieces to just a few at first to help your child focus his attention on you. See what action your child does with the item first, and then imitate it back with your object, adding simple language to narrate the activity. After a few rounds of imitating your child's actions, elaborate or vary the activity by now showing your child something new to do with the object. For example, your train can crash into your child's or fall off the track. You might need to repeat your action a couple of times and make a big display to help your child appreciate the fun factor. Then pause, wait, and (if needed) help your child imitate the action—he crashes his train into yours or knocks a train off the track. Go back then to the original action your child was doing with the object if this is needed to maintain interest and attention, and after a few rounds, model the new action again and help your child imitate it. Follow this formula of imitating your child's preferred action, then showing your

Helpful Tips

- What if your child wants your toy? No problem: Hand it over and pick up another, or trade yours for his.

- What if your child is so focused on her own toys that she does not pay attention to your toy? You can try spending more time precisely imitating what your child is doing. Most kids, over time, will be interested in the fact that you are copying them and will start to notice what you are doing with your toy. Give your child more time to learn about the mutual imitation game. You can also put your own toys away and take turns using your child's object to imitate each other back and forth. So, for example, you would take the object from your child, briefly imitate her, and then give it back for your child to do. In your own turns, alternate between two or three rounds of imitating your child's action (to keep it fun and motivating) and modeling a new action for your child to imitate with your help, if needed.

- Be aware of how many turns you take (keep them balanced with your child's), as well as the length of your turn (short!). If your child likes the effects you are creating, then you have more leeway to take more frequent turns. If not, keep your turns short, keep the turns balanced, and be sure to imitate what your child does often, to keep the child engaged in the activity.

new action (and it can be different things—crashing, rolling, circling the train), and helping your child quickly imitate it.

> "This type of activity worked really well for us. My son loved seeing new, fun things to do with his cars (like racing them fast up the sides of furniture or crashing them down again). Because he thought the activities were fun, he was very interested in copying them."

- Expand beyond playtimes. Imitation with objects is an activity that can occur any time your child is holding an object. There are lots of opportunities for imitating your child at mealtimes (taking bites with spoon, using hands, drinking from a cup, banging a spoon on a tray, etc.). Children are also often vocal at mealtimes, so there should be opportunities to imitate your child's sounds as well. Bath time offers lots of opportunities too—activities with bath toys, as well as activities with water (splashing, pouring, bubbles, washcloths). Toddler books that elicit actions (holes to poke in, doors to open, etc.) can also be used.

> **Helpful Tip**
>
> Read toddler books in simple language—label actions and objects. Don't try to read whole sentences to children who don't yet speak. They will get more from the book if you label what they are looking at and doing.

Summary of Step 2

If you have followed along and carried out the preceding activities, you will have found ways to use toys and household objects to imitate your child and to begin teaching your child how to imitate your actions with objects. See if you agree with most of the statements in the following checklist. If so, you are now armed with important skills for teaching imitation of new actions to your child—knowledge you will use in **Step 3**. If not, start experimenting during play and caregiving routines until you have found some methods that work for each statement.

Activity Checklist: Imitating Actions with Objects

_____ There are double sets of toys or multiple objects that I can use with my child.

_____ I frequently imitate my child's actions with objects.

_____ I sometimes model variations on my child's actions as well as different actions in play, and prompt my child to imitate my actions on objects.

_____ My child and I can trade an object back and forth when we are taking turns with it.

_____ I am aware of my child's attention to my actions, and can "feel" when I can take longer turns and when I need to keep my turns very short.

_____ I have found opportunities to imitate my child across most of our daily activities; it feels almost automatic now to do so.

What about Claire? *Claire's dad has continued to make animals out of play dough to work on Claire's vocal imitation skills. Her favorite animals to make are a dog, cat, and cow, and she will now attempt to imitate sounds back. Claire's dad would like to help her learn to use objects during the play dough routines instead of just watching him, so he sets out a few different utensils (pizza cutter, rolling pin, and fork) next to the dough and cookie cutters. He knows that Claire will be more likely to imitate new actions if they are part of her favorite game—watching Dad make animals. He makes an animal, and when Claire shows that she is ready for the next* *one, Dad takes out the rolling pin and smooths out the dough. Then he takes the cow-shaped cookie cutter and hands it to her, helps her make the cow, and then makes the animal noise she loves. He rolls out the dough again and offers her the cat. She takes it and moves it to the dough. He quickly gives her hand a little push so the cutter goes in, and then he pulls out the cat and makes that noise. They continue with the game, with Claire now putting the cutters onto the dough when he gives her one. In the next few days he will help her add the rolling pin step to the routine.*

What about Malik? *Remember Malik? He's the little boy who tends to mouth objects rather than playing with them, and his mom has been practicing mouth games to encourage sounds from Malik. So far, Mom has found that the games help Malik make "bbb," "ooo," and "aah" sounds. Even though Malik doesn't play with objects, Mom hates to skip over this step. After Mom thinks about it, she decides that using one toy to take turns with rather than double sets may minimize Malik's mouthing on objects and possibly help him learn how to imitate actions. Mom considers different toys to use and decides that if a toy does something when pushed or pulled, it might captivate Malik enough not to want to chew on it. She takes out a rocket toy; when she pushes its button, a circle spins from its top and lands on the floor.*

Mom sets the rocket on the floor between her and Malik. She tells him, "Watch this. Push." Meanwhile the circle shoots straight up and lands a few feet from Malik. Mom says, "Let's get it," and takes him by the hand to pick up the circle and set it on top of the rocket. Again Mom says, "Watch this. Push," and sets the circle off into the air. This time Mom points to where the circle landed and tells Malik, "You get it." Malik looks at the circle but doesn't get up immediately. Instead of getting up herself, Mom waits and encourages Malik to pick up the circle by pointing toward the circle and saying again, "You get it." This time Malik gets the circle but doesn't take it over to Mom. However, he doesn't put it in his mouth either, so this is an improvement. Mom moves the rocket closer to Malik and says, "Put on," referring to the circle. She then helps Malik with the action and next tells him, "Push," as she helps him launch the circle. After it lands, Malik runs over to get the circle and brings it back to put on the rocket. Mom helps him, and together they push the button.

They now have a turn-taking game with an object, and Mom never thought this would be possible. She's realized that using a toy that the two of them can take turns with and share may be the best strategy for building up his play repertoire, at least until he develops more skills. Mom is so excited about this development that she adds one new action to the game. She holds the circle up to her eye and says, "Boo, I see you," and then tickles Malik. He likes to be tickled and enjoys the variation to the game. Mom peeks through the circle the next time it lands on the floor and tickles him again. Then she helps Malik hold the circle up to his eye and says, "You see Mommy." Malik doesn't imitate this action yet by himself, but he stays involved with the activity and likes the action that follows—being tickled—so Mom decides to make tickling another action he can imitate back. Now they have multiple actions within a game with an object that Mom and Malik can do together.

Step 3. Imitating Hand Gestures and Body/Facial Movements

Rationale. At this point you have developed interactive games for teaching your child to imitate sounds and actions with objects during various activities. The next step is to teach your child how to attend to and imitate the hand gestures and physical motions that are part of your songs and sensory social games. Remember that in Chapter 6 we talked about how to build fun little social routines with special actions and words (peekaboo, "so big") or songs with finger plays or other kinds of movements ("Itsy-Bitsy Spider," "London Bridge," "If You're Happy and You Know It"). Now it's time to teach your child how to imitate some of the different gestures, body movements, and physical actions that you've been doing naturally during these routines. Practice the strategies presented next during familiar and pleasurable sensory social routines, to teach your child to associate some of the words and rhythms of the songs and games with the important movements that are part of the game. For instance, "The Wheels on the Bus" is associated with the movement of twirling your arms; peekaboo is associated with hiding your face behind your hands and then opening them when you say "Boo!"; and so on.

Activity: *Teach Imitation during Finger Plays and Songs with Actions*

Remember that up until now you and your child have been participating in face-to-face social games in which you start a physical game (tickle) or sing a song ("Slippery Fish") and gradually pause in midverse or before performing the action, waiting expectantly for your child to signal you to continue the game (saying "tickle" or looking up at you). You have been doing this for a while now, so it's likely that your child now easily communicates to tell you to continue or "do it again" with eyes, gestures, expressions, or sounds. Once your child is easily and frequently communicating this goal, you can begin to focus on teaching your child to imitate one of the key movements used in the song or game.

Here is the sequence for teaching your child to imitate gestures/movements:

- Pick a favorite, well-practiced song or game, and then pick a movement that is very easy to do (hands up, hands together, clap hands, etc.) from a routine that your child really enjoys!

- Teach your child to imitate this gesture by starting the song; then, when it is time for the gesture in the song, begin the gesture and then stop and help (prompt) your child to make the gesture. **Prompting** means giving your child some help in order to bring about the action you want him to perform. The prompt could be a gentle touch on the body part you want your child to use (touching the elbow to prompt raising hands in the air), or, if needed, physically guiding your child's body through the action (taking his hands and bringing them up in the air). Over time, the goal is to reduce the prompt gradually. For example, if you have been guiding your child's hands through the movement, you would start to fade the amount of guidance until you are only briefly touching his elbows to encourage him to raise his hands in the air or pointing toward his arms. Eventually, you want to remove the prompt altogether so your child will do it all by himself in imitation of you.

● Once your child has imitated the action with your help, continue the routine so that your child experiences the pleasure of the routine as the "reward" for imitating the movement.

Helpful Tip

Be careful not just to move the child's body through the motions day after day. This does not teach imitation. You teach imitation by demonstrating the movement first, and then waiting for and encouraging your child to imitate you. If your child does not produce some version of the gesture, then physically help your child to do it. But give as little help as possible to get some version of the gesture, and give less and less help over time. This is called **prompt fading**, and it is really important to your child's learning to make the movement on his own. Making a sloppy imitation all by himself is *much* better for your child than making a perfect imitation because you have helped him.

● Try not to manipulate the child's hands after the first few prompts. Rather, prompt her from the wrist, arm, elbow, or shoulder, so your child does not think that what is expected is to give you her hands for you to move.

● Always continue the song after the child has made the gesture, either with or without help. That is the **reinforcer**, or reward.

● Teach only one gesture at a time. For instance, if you are teaching "Itsy-Bitsy Spider," you might teach the "spider" gesture by having your child bring the fingers of both hands together several times. You would have your child imitate this gesture each time you use it. But you won't start teaching your child a second gesture ("Down came the rain") until he can produce the "spider" on his own. You will still sing the song and use all the gestures yourself every time, but you will teach your child one gesture at a time until your child produces some version of it independently, often, and easily.

● Don't be a perfectionist. The sooner your child makes some gesture independently, the better. Don't be concerned if the gestures are partial, "sloppy," or rough approximations at first. In the same way that you have encouraged your child to imitate vocalizations by responding to any sound, you want to encourage your child to imitate gestures by positively responding to any movement with the right body part first (e.g., slightly wiggling fingers when you make the spider gesture). The gestures can get more exact later.

● Some gestures are used frequently in a lot of songs. For instance, hand claps figure in pattycake, "Open, Shut Them," and "If You're Happy and You Know It." Once your child is beginning to imitate clapping hands in one of the songs, prompt her to do it in the other songs that use it, too. The more imitation practice and use your child engages in, the better.

Here are some additional activities for developing gesture imitation:

● Add facial expressions (smiles, pouts, fake crying, surprised faces) to your sensory social routines. Exaggerate emotions to cue your child to pay attention to your face, and encourage your child to imitate you. Obviously, you can't physically help your child make a smile or frown, but you can give the expression meaning with your language and actions. You can touch your child's face as a prompt, however.

● For facial imitations, you will need to use exaggerated and somewhat slowed-down movements. For instance, with a balloon or bubbles, get close to your child—on the floor, face to face. Puff your cheeks up really big, and blow slowly and dramatically. This dramatic setup of the game tells your child what is coming and helps your child notice and read your nonverbal communications. However, it also puts your facial actions into your child's spotlight of attention. As your child comes to know the meaning of the action, pause while making it, model the action for your child, and wait to see if your child will imitate it to request the action. Again, at first, you don't expect exact imitations. If your child slightly opens his mouth when he sees you making the blowing gesture, that's terrific!

> *Two-year-old Amber loves the balloon game. Her mom begins to blow up a balloon, slowly and dramatically, and then takes her mouth off the balloon, looks at Amber, and makes the blowing gesture with big cheeks. She pauses, waiting expectantly to see if Amber will imitate the gesture. Whether Amber imitates or not, Mom says, "Blow balloon," puffs her cheeks dramatically, makes some blowing sound effects, and blows it again and lets it fly for Amber to chase. In a few days, Amber comes to expect the puffed cheeks and imitates the gesture*

(approximately) during the expectant waiting pause. In a few more days, she is also saying an approximate version of "Blow."

● Playing face imitation games in front of a big mirror often helps your child learn facial imitations like blowing, raspberries, making a popping sound with your lips, kissy faces, and the like and becomes a very fun activity.

Here are some ideas for using other daily activities to develop face and voice routines:

● During diaper changing—when your child is lying in front of you, focused on your face—is a great time to develop silly face and voice routines, like animal faces and calls, alphabet song or number songs, tongue wiggles, and raspberries. Put a kazoo on the changing table, and use it to make silly noises while you change the diaper. This is also a time to buzz a belly, play creepy fingers or peekaboo, and so forth.

● Dressing also allows for peekaboo with shirts; sound effects for "stinky shoes, stinky socks, stinky feet" routines; buzzing bellies; "This Little Piggy"; and so on.

● Mealtimes also offer times for big face and voice effects—"yum" faces and sounds for delicious foods; "yucky" faces and sounds for food your child rejects; drinking sounds and gestures; eating sounds and gestures; licking something good off a finger; using your tongue on an ice cream or a peanut-buttered carrot. If your child is in a high chair and you are sitting pretty much in front of her, you are in the best possible position for drawing your child's attention to your face and voice.

● Label and react big-time to unexpected events that happen during the day. Use a big "uh-oh" and a startled expression when something falls. Use "oh, no" and a big expression when you build a tower and it falls. Use a big "crash" when cars crash. When your child gets hurt, say, "Owie, you got an owie," with a big expression as you examine the owie and give comfort. Then put a big, noisy kiss on the owie with a big display of "all better."

● **Caution!** Imitating facial movements and sounds is a lot harder for young children with autism than imitating actions on objects is. You are likely to see your child imitate your actions on objects before she imitates body and facial movements or songs. Don't worry about this—it's the usual way that imitation develops in most young children with ASD. Just keep the various sensory social routines up, adding new ones each week, keeping up the old ones, and sooner or later your child will start to imitate some actions or sounds in them. Don't forget to expect that your child will imitate these someday. Continue to wait, help your child imitate, and then continue the fun game.

Summary of Step 3

If you have followed along and carried out the preceding activities, you will have found gestures, body movements, and maybe some facial expressions that you are helping your child to imitate during sensory social routines and daily activities. See if you agree with most of the statements in the following checklist. If so, you are now armed with important skills for varying imitation inside toy and social games—knowledge you will use in **Step 4**. If not, start experimenting during play and caregiving routines until you have found some methods that work for each statement.

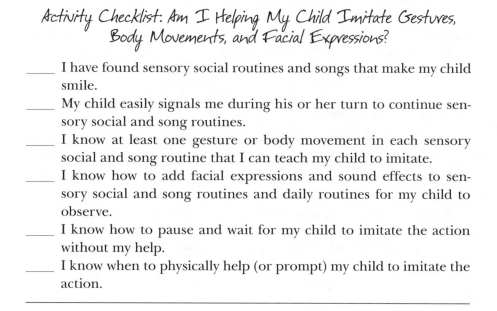

Activity Checklist: Am I Helping My Child Imitate Gestures, Body Movements, and Facial Expressions?

_____ I have found sensory social routines and songs that make my child smile.

_____ My child easily signals me during his or her turn to continue sensory social and song routines.

_____ I know at least one gesture or body movement in each sensory social and song routine that I can teach my child to imitate.

_____ I know how to add facial expressions and sound effects to sensory social and song routines and daily routines for my child to observe.

_____ I know how to pause and wait for my child to imitate the action without my help.

_____ I know when to physically help (or prompt) my child to imitate the action.

What about Malik? *Mom has a few songs she sings to Malik ("Twinkle, Twinkle, Little Star" and "Open, Shut Them") every day during dressing, diapering, and bath time. Mom begins singing "Twinkle, Twinkle, Little Star" while opening and closing her fingers during each verse. She decides that this might be a relatively easy gesture for Malik to learn how to imitate. After singing the song in its entirety one time through, she starts the song again and pauses at the end of the first line with her hands open and out in front of her. Mom waits to see if Malik will move his hands in some tendency to imitate hers (lift up his hands, reach his hands toward Mom's, open and/or close his hands, etc.). He doesn't do any of these movements, but continues to look at her with great interest. Mom takes her hands and pats her palms against his palms several times. Then she continues the song. When she gets to the end of the song, where the words "Twinkle, twinkle, little star" are repeated, she again lifts her open hands in front of him and waits for him to pat hers. When* *he does not, she opens his palms and pats them with hers. For the next few days she does this repeatedly, and within a few days Malik reaches his palms to hers when she puts her hands in front of him. Mom is thrilled and pats his palms a couple of times as she sings the line. Over the next few days, he not only reaches to her palm, but also starts to pat. She's ecstatic that he's trying on his own to imitate a new gesture, even if it's not perfect. He is really learning!*

Step 4. Imitating and Expanding on Actions

Rationale. Developing variations in the imitative turn-taking games keeps the games interesting and less repetitive for longer periods of time. It supports your child's longer periods of attention to you. It also teaches your child to use objects in a variety of ways. This expands the number of things your child can do with objects, and replaces repetitive play with flexible and more complex play with toys and social games. Each time your child imitates a new action, it makes future imitation easier and easier for your child and more automatic.

Activity: *Add Variations*

Once your child easily and consistently imitates a familiar action that you model, you can start expanding the actions so that the initial action or theme doesn't become boring or repetitive after a few turns for you or your child. Adding a variation often makes the imitation fun and surprising for your child. How will this look? Your first imitative action back and forth two or three times in the play establishes the theme, the main action. After this, you will introduce something new into the imitation—a variation—to keep it interesting and keep the turn going longer. In doing so, you will also teach a different action imitation, making the routine a little more advanced.

Here are some ideas for introducing variations:

- Earlier we talked about copying your child's use of an object to create a turn-taking imitation game. Once your child does this easily—copies you copying him—show your child a new, easy, and very interesting action to perform with the object. It might be showing your child how to stomp bubbles you've just blown, how to hit an inflated balloon up into the air, how to turn around while playing "Hokey-pokey," or how to crash a car into a tower of blocks after building them. You model it first, then hand over the object to your child so he can imitate you. If your child doesn't begin to imitate, then prompt him to imitate you, show enthusiasm for your child's success, and then let your child play with the object any way he wants to for a minute. Then repeat the whole sequence: modeling Action 1; giving your child the materials to imitate; then taking your turn and modeling Action 2; then giving your child the chance to do Action 2; and cheering or clapping and letting your child have the toy. The reinforcer for your child's imitation is to have the desired object for a bit without any demands. Of course, your happy cheers are also a big reward.

● Variations are often more interesting to your child if they involve simple, but unusual and interesting, actions on objects: sticking a stick into a play dough ball, tapping a shaker with a stick, or putting a ball in the bottom hole of a maze instead of the top. You will teach your child to imitate these new actions in exactly the same way we have discussed before: showing your child while labeling your act, waiting expectantly, prompting if needed, cheering your child for trying to imitate, or helping your child imitate if she doesn't try and then cheering. Excellent materials for working on theme and variations include play dough, art activities, musical toys, and complex arrays of things (train tracks and cars; sets of blocks; building sets, and pretend play props like glasses, hats, necklaces, bracelets, brush/comb, etc.).

● Theme-and-variation imitative play is a great way to introduce new toys or objects for which the child has no set ways of playing, so that everything you model will be new. Materials that don't work well for teaching new object imitations are those that the child has a very set and repetitive way of handling.

Summary of Step 4

If you have followed along and carried out the preceding activities, you will have developed all of the stages or steps in how to teach different kinds of imitation (verbal, actions with objects, gestures, body movements, facial expressions) to your child in toy play and sensory social routines. You know how to take turns with your child and develop an initial theme for imitating one action, and after several rounds you know how to vary or expand the activity to include other types of imitation that your child can do. If so, you are now armed with important skills for taking turns and teaching during joint activities. If not, start experimenting during play and caregiving routines until you have found some methods that work for each statement.

Activity Checklist: Am I Expanding My Child's Imitation?

_____ I know how to develop a theme during imitation with my child during toy play and sensory social routines.

_____ My child can easily imitate at least one kind of action without my help during toy play and sensory social routines.

_____ I know how to vary or expand the joint activity to teach other kinds of imitation to my child during toy play and sensory social routines.

_____ I know how to create interesting and new spectacles that my child will imitate during toy play and sensory social routines.

_____ My child thinks these variations are fun and attempts to imitate actions back.

Step 5. Putting Imitation Games into the Joint Activity Frame

In Chapter 6 we discussed at length the four parts of a joint activity routine: setup, theme, variation, and closing/transition. You can probably see now how well imitation games fit into this framework. You may even have been using this four-part framework already, either intentionally or automatically, as you have been focusing on imitation activities and variations within them.

The play frame that we have been talking about all through this chapter on teaching imitation is the joint activity frame, with a beginning (materials come out), a theme (the first action is imitated), and one or more variations. We have not discussed closings/transitions yet, but ideally the closing is an organized ending, as you have practiced in Chapter 6. In the rest of this book, we continue to suggest ways for you to use the joint activity framework and imitation strategies to teach other kinds of developmental skills to your child. Imitation and turn taking during object-focused joint activities and sensory social routines, as well as during various caregiving routines, are fundamental processes by which young children learn from others about language, social behavior, and how objects work. If you learn the concepts we have introduced so far, you will already have the most important teaching skills you can have for helping your child move ahead, even if you go no farther than this chapter.

Activity Checklist: Am I Putting Imitation into the Joint Activity Frame?

_____ My imitation activities typically involve a setup period, in which my child and I identify a theme of the activity.

_____ We take a few turns sharing the theme by imitating each other in turn or playing it in unison.

_____ After a few repetitions, either my child or I typically vary or expand the theme to include additional actions to imitate.

_____ When my child's attention is beginning to wane, or when the routine feels too repetitive, we typically do an organized closing/

transition—putting things away, making a clear transition together, or making another choice.

_____ I am using the four-part structure of joint activities at least sometimes during meal, dressing/changing/bathing/bedtime, and I see my child beginning to anticipate the steps in more of these routines.

What about Claire? *Claire and her grandma have developed several toy games and sensory social routines that include different acts of imitation. One of Claire's favorite activities is when Grandma imitates her rolling a toy car back and forth on the coffee table. Grandma takes a second car, faces Claire from the other side of the table, and imitates the rolling, saying "zoom, zoom, zoom" as she rolls. Then she pauses. Rolling is the theme of the imitation game, which Claire has set. Claire stops and looks up during Grandma's pause, and Grandma takes that as a cue and rolls again, which Claire imitates with her own car. Grandma repeats this whole round again. But Grandma can tell that Claire is losing interest in this game, because she's not responding or participating as energetically as before. Also, this is a skill that Claire performs easily. So Grandma makes a variation. She puts a long wooden block on the coffee table, with one end of it on a stack of books, and she sets her car on the high end and lets it roll down. Claire watches this with great interest and then rolls her car on the table again. Grandma gets her attention, rolls her car down the hill again, pauses, and then prompts Claire to do the same by helping her place her car on top of the block. Claire's car rolls down, and Grandma cheers. Grandma rolls her car again and then starts to help Claire, but Claire now does it herself, and Grandma cheers again. This is now appealing to Claire, who shifts her focus to this new game, and the two imitate each other for a few more rounds on the hill.*

Grandma realizes that she and Claire have built theme and variation in their imitation game. She also notes the number of imitations, including new acts, that Claire is now making; the length of Claire's attention to the play routine; and the number of practice turns (learning opportunities) that Claire experiences. This strategy has allowed Claire's grandmother to do more teaching in the play than she could have if she had only stayed with the theme. Claire likes the variation described above and has learned to imitate it after a few experiences with it, which Grandma realizes may be necessary to show a new idea and have it become interesting to Claire. If Claire doesn't like a variation after a few examples, Grandma can go back to the rolling game for a turn or two and then try a different variation—like crashing the cars or rolling them off the coffee table. Grandma understands that the overall goal is to extend the length of the joint activity routine, to have as many back-and-forth imitative exchanges as possible, and to weave in opportunities for varied imitation. Once the cars begin to lose Claire's interest, or if the game loses its social nature or becomes overly repetitive, Grandma is ready to suggest "all done" and model putting her car in the car box, gesturing for Claire to do the same—a nice ending to this well-done joint activity routine!

Chapter Summary

This chapter has focused on ways to help your child increase his or her imitation of you and others. We began by discussing the importance of your imitating your child—his or her actions and sounds. We then discussed several different types of imitations: imitation of actions on objects (the easiest for most children with ASD), imitation of sounds, imitation of varied actions, and imitation of gestures and facial movements (the hardest for many children with ASD). If you have followed along, you have increased the imitative opportunities your child has throughout the day. We then discussed the importance of adding variations to imitations to keep them from getting too repetitive. We pointed out how well imitation routines fit inside the four-part structure for joint activity routines: setup, theme, variations, and closing/transition. And, finally, we mentioned how imitative joint activity routines can fit into all your child care routines—not just toy or other object play and sensory social routines (including songs), but also meals, different types of caregiving, book routines, and household chores. Each imitation is a learning opportunity, and by embedding these kinds of games throughout all your activities with your child, you can dramatically increase the number of learning opportunities your child has.

Refrigerator List

Goal: To teach your child how to imitate different actions.

Steps:

✓ **Imitate your child's play with objects and expect your child to imitate back.**

✓ **Imitate your child's vocalizations and sounds and expect your child to imitate back.**

✓ **Use prompts to encourage imitation, but fade them fast!**

✓ **Don't expect perfection; accept your child's approximations.**

✓ **Make your imitative games turn-taking games— mini-conversations.**

✓ **Use the four-step joint activity structure to vary the imitations.**

✓ **Use songs and sensory social routines to build gesture imitations.**

✓ **Stay in your child's spotlight.**

9

Let's Get Technical

How Children Learn

> **Chapter goal:** To explain the basic principles and underlying strategies for helping your child engage, communicate, and learn, so you can apply these in new ways to boost your child's learning.

Chapters 4–8 have provided the building blocks that form the foundation for your child's learning. If you have followed along and practiced these strategies, you have already accomplished a lot and have likely seen a noticeable increase in your child's ability to engage, communicate, and learn. Good for you! Now we want to provide some background on how kids learn, so you can use these underlying principles flexibly in new situations as your child moves forward and meets new learning challenges.

With an understanding of *a*ntecedents (events that immediately precede a behavior), *b*ehaviors (your child's goal-directed actions), and *c*onsequences—the ***ABC's of learning***—you can motivate and teach new and even more sophisticated behaviors you want your child to learn, from pretending to starting to speak. These principles are based on the science of ***applied behavior analysis (ABA)***. In Chapter 1 we have explained that ABA is the application of the science of learning to help people learn new behaviors or change existing ones, including. reducing the frequency of problem behaviors. We use these principles—the ABC's of learning—throughout the chapters of the book.

Why Applied Behavior Analysis Is So Important

We have defined what ABA is, but you may not know that it isn't one specific intervention approach. This is a common misunderstanding. ABA is *applying* the science of learning to understanding and changing specific behaviors, and it underlies many different early intervention approaches for children. Discrete Trial Training, Pivotal Response Teaching, the Early Start Denver Model, Reciprocal Imitation Training, Milieu Teaching, and Incidental Teaching all use the principles of ABA.

You've been using them too! If you've been following the chapters up to this point and trying the strategies from each one with your child, you have taught your child a number of skills. In other words, you've encouraged new skill learning in your child by making it worthwhile for your child to learn what you're teaching. Because we've found it so helpful for parents to learn new habits of interacting with their children, we've been walking you through the use of these without using the technical terms of ABA, to help you get started. But the truth is that even your own behavior has been shaped by the principles of learning! You've been following the "rules" of learning new behaviors too; you've been trying new strategies, and the rewarding consequence of your applying these strategies has been experiencing the delight of seeing your child learn from you, right before your eyes. Pretty motivating, isn't it?

Now is a good time to understand the "rules" of learning in a more technical way, because this is likely to help you become more aware of many things:

1. Your own behavior
2. The meaning and goals that underlie your child's behaviors
3. How various situations lead to, or cue, your child's behaviors
4. How various events that follow your child's behavior reward your child for behaving in certain ways

Once you understand how the ABC's of learning work to build and maintain your child's current set of behaviors, you will have the tools you need to (1) teach your child new ways of behaving that are more age-appropriate or more acceptable (encouraging desirable behaviors and discouraging undesirable ones); (2) increase the number of learning opportunities for your child that are potentially present in every daily activity; and (3) help your child take full advantage of these learning opportunities you are providing.

What's Happening in Autism?

Children with autism respond to the ABC's of learning just like everyone else, but three aspects of autism demand a much more explicit focus on their learning than we need for other children:

1. **Children with ASD are not as interested as other children in pleasing other people.** Most children appear quite aware of their parents' pleasure, or displeasure, in response to what they say and do. Thus their parents' approval or

disapproval naturally serves to shape children's behavior, since children are motivated to gain parental attention and approval. Children with autism, however, are usually not so aware of or affected by the subtle (or even not so subtle) social consequences of their behavior, and therefore aren't as likely to do what adults want them to do just to please them.

2. **Children with autism are less interested than other children in sharing their experiences with others.** Most small children share with others by making eye contact, smiling, giving or showing objects, and pointing out interesting objects to their parents. For example, by the age of 12–18 months, most children will start pointing to things they find interesting, labeling them, and then looking toward their parents to share or show what they are noticing. They want their parents' attention and response. However, these child behaviors—*joint attention behaviors*—are quite infrequent in young children with ASD. And without these tools in their repertoire, they miss out on an enormous amount of language learning, social learning, and interpersonal connectedness. This is why you've been developing ways to promote what is known as **shared attention**, or **joint attention**, with your child in many of the strategies you've already learned. We focus very specifically on teaching joint attention in Chapter 10.

3. **Children with autism imitate others less than other children their age**

"My son was less interested than others in being independent but became more and more interested in being like his sister or like friends as he saw them doing appealing things. I first noticed this when his sister was hopping around pretending to be a frog. He realized that she was having a great deal of fun and started hopping with her, even though he may not have understood the pretend play aspect at the time (he does now, at age 3½). Having his sister or other role models demonstrate fun activities, I think, has helped his overall ability to care about and model his behavior after that of peers. He is still less motivated than other children to do things that don't seem as obviously fun, such as washing his hands, but I think even that motivation is improving as he understands that he can learn from them. He is doing more and more things that are expected behaviors rather than just fun behaviors (he has been able to start a taekwondo class recently, due to his improved ability to model others and show appropriate behavior in a class!). Many of the activities mentioned in previous chapters can be used by other children (especially when the children are slightly older) to encourage cooperative play and imitation."

do. Other children seem to have an internal goal of being like others, and to find their own personal pleasure in doing what others do and doing so independently. A child without ASD wants to handle a spoon alone, put on her own socks and shoes, do what her big brother or sister can do. We've heard many parents of children with autism say, "I think he would happily have me dress [or feed, diaper, etc.] him forever; he doesn't seem to have any desire to be independent or to do things for himself." Children with autism may imitate another person to make a toy work or to get to the cookie they want—in other words, to achieve a goal—but usually not just to "be like" another. Without that powerful goal, a child with autism does not practice skills he sees others use, and so he misses out on learning social and adaptive behavior from observing others. That's why we spent so much time on teaching imitation in Chapter 8: to help your child build up motivation to do what others do.

Why Is It a Problem?

Because children with autism are less interested in pleasing others, sharing their experiences with others, and imitating others, they miss out on many ABC learning opportunities that are present in the daily caregiving and play that provide most children with constant learning opportunities. These missed opportunities are reflected in the developmental delays—in language development, gestural development, self-care skills, and social play—that are part of the profile of early autism. Since children with autism have difficulty using existing social interactions as learning opportunities, those around them need to make those opportunities more explicit. That's the good news: It is possible to teach a child with autism to enjoy the praise of others, to enjoy sharing and imitating others! To make this happen in a wider set of circumstances and with a wider set of behaviors, you need to know the basic principles that are operating when learning occurs.

> *When Molly sees big sister Tina get some milk from the refrigerator, she screams and grabs at Tina to get the milk. Dad says to Tina, "Your sister wants some milk. Give it to her and get more for yourself." Tina cooperatively hands Molly the glass of milk and gets another. What has happened here? Molly's behaviors involve screaming and grabbing (occurring in response to the antecedent of seeing another person with some milk) and have resulted in a positive consequence, or* **reinforcement**: *She has achieved her goal and gotten the milk she wanted. Next time Molly sees someone with a glass of milk and she wants it, she will be more likely to scream and grab. A well-meaning father, who cares about his daughter and understands her desires, has inadvertently rewarded her unwanted behavior by having her sister hand over the milk. As you'll see, applying the learning principles described in this chapter can dramatically change the outcome of situations like this.*

➤➤➤➤ What You Can Do to Understand and Teach the ABC's of Learning to Your Child

There are six specific steps you can carry out to increase your understanding of the ABC's of learning and teach your child new skills and appropriate behaviors:

Step 1. Pay attention to what your child *does*: B is for behavior.

Step 2. Choose the reward: C is for consequence.

Step 3. Identify what came first, right before the behavior occurred: A is for antecedent.

Step 4. Put the ABC's of learning together.

Step 5. Use the ABC's to increase your child's learning opportunities and teach your child new skills and behaviors.

Step 6. Change unwanted behaviors.

Step 1. Pay Attention to What Your Child *Does*: B is for behavior

Rationale. All behavior is *lawful*. In other words, all children do the things they do for a reason. Behind every single action your child (or anyone else) performs is a reason—a goal for that behavior—and no matter how unusual the action is, there is a logic to it, a reason why the person is doing it. This goes for what people say as well as what they do; it also goes for what they don't do. When you see your child doing something that makes no sense to you, stop and ask yourself, "What is her goal?" It will often be clear, and then you will see the purpose, or function, of that puzzling behavior. All behavior is functional—it functions for the person; it generally results in some positive consequence for her. We'll come back to this later in more detail, but for now, consider the following rules to help you understand the reasons or goals behind your child's behavior.

➤ *Rule 1.* We focus on what children *do*—their behavior—not on what they "know." We do not measure our success at teaching in terms of what children end up knowing, but rather in what they do routinely. Why? Because little children cannot tell us what they know, and because what we want to teach are the behaviors that are difficult because of autism—the way they act toward others, communicate with others, play with objects, and participate in daily activities. It is common for us to ask a question like "Does she use a fork?" about a child and to hear a parent answer, "Yes, she knows how to use it. She prefers to use her hands, but if I make her, she will take a bite with a fork." We'd argue, then, that the correct answer to the question is no, because knowing how to do something is not the same as doing it, and the kinds of skills that young children with autism need to learn are those that are used all the time, independently, without someone having to make them use them (skills like speech, gesture, sharing, play with others, greeting others, sharing emotions, etc.). So when we focus on what children with autism do, we are talking about observable, consistent behavior. And there are always reasons, goals, or functions that lie underneath their behavior, built up from their previous experiences of the physical or social consequences of the behavior.

→ *Rule 2.* People do what they do to (a) get something they want, something that pleases them; or (b) avoid something they don't want, something that is unpleasant to them. It seems too simple to be true, but these are the only two primary reasons, goals, or functions for behavior. Your child behaves the way he does because in the past the behavior has worked for him either to obtain something rewarding, or to escape or avoid an experience he didn't like or something that prevented your child from achieving his goals.

♟ Activity: *Observe Your Child's Behavior*

We suggest you find some time over a couple of days to observe some of your child's behaviors and consider the goals or functions behind the behaviors. Try to do a few observations in most of the six types of target activities: toy or other object play, social play, meals, caregiving (bathing/dressing/changing/bedtime), book activities, and household chores. This does not mean that you must sit down with a notebook on the sidelines and observe. It means spending a little time paying attention to your child's

Helpful Tip
Remember, a behavior is an observable, intentional action: *yells, cries, grabs, reaches, speaks, looks.* It is not a feeling or state: *frustrated, angry, distressed, in pain,* or *tired.*

behavior and what is happening around your child for 15–20 minutes here and there. Observe and jot down some specific behaviors that your child demonstrates, and also those that you'd like to see more of (e.g., saying "Mama," giving you a smile, or coming to sit in your lap). Also, note the behaviors you don't like, the ones that you would rather see decrease.

Remember the assumption that all intentional behavior is functional and goal-directed. Then ask yourself: What is your child's goal when your child is screaming, looking and smiling at you, or leading you by the hand to the refrigerator? On the next page is a form to use to take some notes so you can develop an eye for looking at your child's behaviors and thinking about the underlying goals. Try to include both positive behaviors and some negative behaviors. The form includes some examples to get you started. Make extra copies of the form if you need more space.

Seeing the Goals in Behavior

Child's behavior	Child's goal
Reached up and looked at me	Wanted to be picked up
Pointed to the dog	Wanted to hear me say "Woof woof"
Said "Help" and put toy in my hands to fix	Wanted the toy to work again
Screamed and clutched toy when sister approached	Wanted to hold on to toy and not lose it to sister
Cried and looked at cupboard	Wanted a cookie from the cupboard

Summary of Step 1

If you have followed along and carried out the preceding activities, you now know how to "see" the goals that underlie your child's behaviors. This step begins the process of understanding the function of your child's behavior, situation by situation. The next steps will address how to "see" the antecedents and consequences that cue and reinforce your child's behavior in each of these situations, but for now, see if you agree with most of the statements in the following checklist. If so, you are now armed with important skills for understanding the relationships between goals and behavior—knowledge you will use in **Step 2**. If not, review this section, spend more time observing, and discuss your observations with a supportive other. Stay with this until you can easily see the goal underlying your child's behavior in a variety of situations.

Activity Checklist: Am I Effectively Observing My Child's Behaviors?

_____ I have spent some time observing my child and have made a list of my child's behaviors.

_____ I understand the difference between an observable behavior and an interpretation of a state (e.g., whining = behavior, tired = state).

_____ All the behaviors on my list are observable behaviors, not states.

_____ I understand the goals underlying some of my child's requesting behavior.

_____ I understand the goals underlying some of my child's undesirable behaviors.

_____ I have observed some behaviors in most of the six types of target activities.

Step 2. Choose the Reward: C is for Consequence

Rationale. ***Consequences*** are environmental responses to a child's behavior. They influence whether a child is likely to use the same behavior again to achieve a particular goal. Look at the examples in the form on page 203. For the first example, the child is approaching with upraised arms and face. The child's goal is a pickup. If the parent responds with a pickup, the child's goal has been met. A positive consequence (***reward***, or reinforcement) has resulted. His behavior has been successful at getting him to his goal. The reward (being picked up) that is obtained as a result of the raised arm gesture increases the chance (reinforced) that the child will use this gesture again to be picked up. A learning opportunity has occurred. A desired behavior (B)—a clear gesture, in this case—has been followed by a positive consequence (C). In other words, the behavior has been rewarded, or reinforced, by the pickup, the delivery of the child's goal. When we use the term *learning opportunity* in this book, this is what we mean: an occurrence in which you have helped your child produce a desired behavior or skill, and you have made sure that this is followed by a rewarding consequence—usually the goal your child has been seeking.

There are also environmental consequences for unwanted behavior. Rushing to your child and providing comfort and attention when she screams is a typical parental reaction. However, if your child's goal in screaming is to get your attention, then meeting your child's goal by delivering the positive consequence of getting attention rewards, or reinforces, your child's screaming. It gives your child the message that screaming is a powerful way to get your attention. Your child will be more likely to scream for your attention next time she wants it, because it has been successful this time. Taking a look at the consequences that follow your child's behaviors is the second step toward understanding why your child does what she does.

Whether behaviors are ones we appreciate (playing nicely, using language) or ones we don't appreciate (yelling, whining, repetitive behavior, screaming, running away, throwing things on the floor, hitting), behaviors are maintained by reinforcing consequences. The technical term for a consequence that increases the chances that the behavior will occur again is *reinforcement*. As in the preceding example of screaming to get attention, sometimes consequences that we think of as "negative" can act as reinforcement. But responding to a screaming child is actually *positive reinforcement*, if the child has attained her goal.

Now let's look at another situation. We'll continue to focus on screaming. In this situation, the parents of 4-year-old Jordan, the screamer just described, are trying to brush her teeth. They come to her with the toothbrush in hand. She screams the minute they touch her and puts up a huge fight when they try to get the toothbrush into her mouth. They cannot brush her teeth, and her parents give up in dismay. What has happened here? Jordan's goal is to escape from toothbrushing. Her screams and fighting are rewarded by her escape. Remember from our earlier discussion that that there are basically two functions for behavior—achieving something desirable and avoiding something undesirable. This is an example of escape as a reward. The technical name for this is *negative reinforcement*. The consequence is still reinforcing—Jordan has achieved her goal—but it is through the *removal of an aversive stimulus*; hence the term "negative." The earlier example, when Jordan achieves her parents' attention through screaming, is an example of "positive" reinforcement: She has attained a desired consequence. Both attaining something pleasant and avoiding something unpleasant reinforce, or strengthen, the behavior your child uses to try to achieve her goals. Here's an important rule to consider when you are observing what consequences follow your child's behavior:

➔ *Rule 3.* Learning new behaviors occurs in response to their consequences. You have been using this rule to teach your child in each of the earlier chapters in Part II of this book. Every time you have given your child a choice and he chooses something, your child has told you what his goal is: to have that thing. When you were teaching your child to extend his arms to request being picked up, you first saw that your child had that goal in mind, because he approached you and indicated in some way that that was what he wanted. Then you extended your arms and got your child to extend his arms (the new skill you were teaching). After he raised his arms (the new skill), you picked him up. In doing so, you made sure he attained his goal. Your pickup was (and is) his reward, the reinforcement, for the new behavior, extending his arms. And it is a reinforcement because he wants it—it's his goal.

♟ Activity: *What Behaviors Do You Want to Reward?*

Every time you provide a toy, a food, or an activity that your child wants, you are rewarding whatever action your child has done just before you hand it over. If she has cried just before, you are rewarding that. If she has looked at you, you're rewarding that. If he has not looked at you, you're rewarding that. If she has grabbed something, you're rewarding that. You strengthen whatever action, or behavior, you reward. Keeping this idea in mind as you interact with your child will help you be a more effective teacher for your child. Try to make sure that your child experiences positive consequences for desired behaviors. Try to make sure that your child does *not* receive positive consequences for undesirable behaviors.

➔ *Rule 4.* Behaviors that are not reinforced will decrease over time. Removing all the positive consequences, or rewards, of a behavior will weaken it over time (reduce its frequency) through a process called ***extinction***. Extinction occurs once all possible benefits of a behavior are eliminated.

> **What about Molly?** *Molly's father decides that he will no longer reward her screaming for her sister's possessions. He instructs Tina to turn her back on Molly and walk away when Molly screams and tries to grab something. Tina appreciates the change; she walks to her room and closes the door if Molly starts to scream. Over the course of the week, Molly stops heading toward Tina for things, and instead begins to go toward her parents and pull at them to get her what she wants. The parents decide that this is a better form of communication and allow her to lead them to the cabinet or fridge. We see that over the week Molly's screaming and grabbing at her sister has been extinguished. The behavior is no longer successful at achieving her goal, and so she gives it up and finds a new behavior that is more functional for her, one that is more successful at helping her reach her goal—dragging her parents to what*

she wants. They follow through by fulfilling her desires, so this new behavior is now being rewarded via the positive consequences that result.

Extinction can also reduce desirable behaviors. Here is a very common example.

Alycia is the mother of Max, who has ASD, and his younger sister, Kerry. Alycia tells Max to ask Kerry for a turn with a toy instead of grabbing it from her. So Max asks Kerry for the flashlight. Kerry ignores his request. So Max is not rewarded for asking. After three tries, Max grabs the toy and takes a turn. His grab is rewarded by getting the toy; his request is ignored. If this continues, he will not continue to request. His requests will quickly be extinguished because they are not successful at helping him attain his goal, and he will continue to grab, because it is successful.

Here is one way this could play out differently:

What about Kerry and Max? *Max asks Kerry for the flashlight. Kerry ignores him. Alycia steps in, guides Kerry's hand and flashlight to Max's hand, and makes sure he gets the flashlight. Max's request has been rewarded. But what about Kerry? She also needs to be rewarded for giving it to him. Fortunately, Alycia has another flashlight right there and offers it to Kerry right away. Kerry takes it and is happy. So Kerry has been rewarded for giving the flashlight in response to Max's open hand and request. Each child has been rewarded for a mature behavior.*

Realistically, it isn't always possible to have another item available (you don't necessarily know in advance that a struggle will develop over a flashlight, a fork, a plate, or a toy), and asking the older sibling to help by giving up the flashlight or other object can lead to a lot of resentment in the older sibling. It is helpful to get "buy-in" from other siblings at home to get their cooperation. Explain what you are doing to help their sibling with ASD learn to communicate and why it is important. That way, if they do give up an object, they feel proud (a reward) and are praised by you (another reward). Alycia could also try giving a different, appealing toy to Kerry (or Max), along with lots of verbal praise and hugs when the requested object is handed over (a positive consequence).

→ *Rule 5.* There is one other way that consequences change behavior over time: When a consequence (usually a negative consequence) follows a behavior and results in a decrease in frequency of the behavior, it is called ***punishment***. Punishment in this case doesn't mean sitting your child in the corner or something similar. It simply refers to a consequence that is unwanted by the child (or adult) and therefore leads to a reduction of the behavior that has directly preceded the punishment.

"*Unfortunately, siblings don't always want to reward nice, polite requests to share. I have encouraged my older daughter to encourage her brother to share, but it can be hard for her to give up toys she values, even when he asks very nicely. I want him to be rewarded in some way for his polite requests, though. We've worked out a system that seems to help. If my daughter has a toy that she absolutely does not want to share under any circumstances, then she is expected to keep it in her room or out of sight of her brother. If she is playing with a toy anywhere else in the house, then she is expected to share. If my son grabs a toy, he can't have it; I take it away so that my daughter is not the one engaging him in a fight (we have a rule that neither child is allowed to grab toys, even if the other one has taken a toy inappropriately). If he asks nicely, then she is expected to let him see it, but she can ask for it back right away (for instance, if she is in the middle of a game and doesn't want to be interrupted). If she asks nicely, then he is expected to cooperate and to return the toy. My son has become very good at sharing even his most valued toys.*"

What about Kerry and Max? *Let's imagine that after asking nicely to share the toy and being ignored, Max grabs for the toy. Kerry quickly leaves the room with the toy, not allowing Max to have it. Max begins crying and goes to Alycia, who says, "That's what happens when you grab." Max is less likely to grab next time, because his grabbing has resulted in an unpleasant, or negative, consequence—he has lost access to the toy. In technical language, his behavior has been punished.*

Punishment and extinction both result in decreases of behavior over time. Any unwanted consequence is technically punishment. For a child, being told "no" or "not now," having a parent put away an object that the child wants, or having a sibling take something away or push her down when she approaches to

---

Helpful Tip: Quick Terminology Review

When a behavior is followed by goal achievement, a positive consequence, it is **reinforced**. When it is routinely not followed by any goal-related event, it is **extinguished**. When it is followed by an unwanted event that results in goal loss, it is **punished**.

Extinction and punishment weaken the behavior being used to seek that goal. Reinforcement strengthens it. Children's intentional behaviors are strengthened or weakened by the consequences that follow their responses.

play can all be punishing consequences—unwanted consequences that follow an intentional behavior.

Activity: *Continue to Observe Your Child's Behavior*

For this exercise, take a day or two to find some observation times to pay attention to the consequences of your child's behaviors, considered in terms of your child's goals. Think about whether the consequence of the behavior met your child's goals, and thus was a reinforcer (R); whether it provided an unwanted consequence/punishment (P); or whether it had no consequence at all related to the goal, and thus resulted in extinction (EX). In the form on the facing page, be sure to include some examples of both socially desirable behaviors that your child uses (eye contact, gestures, sounds, or words) and socially undesirable behaviors (e.g., screaming and throwing). For all of these, remember that a reinforcer is the achievement of the child's goals. Sometimes even a behavior that on the surface seems like a negative response to the child's behavior (correction, scolding, etc.) can be a reinforcer if it helps the child achieve her goal (e.g., an older sibling's getting upset might serve as a reinforcer for a younger child who enjoys seeing the sibling upset). Make extra copies of the form if you need more space.

Summary of Step 2

If you have followed along and carried out the preceding activities, you now know how to "see" the consequences that follow and reinforce, punish, or extinguish your child's behaviors. This step continues the process of understanding the function of your child's behavior, situation by situation. The next step will address how to "see" the antecedents that cue your child's behavior in each of these situations, but for now, see if you agree with most of the statements in the following checklist. If so, you are now armed with important skills for understanding the relationships between goals and behavior—knowledge you will use in **Step 3**. If not, review this section, spend more time observing, and discuss your observations with a supportive other. Stay with this until you can easily see the consequences and the type of consequence underlying your child's behaviors in a variety of situations.

Activity Checklist: Am I Identifying Consequences of My Child's Behaviors?

_____ I have spent some time observing my child and have made a list of some of my child's behaviors.

_____ All the behaviors on my list are observable behaviors, not states.

Did a Behavior's Consequences Meet Your Child's Goals?

Child's behavior	Child's goal	Consequence: R, NR, or EX
Reached up and looked at me	Wanted to be picked up	Picked up my child—R
Pointed to the dog and looked at me	Wanted me to say something	I said, "It's a doggy. Doggy says bow-wow-wow"—R
Said "help" and put toy in my hands to fix	Wanted the toy to run again	I fixed the toy and handed it back to my child—R
Screamed and clutched toy when sister approached	Wanted to hold on to toy and not lose it to sister	Sister left and child was able to keep the toy—R
Led me to door	Wanted to go outside	Said no and did not let him go out—P
Watched brother with a puzzle and vocalized	Wanted to play with the puzzle	Brother ignored—EX

_____ I have listed the goals and consequences that follow some of my
child's desirable behaviors.

_____ I have listed the goals and consequences that follow some of my
child's undesirable behaviors.

_____ I have been able to classify most of the consequences as reinforcing, extinguishing, or punishing.

_____ I have observed some behaviors, goals, and consequences in most
of the six types of target activities.

Step 3. Identify What Came First, Right Before the Behavior Occurred: A Is for Antecedent

Rationale. We've been talking about two important principles for learning: (1)
The function of a behavior is to gain or avoid certain experiences; and (2) the
consequences that follow the behavior strengthen or weaken its use in that situation in the future. Now it is time for the third key principle for understanding
and changing behavior: (3) The event that occurs right before the behavior happens is the trigger or cue for the behavior to happen—the ***antecedent***, or stimulus,
that cues the behavior.

➔ *Rule 6.* Behaviors occur in response to a stimulus, also called an ***antecedent event***. Antecedents are often observable in your child's environment. Your
child sees something he wants (lollipop) or doesn't want (medicine container).
He hears a noise (the garage door opening) that means Dad is home. He sees a
dog he is afraid of. He walks into Grandma's kitchen and sees the shelf where
Grandma always keeps the chips. Antecedents can also be felt: He is hungry. He
is tired.

Although we often focus a lot of attention on the consequences of a behavior,
we need to focus just as much attention on the antecedents. If we are thinking
about a behavior we want a child to develop, we have to think about what environmental event—what stimulus—should cue that new behavior. Then we have to
make sure our teaching approach is focused on linking the new behavior to the
appropriate cue, or antecedent. That way, we can use the antecedents in various
situations to cue the behavior we want to see. We can also remove antecedents to
help reduce the chances that an unwanted behavior will occur.

What antecedents do we target? It's easy to focus on verbal instructions. We
want children to behave as we tell them to. However, for most of this text, we
have been helping you use nonverbal—or gestural—cues as antecedents as well.
You have been demonstrating the use of toys (A) so your child would imitate (B),
which resulted in an interesting effect (C). You have been pointing (A) so your

child would look at and retrieve something (B) that she wanted or liked (C). You have started a chase game and then stopped (A), so your child would chase you (B) and end up getting caught and thrown up in the air (C). You have started a song your child enjoys and done a finger movement (A1), and a pause (A2) your child imitated (B), and then you continued the song (C). In all these examples, you have used gestures—nonverbal communications—as the antecedents. You are probably quite skilled at this by this point in the book.

Note another important point: Many behaviors we want children to learn are independent skills—skills that other children use without needing an instruction or cue from another. Playing independently, going to the toilet when the need arises, greeting a parent who returns from work, giving a toy to a sister who asks to share—these are a few of many examples in which we expect young children to respond in certain ways without a parental instruction. If you look carefully at each of these complex independent skills, you will see the function, and the reinforcers, in them as well. Children play independently because they enjoy the activity (positive reinforcement). Children use a toilet independently because using the toilet avoids the inconvenient and uncomfortable situation caused by soiling their clothes (negative reinforcement), and also because of the social praise young children receive when they master this complex task (positive reinforcement). Greeting a beloved parent results in an affectionate exchange (a positive reward). Sharing toys avoids conflict (negative reinforcement) and continues pleasant social exchanges (positive reinforcement). These are very well-learned chains of behaviors that children can carry out without instruction, but when they were first learned, there were clear antecedents and direct rewards for each of them. Children with ASD can also learn these complex chains and carry them out independently, as long as there are clear antecedents and reinforcing consequences for them. You are teaching these with every chapter in Part II of this book.

What if you want to teach a new skill but are unsure of the antecedent—the cue—you should use? A good way to figure out what antecedent to use to cue a behavior is to think about what stimulus cues this behavior for most other children your child's age. Whenever possible, we want to use the same antecedents for children with autism that other children use. If you are not sure, observe children at the park, at school, in church, at the grocery store, and in other settings. Or ask friends or family members what their children respond to. Using the same antecedents that other parents use with their children means your child will be able to understand cues that many different people might use. This is why we have been suggesting that you use very typical (though simplified) language and gestures in working with your child. The words and gestures you are using, and the toys, songs, games, and daily routines you have been teaching, are very likely those that other members of your family and your network of friends use as well. Teaching your child these typical antecedents and responses in everyday situations, and with the household objects that occur around you, makes it much easier for your child to learn the antecedent–behavior chains that others will use as well. Your child is learning what he needs to respond to many people, not just a few, and in many situations, not just the "teaching" environment.

> **What about Max and Kerry?** *The stimulus, or antecedent, for Max's grabbing was the sight of Kerry playing fun games with the flashlight. What is the typical behavior that preschoolers use in response to the antecedent event of seeing another child with a desired toy? Yes, grabbing does occur, but ideally, they ask for a turn. So the mom, Alycia, is correct to prompt Max to ask Kerry for a turn with the flashlight. The typical reward for making the request is getting a turn with the toy.*

The goal here is to teach Max that when he sees Kerry with another toy (A—the antecedent), he should request a turn (B—the behavior), and hopefully be rewarded with a turn (C—consequence). Consider the behaviors and their antecedents in the chart on the facing page. Fill in some you have observed for your own child. Make extra copies of the form if you need more space.

Summary of Step 3

If you have followed along and carried out the preceding activities, you now know how to "see" the antecedents that cue your child's behaviors in many situations. This step continues the process of understanding the ABC's of a variety of your child's behaviors, situation by situation. The next steps will address how to put together all that you have learned to build or change behaviors and skills your child uses to meet her goals. See if you agree with most of the statements in the following checklist. If so, you are now armed with important skills for understanding the relationships between antecedents and behavior—knowledge you will use in **Step 4**. If not, review this section, spend more time observing, and discuss your observations with a supportive other. Stay with this until you can easily see the antecedents preceding your child's behavior in a variety of situations.

Activity Checklist: Am I Identifying Antecedents of My Child's Behaviors?

_____ I have spent some time observing my child and have made a list of my child's behaviors.

_____ All the behaviors on my list are observable behaviors, not states.

_____ I understand the antecedents, goals, and consequences underlying some of my child's desirable behaviors.

_____ I understand the antecedents, goals, and consequences underlying some of my child's undesirable behaviors.

_____ I have observed some behaviors and their antecedents in most of the six types of target activities.

Understanding the Antecedent to Your Child's Behavior

Child's behavior	What happened before: Antecedent
Reached up and looked at me	Held out my arms to pick up my child
Pointed to the dog	Asked my child, "Where's the dog?"
Said "help" and put toy in my hands to fix	Asked my child, "Do you need help?" and held out my hands to take toy
Screamed and held toy close to chest	Sister was approaching and showing interest in the toy
Led me to kitchen and put my hand on the fridge	Internal feeling of hunger

Step 4. Put the ABC's of Learning Together

Rationale. We have now discussed the basic ABC principles of learning, and if you have tried the preceding exercises, you've thought through your child's behavior the same way behavior analysts do. Step 4 is to put the ABC sequence together. Each child has unique ways of behaving, responding, and interacting with others. By observing your child's behaviors, and the antecedents and consequences of those behaviors, you learn about your child's goals and the functions of his behaviors—why he acts the way he does. Your child's behaviors communicate what consequences or outcomes he has previously experienced, and what cues or antecedents lead to his behaviors. Unwanted behaviors like tantrums and aggression are part of all children's repertoires of behavior, and they become habitual if these behaviors have repeatedly led to goal achievement—to positive consequences. These are not "naughty" behaviors; they are functional behaviors for a child who uses them. They are the child's best efforts to attain his goals. Desirable behaviors, like giving a hug or kiss, occur for the same reason: They result in positive consequences for a child. All of your child's intentional behaviors follow the same rules. They are the most effective means your child has found for achieving his goal in a situation signaled by an environmental cue. Desirable or undesirable, they are functional—they work.

♟ Activity: *Observe Your Child's Socially Desirable and Undesirable Behaviors, Their Antecedents, and Their Consequences*

This exercise will help you see and describe the whole sequence underlying some of your child's habitual behaviors. It is so important to begin to see the ABC sequences that underlie your child's current repertoire of desirable and undesirable behaviors that we encourage you to spend the next few days learning to see them. If you learn this skill well, you will be able to use it effectively throughout your child's life to teach new behaviors, increase desirable behaviors your child already does, and reduce the frequency of your child's unwanted behaviors. These principles work in the elementary school period, during adolescence, and in adulthood. Once you learn to see them, they will start to "pop out" at you, which will give you many more ideas for ways to teach your child new or different responses to situations and experiences. Start by jotting down examples of your child's behaviors (B's) and goals. Those are the keys to defining the antecedents (A's) and consequences (C's). Once you have the B's and goals down, note the consequence and the antecedent, just as you have done earlier. These are probably getting easier and easier to see. Be sure to write down some desirable behaviors that your child demonstrates, and also some undesirable behaviors—things you wish your child did not do.

Summary of Step 4

If you have followed along and carried out the preceding activities, you now know how to "see" the goals, antecedents, and consequences that underlie a number of your child's desirable and undesirable behaviors. This step continues the process of understanding the function of your child's behavior, situation by situation. The next step involves using this knowledge to teach your child new skills and to increase the number of learning opportunities you provide for your child. See if you agree with most of the statements in the following checklist. If so, you are now armed with important skills for understanding the relationships that support your child's various behaviors: goals, antecedents, and consequences—knowledge you will use in **Step 5**. If not, review this section, spend more time observing, and discuss your observations with a supportive other. Stay with this until you can easily see the antecedents, goals, and consequences underlying a variety of your child's most desirable and most undesirable behaviors in many situations.

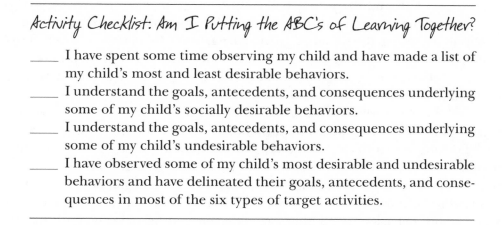

Activity Checklist: Am I Putting the ABC's of Learning Together?

_____ I have spent some time observing my child and have made a list of my child's most and least desirable behaviors.

_____ I understand the goals, antecedents, and consequences underlying some of my child's socially desirable behaviors.

_____ I understand the goals, antecedents, and consequences underlying some of my child's undesirable behaviors.

_____ I have observed some of my child's most desirable and undesirable behaviors and have delineated their goals, antecedents, and consequences in most of the six types of target activities.

Step 5. Use the ABC's to Increase Your Child's Learning Opportunities and Teach Your Child New Skills or Behaviors

Rationale. *Every interaction you have with your child is a potential learning opportunity.* To mobilize more of the many opportunities you have, you need to be aware of all the potential reinforcers that present themselves. Often these are things your child desires—food and drink; attention; favorite objects; comfort and affection; safety and security; interesting sights, sounds, and events; pleasant touch and movement. Or they may be unpleasant stimuli your child wants removed, such as hunger or thirst, noxious sounds (e.g., vacuum cleaner), unpleasant sensations (e.g., sticky hands or a messy diaper), frightening stimuli, or barriers to your child's goals (e.g., fixing a broken toy, opening a cupboard or refrigerator).

♟ Activity: *Make Sure Your Child Is Communicating Goals as Maturely as Possible*

You can corral these opportunities to work on your child's behalf by asking yourself these questions every time you deliver something your child wants or remove something your child dislikes: How is my child communicating her desires? Is she using the most mature communicative behaviors she is capable of to indicate her goals? Or am I providing all these reinforcers to a child who is doing little to communicate her goals? *These are really important questions.* One parent who asked herself this question said, "You know, he is like the Little Prince. He doesn't have to do a darn thing—we all meet his every need without him exerting any effort at all!" It was a big insight for her. She was not asking of her son what we typically expect other children to do: *to communicate as well as they can.* How often have we all said to a whiny child, "Use your words," or cued a child who said, "I want more milk," to add "please" to that demand? Or to correct a child who grabs by taking the toy away, giving it back to the first child, and telling the grabber to "ask nicely"? We expect children to use their current communicative ability to achieve their goals, and we cue them, or *prompt* them, to use the desired behavior.

So think about what communications your child is easily capable of: Reaching? Pointing? Vocalizing with intent? Imitating sounds? Making a choice between two? Looking at you to communicate? Whatever communications are currently present in your child's repertoire and are easy for your child to do—that's how your child can be communicating his goals. When he is using undesirable behaviors to communicate, such as whining, screaming, or tantrums, do these things: Ignore those behaviors (extinguish); cue the desired behavior by modeling or prompting an appropriate behavior that will allow the child to achieve his goal (a reach or a verbal request); expect your child to use the appropriate behavior; and then allow your child to reach his goal (reward).

Make a list of your child's current communications, both verbal and gestural. These are the tools your child has for communicating her needs and desires. Now keep those in mind when you next start to provide your child with something you know she wants. Clearly show your child it is available; that is the A—the antecedent. But hold back and wait to deliver it until your child has communicated for it, using one of the communications you have listed. Wait for the B—the behavior—and cue it if your child needs some help. Once your child communicates well, *then* deliver the C—the consequence, the reinforcer for your child's communication.

What if your child does not produce the communication or uses an unwanted behavior, such as whining? Ignore the unwanted behavior and prompt the behavior that is appropriate. Help your child do it. If your child can say a word, model the word. If your child can reach, put the object within reaching distance. If your child can point, model the point. If needed, physically guide your child through the response you are teaching. After your child acts, deliver. You have provided a *learning opportunity*—a full ABC sequence.

Let's say the situation involves giving your child a peanut butter sandwich, and your communicative goal for your preverbal child for her to use her voice to communicate requests. Let's say you have cut the sandwich up into eight tiny bite-sized pieces for your child. If you hold the plate toward your hungry child (A), and your child reaches and says "Mmmm" (B), and you hand the plate over (C), you have provided one learning opportunity for your child.

Now let's say you are sitting at the table as well, and when your child reaches and says "Mmmm," you provide one piece of the sandwich. Your child stuffs it into her mouth and reaches and says "Mmmm" again. You deliver another piece. Your child's drink is also beside you, out of your child's reach. Your child reaches for the cup. You hold it up and say "Drink?", and your child reaches and says "Mmmm." You give the cup over, your child has a drink, *and you take it back.* Over this meal, with the sandwich, the drink, and a few pieces of banana that you have also cut up, you have provided 15 or more learning opportunities for your child to learn to use her voice to request. And that doesn't take into account the number of times you have also imitated your child by taking a bite of your own sandwich, saying "yum yum," and having a little imitation exchange (more learning opportunities).

So here is an important way to start to build more learning opportunities into your child's day—by being aware of the many antecedents that precede the behaviors you are teaching, the many times you deliver reinforcers by meeting your child's goals, and the many ways you can help your child develop and practice an appropriate communicative behavior of some type before you deliver.

Activity: *Observe Your Child's Behavior for Occurrences of the ABC's*

Spend some time reviewing your day with your child. Think about the times today you gave your child something you knew he wanted. Think about the times you removed something or changed something you knew was bothering your child. List them in the left-hand column of the form on the next page. Those are the reinforcers, or potential reinforcers, that you provided your child. For each one, remember what your child did that resulted in your action—how your child communicated his need or desire. Write that on the right-hand side. Here are the learning opportunities that you provided your child in these situations. If there was no child behavior that preceded your rewarding action, write down "None" in the right-hand column. There was a missed opportunity for learning. Over

Observing the ABC's

Reinforcer I provided	Child behavior that was reinforced

the next few days, see if you can become more aware of these potential missed opportunities, and instead wait for a child communication or prompt your child to communicate in some way before you provide the consequence, *so that you are turning missed opportunities into learning opportunities.* Make extra copies of the form if you need more space.

Step 6. Change Unwanted Behaviors

Rationale. All little children (and most adults as well) have habits that are not very pleasing or attractive. In the lists you have just made, you may have identified some of your child's behaviors that you are not so happy with. Your child may scream to communicate a desire, or drag you by the hand, or bite to avoid someone or to gain access to a desired object. Your child may fall on the floor and bang her head when her brother takes a toy or when you refuse to give her another candy bar. Why does your child do these things? You may have already figured that out: In completing the activities earlier in this chapter, you may well have run into some of these unwanted behaviors. By analyzing the ABC sequence of these behaviors, you have "evaluated" them. You have learned the functional relations that supported the behaviors—the A and the C. If your child has some unwanted behaviors and you have not yet identified their ABC sequences, now is the time to do that. In this final step, we are going to explain how to help your child learn more acceptable behaviors to replace these unwanted ones.

♟ Activity: *Identify an Unwanted Behavior and a Possible Replacement*

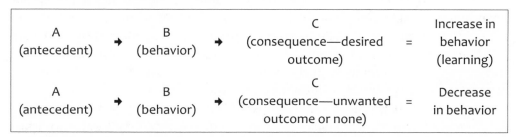

Choose one of your child's unwanted behaviors that occurs often and that has a clear ABC frame—a behavior you would really like to change.[1] Now remember

---

[1]Keep in mind that sometimes unwanted behaviors, such as crying, screaming, and tantrums, are signs that your child doesn't feel well. Remember that in Chapter 1 we have discussed the fact that children with autism sometimes experience gastrointestinal problems, food sensitivities, lack of sleep, and other health-related problems. Recall also that sometimes it is difficult for children with autism to tell us that they are in pain or where the pain is occurring. If your child shows a sudden change in behavior, such as suddenly becoming more fussy or aggressive, and it doesn't appear to be linked to a specific antecedent or consequence, consider

the ABCs of learning. Look at your child's goal without expecting that your child will change goals. Ask yourself: "What does he want? What is his goal?" *After you have answered that question, ask yourself:* "What do I wish he would do instead to ask for what he wants or achieve his goal?" If he screams to get out of doing something he doesn't like or to get a toy, what do you wish he would do instead of screaming to request that you stop what he is being asked to do or to have access to the toy? If he bangs his head on the floor when you take his pacifier away, what do you wish he would do instead to achieve his goal? The behaviors you wish to see instead of the unwanted behaviors are called ***replacement behaviors***.

➔ *Rule 7.* A good replacement behavior must be as easy for the child to do as the unwanted behavior, and must result in the same reward as quickly as does the unwanted behavior. The replacement behavior will work only if it is as functional—as efficient, as effective, as easy—as the unwanted behavior. The replacement behavior already has to be in your child's repertoire, and you have to be able to prompt it easily.

♟ Activity: *Teach the Replacement Behavior*

So, with Rule 7 in mind, focus on the unwanted behavior you would like to see changed, and think about what else your child could do—now, easily, efficiently—to achieve the same goal. That is your ***replacement behavior***. Write down how the sequence will look: What is the antecedent (A); what is your replacement behavior (B); what is your child's goal; and what is the consequence (C), or reward, for using the replacement B? Got it?

Here is an example. A = your Pepsi. Unwanted B = grabbing. Replacement B = pointing. Child's goal = your Pepsi. C = your Pepsi. Now think about how you are going to prompt your child to do the replacement B as soon as the A occurs and *before* the unwanted B occurs. Get ready to prompt the replacement B, and then deliver the C right away. If the unwanted B is already under way, ignore it, prompt the replacement B, and then provide the positive C.

Example: You get your Pepsi and sit down on the couch. Your daughter appears and heads for the Pepsi. You pick it up, and as she looks at it, you say, "Want a drink? Point. Point to Pepsi." You model, she points, and you give her a sip, but not the whole can. You take it back and get a drink. She reaches and you say again, "Point." She points and gets a sip. This goes on a few more times, until she is pointing without any instructions. No grabbing has occurred at all.

---

having your child's health status evaluated by a pediatrician. Similarly, if your child is not sleeping well or is eating poorly, it will be much more difficult for her to refrain from being irritable and fussy. By making sure that your child is healthy, you set the stage for your child to be more cooperative, show fewer problem behaviors, learn more easily, and generally be a happier and more engaged child.

What about Molly? *As described earlier, Molly screams and grabs when her sister gets a glass of milk, and Dad tells her sister to give it to Molly and get another. A = sight of milk. B = scream and grab. Goal = wants milk. C = gets milk. Dad has to think of a replacement behavior for screaming and grabbing, and Molly has not yet learned to speak. What behavior can Molly use to request a glass of milk? Pointing to the milk? Signing "drink" or "please"? Vocalizing and making eye contact? Molly's family has to decide what kind of appropriate communication Molly should use when she wants something from someone else. They decide on a simplified "please" sign that their speech therapist has suggested—her hand held against her chest. Now her parents need to create the learning opportunities for her to learn this replacement communication.*

The antecedent occurs: Molly sees big sister Tina get a glass of milk from the refrigerator, and Molly screams and grabs at Tina to get the milk. Dad goes to Molly, takes her hands off Tina, puts her hand to her chest to make the "please" sign, and says to Molly, "Please." As soon as Molly finishes making the sign, with Dad's help, Tina cooperatively hands Molly the milk and gets another. Although this is a step in the right direction, Dad thinks this through later and notices two things he would like to improve on: (1) Molly is still screaming and grabbing, and (2) Tina is still losing her original glass of milk. The next time, Dad is ready. When Tina asks, Dad encourages her to get two glasses of milk, and Dad moves right beside Molly. Tina gets the glasses of milk, and when Dad sees Molly look at the glasses of milk, he immediately walks her to Tina and helps her sign "please." Then Tina gives Molly the second glass of milk, feeling very proud that she has helped her little sister learn to communicate. Now Dad has assured that Molly receives the milk for making the sign and not the scream.

See what has happened? The same antecedent (seeing Tina with the milk) is now being linked with a desired behavior—an appropriate communication—which results in the same reinforcer (the milk) that has previously supported the unwanted behavior. Over time, if the family is consistent with this new routine, the "please" sign will become linked to the sight of the milk (and all other objects she wants from another person), because that is the only way Molly will get the milk. The glass of milk will support a positive behavior rather than an unwanted one, while Molly learns a more useful and acceptable communication, and she still gets the milk.

With this example in mind, go back to the unwanted behavior you have zeroed in on for your own child and consider how you will help your child use the replacement behavior for attaining her goal. Imagine how you will help your child, or prompt your child, to carry out the replacement behavior and then deliver the reinforcer. Start practicing as soon as you can imagine it.

Caution! A coping strategy that families sometimes use in the face of unwanted behaviors is to try to avoid problem behaviors by placing fewer and fewer demands or expectations on the child. Although this is a very natural response to tantrums or aggression, it backfires in two ways, both of which over time reduce the child's learning. First, it takes away learning opportunities. If the child does not have to do anything to gain what he wants, then no new learning is taking place. Second, it reinforces either very immature behavior, like whining or grabbing, or unwanted behavior, like Molly's screaming. Avoiding the problem behavior by giving in earlier does not change the use of unwanted behavior. Only by actively teaching a more desirable response can you really change your child's behavior. Your child can learn a more desirable response. Your child has learned one way of responding, and your child can learn a more desirable way as well.

Summary of Step 6

If you have followed along and carried out the preceding activities, you likely have learned how to use your everyday interactions to support your child's more desirable social and communicative skills. You also know much more about why your child does all those things you wish she wouldn't do, and you know what consequences, or rewards, are supporting your child's use of those unwanted behaviors. You have developed some ideas about how to replace them with more socially desirable behaviors, and you have some ideas about how to avoid rewarding those unwanted behaviors. You have tried to prompt your child to use a replacement behavior before the unwanted behavior even occurs, and you have been able (we hope) to reinforce the replacement behavior. See if you agree with most of the statements in the following checklist. If so, you are now armed with (1) knowledge and skills for providing more learning opportunities within your everyday activities with your child; and (2) strategies for replacing your child's unwanted behavior with more socially acceptable, communicative behavior. If not, review this last section of the chapter, and discuss these concepts and your observations with a supportive other—ideally, someone who also understands the basics of behavior, like one of your child's professional team members. Mastering these concepts will help you help your child for many years to come (and your other children as well!)

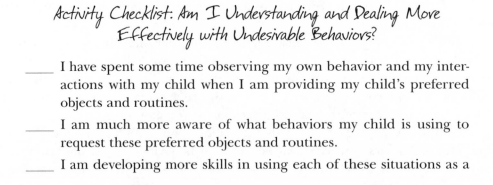

Activity Checklist: Am I Understanding and Dealing More Effectively with Undesirable Behaviors?

_____ I have spent some time observing my own behavior and my interactions with my child when I am providing my child's preferred objects and routines.

_____ I am much more aware of what behaviors my child is using to request these preferred objects and routines.

_____ I am developing more skills in using each of these situations as a learning opportunity, by either rewarding or cuing my child's use of more mature communicative behaviors.

_____ I have had some successful experiences in replacing one or more of my child's unwanted behaviors with a more desirable communication or behavior.

_____ I am much more aware of my tendency to provide positive consequences when my child uses an unwanted behavior, and I am doing it less.

_____ I am seeing positive effects of my new knowledge in my child's progress in learning to communicate to reach his or her goals.

_____ I am seeing positive effects of my new knowledge in my child's decreasing use of unwanted behaviors that I have focused on.

_____ I am creating more learning opportunities during daily play and caregiving activities by using the ABC's of learning.

_____ I am creating more learning opportunities in most of the six types of target activities.

Chapter Summary

Behavior can be understood in terms of what takes place before the event (antecedents), as well as what follows it (consequences). This relationship or understanding of antecedents, the behavior itself, and consequences can be thought of as a set of linked actions, events, and circumstances that occur together in an environment. Understanding antecedents and consequences and their combined influence on behavior allows us to understand how a behavior functions for a child, and thus helps us know how to teach new behaviors and reduce unwanted behaviors in a systematic and effective way.

- Pay attention to times when you find yourself delivering positive consequences for behaviors that you would rather not reinforce: screaming, throwing, crying, grabbing, fussing, whining, not using words/gestures.

- Pay attention to times when your child ignores your instructions or requests and continues to do what he was doing. In these situations, your child is being rewarded for ignoring you (by getting to do what he wants to do).

- Pay attention to all the times you see your child wanting something and, through your skillful teaching, communicating nicely and receiving what he wants. You are providing great reinforcement for good behavior and an important learning opportunity.

- Pay attention to all the times your child communicates in an unwanted way, through immature behavior or unwanted behaviors, and you hold back on providing what he wants (and thus help extinguish the unwanted behavior). Instead, you prompt your child to request or behave in a desired way and then deliver the reward, supporting your child's learning.

Every time you reinforce a desired behavior, you provide a learning opportunity for your child. Every time you prompt your child to use a more mature or appropriate skill and reinforce that new skill, you provide a learning opportunity. Every time you model a desired behavior and your child imitates you, you provide a learning opportunity. And every time you make sure an unwanted behavior is not reinforced but rather replaced by a more desirable behavior or skill, which gets your child what he wants, a learning opportunity has occurred.

Children with autism need to learn and are very capable of doing so. Teaching them is about creating learning opportunities. Understanding the ABC's of learning helps you think about how to create learning opportunities to stimulate development and build more mature behavior.

Refrigerator List

Goal: To use the ABC's for understanding and teaching new behaviors.

Steps:

✓ Everything happens for a reason! Identify your child's goals.

✓ What happens after your child's behavior solidifies it.

✓ What is your child doing to achieve his or her goals? Is it what you want?

✓ Be aware of the rewards you are providing and what behavior you are rewarding in the process.

✓ Use your child's goals in everyday activities to teach new skills.

✓ What do you wish your child would do instead? Answer this question and replace unwanted behaviors with more acceptable ones.

✓ Replacement behaviors need to be at least as easy, efficient, and effective as the behaviors you are trying to replace.

✓ The rewards that follow your child's new skills are what will make them stick.

10

The Joint Attention Triangle

Sharing Interests with Others

Chapter goal: To help you teach your child how to share interest in objects with you.

Why Sharing Interests and Attention (Joint Attention) Is So Important

So far we've been emphasizing how to increase your child's interest in paying attention to you. You've now learned (and, we hope, are using) methods for encouraging your child to pay attention to your face, voice, and actions. By teaching and promoting turn taking, imitation, and nonverbal communication, you've been showing your child the power of two people communicating directly with one another. Your child has learned that looking at you, coming to you to express his needs and desires, following your lead (and seeing you follow his), and enjoying activities with another person all have rewards that your child may not have grasped as easily as other children do. The importance of this is huge for your child's learning potential, both in structured educational settings and in the all-important social world, where children gain so much new information and understanding by interacting with others.

But these *dyadic* (back-and-forth) interactions aren't enough. Now it's time to teach your child how to share his attention to objects and other interesting events in the world with others. This capacity to share attention with others is called *joint attention*, or *triadic attention*. *Triadic* means "three-way" and refers to the three points of the attention triangle—your child, you, and your child's focus of interest. Joint attention allows people to share information, emotion, or meaning about an interesting event.

Think about a time when you were at lunch with a friend and you noticed something unusual or interesting. You likely looked at the interesting spectacle and then were naturally motivated to share what you were seeing with your friend. After first looking at the interesting spectacle, you looked back to your friend, then commented on or pointed at the spectacle, and then looked back again at your friend to see if she was looking at it too and to notice her expression. You were sharing your attention with your friend. This ***triangle of attention***—the three-way interaction involving two people and an object or event—is joint attention. And it is a fundamental building block for young children's communication and language learning. Studies we authors and our coworkers have carried out, as well as other studies, have shown that children's joint attention skills are strongly related to their later language abilities.[1]

Parents and their young children often share moments of eye contact, smiles or other expressions of interest, gestures (pointing, showing, and giving), and sounds or words to communicate about something one or the other has noticed. They might communicate about things like these:

- The names of objects: Mom holds up a round blue object in her hands and, as her daughter reaches for it, says, "It's a balloon."
- Actions happening in play: Dad points to the open spot in the puzzle and tells his son, "The tiger goes here."
- Instructions: A toddler finishes her drink and then hands her empty cup to Grandma while she looks at her and vocalizes, clearly communicating "I want more."
- Experiences to share: A child points to a dog across the street, and Mom looks and answers, "It's a doggie."

A fundamental skill required for joint attention is the child's ability to shift her gaze back and forth between you and the object. Before joint attention develops, children focus their attention mainly on either an object *or* a person during play, but they aren't yet able to shift their attention back and forth, to focus on both the object and the person. At about 6 months of age, children learn to shift their gaze back and forth between an object and a parent's face. This skill contributes greatly to the joint attention skills and the related social, communication, and language learning that comes from it.

What's Happening in Autism?

Two difficulties seem to interfere with joint attention development in ASD. First, as we have said earlier, children with ASD are a little less socially oriented to

---

[1]Toth, K., et al. Early predictors of communication development in young children with autism spectrum disorder: Joint attention, imitation, and toy play. *Journal of Autism and Developmental Disorders*, *36*(8), 993–1005, 2006.

Thurm, A., et al. Predictors of language acquisition in preschool children with autism spectrum disorders. *Journal of Autism and Developmental Disorders*, *37*(9), 1721–1734, 2007.

begin with. They seem to be less motivated to share and engage socially than other children are. Second, children with autism have difficulty learning to shift their gaze from people to objects easily and frequently. They tend to focus on objects more than people, and they may sustain their attention to objects for a long time. They may struggle to attend to multiple people or things in an environment, even when no demands are imposed. Sometimes their attention gets "stuck" on the first thing they are noticing, and they have difficulty flexibly disengaging their attention from the first object and moving on to the next. Most early intervention approaches focus one way or another on teaching young children with ASD to shift their gaze from objects to people and back. Our goal in helping you teach your child joint attention is to help him communicate with others about his shared experiences in the world. Without intervention, developing spontaneous joint attention skills is one of the harder skills for young children with ASD to learn.

Why Is It a Problem?

Without joint attention, children with autism tend not to share their thoughts and emotions about objects and events with important others, and so they lose out on these learning opportunities that contribute greatly to enhancing language, social, and cognitive development. Joint attention also involves reading another person's cues and understanding the partner's desires or feelings about the object—in other words, reading the partner's mind. When joint attention is limited, so is the ability to understand the meaning behind any situation (what something is called, how an object works, or what should happen during an activity) by looking at and following people's eye gaze and gestures.

Equally important, joint attention appears to strengthen children's desire to appreciate, value, and seek out social attention and praise from others when something fun and enjoyable happens. Remember how excited you were to share something you did with Mom and Dad when you were a child? It might have been a drawing you completed that day at school, or a great move you made during a board game, or when you tackled a new feat that you thought was impossible to do. Chances are that you looked right into your parents' eyes, gave a huge smile, and beamed with delight as they congratulated you on your success. This experience does not have to be different for children with autism. We want them to enjoy the excitement, praise, and pride that can result from social interactions. But to make this happen, they need to understand and use joint attention.

▶▶▶ What You Can Do to Increase Your Child's Joint Attention Skills

In its most basic form, joint attention involves the ability to shift eye contact or gaze between a social partner and an object or event. Once gaze shifts occur easily, children start to use three main gestures to share attention—giving, showing, or pointing at the object or event—while making eye contact. Joint attention also involves sharing feelings about an object or event through gaze and facial expressions. The child looks at the object and then looks at the adult with a smile or frown, communicating her feelings about the object or event. How can you work with your child to develop joint attention? You are already doing some of the work, by doing things you have learned in earlier chapters:

1. Drawing your child's attention to your face and eyes (Chapter 4)
2. Positioning yourself in front of your child for all activities to assist with eye contact (Chapter 4)
3. Pausing and teaching your child to use her body (talking bodies) to communicate her needs to you (Chapter 7)
4. Developing a number of sensory social and object routines that you do together (Chapters 5 and 6)

Once you have increased your child's eye contact and your child's gesture communications, you and your child are ready for the three specific steps toward joint attention skills:

Step 1. Teach your child to give you objects.

Step 2. Teach your child to show you objects.

Step 3. Teach your child how to point to objects to share experiences.

In the following pages, we describe how to carry out each of these steps, give you some ideas for activities to try, and suggest what you can do to solve problems that may come up.

Helpful Tip

When you ask your child to give an object to you during play or caregiving activities, be sure to give it back as soon as you get it. If your child does not get it back right away, she will not be very motivated to give it to you. Remember the ABC's from Chapter 9: If the consequence of giving you an object is losing it altogether, you will not have reinforced giving—quite the opposite!

Step 1. Teach Your Child to Give You Objects

Rationale. Joint attention is a kind of turn taking, and it cannot occur unless your child is willing to hand over an object on request and then get it back. Because your child may not have the built-in motivation to interact in this way, you'll have to teach it "from the ground up," starting with the fact that an outstretched hand is a request for the child to give you an object he is holding. Your earlier work with turn taking (Chapter 6) has provided your child with a foundation for this skill. Continue working on this skill to lay the foundation for joint attention skills.

 ## Activity: *Teach Your Child to Give Objects to Get Help from You*

Teaching your child to give an object to you when she needs help with the object is an important initial step. It motivates your child to learn the gesture, because the action that follows (your help) works in your child's favor! That gesture becomes much more powerful, however, when your child learns to use eye contact as well as giving to communicate a need for help. When your child makes eye contact and gives an object to you for help, your child has made a powerful communication about her goals.

Here are ideas for teaching your child to give you objects to receive help:

- Begin by showing your child a clear container (plastic zipper bag, lidded plastic container) that your child cannot open by himself, and that holds a highly motivating object. This could be a favorite snack during snack time, a favorite bath toy during bath time, or part of a favorite toy during toy play (e.g., the pieces to a puzzle). Your child will see the objects inside the bag and should reach for it when you offer it. Give the container to your child. Your child will likely struggle to open it.

- Then reach your open hand to your child while saying, "Need help?" Prompt your child to give you the container, take it and open it quickly, and give it right back, saying, "Here's the [object name]."

- Repeat this in various activity types across the day—bath toys in containers, food at meals in closed bottles or containers, fun toys in containers during toy play. Always use the same cues: your outstretched hand and the words "Need help?", "I'll help you," and "Here's the [object name]."

- As this becomes a familiar routine over a few days or so, see whether your child will initiate the request. Give the container as usual, but do not offer your hand or ask about help. Wait, looking expectantly at your child. Your child is likely to hand you the bag. Say, "You need help. I'll help," and then "Here is your [object name]" as you hand back the open container. Celebrate! Your child now knows a way to ask for help.

- Once your child spontaneously and routinely hands things to you for help, start to work on encouraging eye contact when he asks for help. To do this, start as described above and wait for your child to initiate the request for help. Wait a little after your child has given you the object. If your child is making eye contact after he hands it to you, open it immediately, with your script. If your child is not making eye contact with you, then do not open the container. Instead, just continue to hold it in your hand and look at your child expectantly. Chances are that your child will briefly make eye contact. When he does this, quickly catch his gaze and immediately open the container. If your child doesn't spontaneously look at you when you wait to open the container, ask, "Need help?" without moving the object. If your child makes eye contact, immediately open it. If your child still doesn't look, move the container near your face while looking at your child and ask again or shake the container. Wait for the gaze and then open it. Notice what is happening here. You have shifted the reinforcer (opening the container) so it now follows eye contact, rather than giving. Over time, this should increase your child's use of eye contact and giving to request help.

- As your child becomes more skilled at giving the object and making eye contact for help, wait for them to occur together before you give help, and reward them consistently when they do by immediately helping your child. Your child will learn that giving plus making eye contact equals a powerful communication.

Here are some ideas for how to set up activities for which your child needs your help:

- Use toys or items that your child cannot activate or act on without you: bubbles, balloons, kazoos, other musical instruments, or spinning tops and gyroscopes. When she gives you the item, blow it, play it, or make it go.
- Divide drinks and snack materials into smaller portions or pieces, and teach your child to offer you the bowl, plate, or cup to request more from you.
- Package pieces of favorite toys (puzzles, blocks, pegs, windup toys, little cars, etc.), in containers, and give them along with the script.

Activity: *Teach Your Child to Give in Response to Your Open Hand and the Words "Give Me" in Many Situations*

Here are some ideas for encouraging your child to give you objects in response to your cues in a variety of situations:

- Ask your child to give you bites of dry cereal, crackers, or other finger foods during feeding activities at the table. Put out your hand, say "Give me," and pretend to eat it. Really ham it up with sound effects and smiles, and then give the food back and thank your child.

- If your child picks up a piece of food and doesn't want it, ask for it back with "Give me." Or, put something on the high chair tray or your child's plate that your child does not want. As your child picks it up to get rid of it, immediately ask your child to give it to you by extending your hand and saying, "Give me," so you can remove it.

- At the end of a meal, have your child "give" a spoon, plate, or cup before you take it off the tray and lift him out of the chair. This is helping with "cleanup," a nice habit to cultivate.

- During diaper changing, hand the diaper to your child and then say, "Give me." Offer your hand, take the diaper, thank your child, and continue the change!

- During bath times, ask your child to give you various toys she is playing with, and then give them right back.

- During dressing, have your child's socks and shoes right there beside your child. Hand the sock to your child (while saying, "Here's sock!") and then say, "Give me sock." Do the same with shoes.

- During object play, ask your child to "give me" a block, a puzzle piece, or whatever little object is part of the play. Go ahead and put it in place, and then give one to your child. This is turn taking, and you are each giving the other an object and a turn. Very nice!

- Practice "Give me" frequently during the day, two or three times in each activity, until it is learned. Then keep it up.

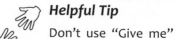

Helpful Tip
Don't use "Give me" or "My turn" as a way to take away things your child is enjoying playing with. If your child is not going to get the object back, then say, "All done with [the object]" instead. If "Give me" or "My turn" leads to object loss, your child will not be motivated to give things to you.

Summary of Step 1

If you have followed along and carried out the preceding activities, you now have ideas for how to help your child give you objects throughout activities. This step begins the process of using joint attention to share things for help. The next steps will address how to expand the skill into sharing thoughts and feelings about the activities, but for now, see if you agree with most of the statements in the following checklist. If so, you are now armed with important skills for teaching one particular type of joint attention—knowledge you will use in **Step 2**. If not, start experimenting during play and caregiving routines until you have found some methods that work for each statement.

Activity Checklist: Am I Teaching My Child to Give Objects?

_____ My child and I regularly take turns during object-based joint activities.

_____ I know how to pause and wait during my turn for my child to look and/or respond to me with a behavior.

_____ I have set up various objects in containers, and my child gives them to me for help.

_____ I provide clear cues for my child to give me objects by stretching out my hand and using simple language in my request.

_____ I make sure to give each object right back to my child.

_____ I have ideas for how my child will need my help during object-based activities (toy play, mealtime, bath time).

Andrew's parents have created several turn-taking games and are now ready to teach their 18-month-old son with autism how to give objects. They decide that creating opportunities in which Andrew will need their help might be more rewarding to him than taking the object out of his hands. With bubbles, Andrew's mom begins by placing the bubbles with the lid tightly closed on the floor, where he can easily see and touch it. As soon as Andrew spots the bubbles, he rushes over with excitement and picks up the container, ready to play; however, he quickly realizes that he cannot open the lid by himself. This is where Mom comes into action! Before Andrew becomes frustrated, she says, "Andrew, you want bubbles? Give me," and extends her hand (palm facing up). She waits a second to see if Andrew will comprehend the action, and when he does not respond, she adds, "I'll open bubbles. Give me," and again moves her hand closer to him. When he does not respond, she quickly helps him place the bubbles in her open hand and without delay unscrews the lid while saying, "Open bubbles" and then "Blow bubbles," followed by blowing bubbles for the two of them to pop. She opens and blows right away to reward his giving.

After blowing bubbles a few times, Mom closes the container lid and hands the bubbles back to Andrew. He tries to open the container and cannot. Again Mom says, "Give me bubbles," and extends her hand toward Andrew. This time Andrew holds out the bubbles, and she helps him place the bubbles in her hand while saying, "Give me bubbles." Again she quickly opens and blows the bubbles for Andrew to enjoy, and together they pop, clap, and stomp on bubbles. She closes them and gives them to him again. This time he puts them directly into her outstretched hand. Within a few more practice sessions, he routinely gives them to her, and even picks them up from the table and offers them to her for help, but not always with eye contact.

Now Mom takes the bubbles from him, but then waits momentarily before opening them to see if Andrew will look up at her. This is a change in the routine, and Andrew does look up at Mom to see what happened. She immediately responds by opening and blowing bubbles, and in doing so she rewards Andrew for combining his eye gaze with the gesture. She doesn't expect Andrew to look at her every time he gives her an object (no child does that), but she does want it to happen more often and become easier for him to do.

Joshua is a 3-year-old with autism who loves playing with trains. His dad has developed reciprocal back-and-forth games with other toy activities and sensory social routines, but does not feel successful when trains are involved. Joshua is protective of his trains and has his own agenda for how the game should be played. This usually involves lining up and rolling the trains on the carpet, and he doesn't want Dad to touch them or change the routine. Joshua's dad thinks that building in opportunities for help might work in his favor for creating a joint activity routine with trains. He decides that using the tracks, which Joshua cannot do alone, may be even more appealing to Joshua than running the trains on the carpet.

Dad begins by connecting some track sections together as Joshua is rolling trains on the floor. He quickly shows Joshua how to roll trains on the track, and them gives them back fast. Joshua loves this! It's a lot easier to roll trains on the track than on the shag carpet. After Joshua rolls the trains back and forth a few times, Dad takes out a piece of track, then another, until there is only one short one left. Joshua wants a longer track and reaches for a piece, trying to fit it in, but he can't. Dad reaches over to help. Joshua wants another one, and Dad helps again. Joshua picks up the next one, but now Dad extends his hand and says in simple phrases, "Need help? Give me." Joshua gives it, and Dad puts it in right away. Joshua then picks up the next piece, and again Dad says, "Give me." After another piece, Joshua looks at Dad

"We found so many ways to use trains and cars to build joint attention and language. My son loves both types of toys. We could hand out cars or trains individually upon request. We could make the trains and cars do fun things that he might not have thought of trying. I found that trying to help with building track was generally too slow to keep my son's attention (he would just find ways to make it work without being properly assembled), but there were many other possibilities, including running cars or trucks rapidly uphill and downhill, building structures into which the vehicles could crash, and hiding vehicles as a game (like peekaboo) without actually taking them away for long. By setting up a game in which a train rushes down a track to crash, I also encouraged joint attention by pausing, so my son would wonder why the train wasn't moving. This encouraged him to use words to ask for the train to move, and gradually to use eye contact more. At this point, he'll look right at my face to find out why I'm not doing what he expects!"

> **Helpful Tip**
>
> If your child doesn't spontaneously make even brief eye contact after several attempts at waiting to solicit eye contact when she gives for help, then try positioning your face very close to the container or object your child has given you—either by holding it up close to your face, or by moving your body so that you are at eye level with the container or object.

and gives a track without any cues from Dad—spontaneously combining gaze and gesture to get help.

Step 2. Teach Your Child to Show You Objects

Rationale. Showing involves sharing interest in an object by getting your partner to look at your object. Children hold things in front of parents, make eye contact, and draw their parents' attention (often by vocalizing), so that the parents will look at the object and make some sort of comment. It's a very important skill, because it gets people to label objects and so builds children's vocabulary. It also opens the door to social attention, praise, commenting, and other intrinsic features that motivate children to want to share things with others. How can you help your child learn about showing?

Activity: *Help Your Child Learn about Showing Objects*

Here are some ideas for motivating your child to show objects:

- First, show your child things. While you are in front of her, say, "Look! *Look* at the [object]," and hold the interesting object in front of your child. This should encourage your child to shift her gaze to the object. As soon as she does, name the object. Do this many times each day with objects your child is interested in.

- If your child reaches for the object after you show it and her gaze shifts to the toy, hand it right over. This rewards your child for looking when you ask her to.

- Think of the toys, materials, and objects your child comes into contact with each day. Since you and your child are already taking turns with these items, start holding them out to show what it's called, how it works, or what new actions can be done with it before you give it.

- During toy play, hold up an object and call your child's name: "Alex, look!" When he looks, name it ("It's a ball," or "See the balloon"), then do something with it (roll or throw the ball, or let go of the inflated balloon). Pairing the concept of "showing" with a fun and interesting effect also rewards the look and is likely to strengthen your child's response. He will understand how fun and exciting it is to pay attention to Mom and Dad when they say, "Look!"

- At meals, while your child is focused on his plate, pick up a container of a highly preferred food and say, "[Name], look" while showing the container. After your child looks, hand over some of the food.

- In the bathtub, show your child different materials or new actions to do. First call your child—"Carissa, look"—and when she looks, hold out the toy ("See the duck") and perform the action (make the duck tickle Carissa or splash the water).

- At bedtime, as you are looking at a book with your child, point to a picture while saying, "Look, it's a [object name]." When your child shifts his gaze to the picture, make an interesting effect (sound effect or action with the book).

Activity: *Teach Your Child How to Show Things to You*

In Step 1, you taught your child how to give for help by making a specific gesture (your outstretched hand), saying, "Give me," and then helping your child give over the object. What you will teach your child now is how to show things to you by building on the "give." Once your child consistently looks when you show him objects, you can begin to teach your child how to show.

Here are some suggestions:

- Find a time when your child is holding an object. Get right in front of her, and then say, "*Show me. Show me* the [object]"—and hold your hand out to your child as if you were requesting a "give" (*your child should be able to give easily before you start working on how to show*). Be sure to emphasize the word "show," because that will be the cue that tells the child that you are not asking her to give it to you, but rather to show it to you. When your child tries to hand the object to you, in response to your request, *don't take it*; instead, admire it very enthusiastically (e.g., "Wow! What a cool bear!") and let your child keep it. Your child has placed the object in front of you, and *your enthusiastic attention is the reward* for showing.

- Practice this many times a day, in many different activities. You can touch the object to admire it, but you don't want to break your child's contact with it. Showing means holding something out for another to see without giving it, and this is what you are trying to teach.

● After your child is routinely holding the object out toward your hand when you say, "Show me," stop offering your hand and see if your child can respond to the words alone. If he does, admire it enthusiastically as before. If not, then offer your hand partway (partial prompt), but not all the way. As you keep practicing, do less and less with your hand until your child is responding just to your words.

● Now, after your child is showing objects to you consistently, wait for eye contact. Ask your child to show, but hold back your enthusiastic comment until your child looks at you. Your child may well look at your face to see why you are not responding. As soon as she looks, admire the object enthusiastically. Continue to wait for the gaze combined with showing to comment; expect your child to show and look at you. If your child doesn't look, then quietly speak her name, make a sound, or draw her hand to your cheek; once you have the gaze, respond enthusiastically! Continue this way, slowly fading your prompts. Your child will likely begin to show while making eye contact and to look more often.

● **Note:** Be sure to name the object as you admire it, every time. For young children, showing is a powerful way to elicit words from parents, and it helps build their vocabulary. A typical response we use is "Car! What a [neat, cool, big] car!" In this response, the child hears the key word twice. Language learning is a secondary goal here (and everywhere).

 Helpful Tip
Do not be tempted to say "Good boy," "Good showing," or another reward phrase. Name the object and admire it enthusiastically! Your enthusiasm is the reward!

● Think about several daily activities you do with your child—breakfast, getting dressed, toy play, snack time, diapering, sensory social routines, lunch, running errands, going to the park or playground, reading books, bath time, and bedtime. How many different objects do you and your child come into contact with? Take advantage of these different activities to help your child learn to show different objects. If you can practice this two or three times in four to six activities each day, you will be providing your child with lots of learning opportunities.

● Be sure to continue to show your child objects and use the "look" instruction all the time you are teaching "Show me." Showing and looking when others show are two sides of the same joint attention act.

● Be sure to continue to use "Give me" throughout the day, so your child doesn't forget about the correct response to "Give me" while you are focusing on "Show me."

Summary of Step 2

If you have followed along and carried out the preceding activities, you will have taught your child to show you objects on request. See if you agree with most of the statements in the following checklist. If so, you are now armed with important skills for expanding your child's joint attention skills—knowledge you will use in **Step 3**. If not, go back to the start of this section and start experimenting during play and caregiving routines until you have found some methods that work for each statement.

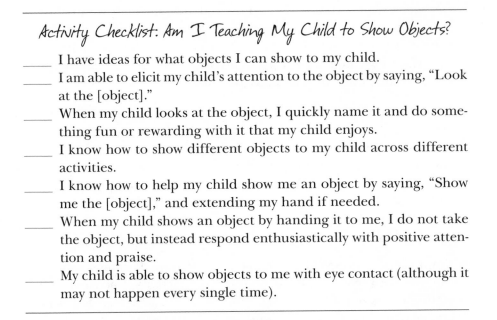

Activity Checklist: Am I Teaching My Child to Show Objects?

_____ I have ideas for what objects I can show to my child.

_____ I am able to elicit my child's attention to the object by saying, "Look at the [object]."

_____ When my child looks at the object, I quickly name it and do something fun or rewarding with it that my child enjoys.

_____ I know how to show different objects to my child across different activities.

_____ I know how to help my child show me an object by saying, "Show me the [object]," and extending my hand if needed.

_____ When my child shows an object by handing it to me, I do not take the object, but instead respond enthusiastically with positive attention and praise.

_____ My child is able to show objects to me with eye contact (although it may not happen every single time).

What about Andrew? *Andrew loves water, and his parents think that bath time might be a fun time to show different objects and actions to him. Dad goes through his usual routine of filling up the tub with bubbles and placing Andrew in it—but instead of dumping in all the toys at once, he decides to show each one to him, starting with a plastic fish. Dad says, "Andrew, look," and when Andrew does, Dad responds with "It's the fish," and hands it over to him. He lets Andrew have a few minutes to play with the fish, describing the actions he does with it and doing fish faces for Andrew to imitate. Next he says, "Andrew, look what I have!" He waits for Andrew to look up before spraying him with the squirting whale, a routine he loves. Andrew laughs and reaches for the toy, which Dad labels, "It's a whale." As he washes Andrew, Dad continues holding up an object every few minutes to show to*

Andrew, and waiting for him to look before naming it. By the end of bath time, Dad is surprised and delighted at how many times he has been able to get Andrew's atten-tion by saying, "Look," and how quickly Andrew has learned the routine.

What about Joshua? *Joshua's mom wants to engage with her son when he plays with trains. She thinks about what she could do that might make him enjoy showing his trains to her, and she decides that adding train sound effects and singing some of his favorite lines from train songs might work. The next time Joshua is holding a train, Mom says, "Show me your train," and holds her hand out. He doesn't want to give her his train, so he ignores her request. Mom repeats her request and lifts his hand in the air a little. She's careful not to touch the train or his hands too long, because she doesn't want him to think she's trying to take it away. As she helps Joshua show the train, she responds with "Ooh, I see the train. It goes choo-choo," and she moves her hands in a circular motion. She makes a little song and dance out of it: "The train goes chug-a-chug-a-chug-a-chug-a-choo-choo!" She stops, and he looks up for more. Then she asks Joshua again to show his train, and again slightly lifts his hand toward her while singing the verse. She decides to elaborate the routine and sing the "Little Red Caboose" song in its entirety with gestures, so that Joshua can enjoy the activity a bit longer before she asks him to show a train to her. Once she has finished, Mom says, "Joshua, show me that train," and points to a different train on the ground. Joshua picks it up and, while he doesn't yet hold it out to Mom, he does look from the train to her. Mom responds immediately, "There's the train! I see it!" and extends Joshua's hand toward her, followed by singing the song. Mom continues the routine, asking Joshua to show her a different train, helping him do the "show" gesture (if he doesn't respond on his own), and responding enthusiastically. She also starts pausing briefly for him to look at her before singing the song, so that she and Joshua can share the excitement.*

Step 3. Teach Your Child How to Point to Objects to Share Experiences

Rationale. Pointing typically develops after giving and showing. It's an impor-tant tool because your child can use it to share interest with you in objects and events that he is not touching—a bird in the sky, the lights overhead, a dog on a leash, a lion at the zoo. It is another means to comment about something your child sees, and therefore another route to a learning opportunity. As with the other gestures, it is easiest to teach your child first to comprehend pointing and then to produce it.

 Activity: *Help Your Child Learn to Follow a Point*

Here are suggestions for teaching your child to follow your point:

● To teach your child what pointing is all about, use your finger to point to, tap, and draw your child's attention to an object very near your child—something your child is looking for or may want. As you point, say something like "Jamie, look. A cookie!" For instance, point to pieces of food on the table in front of your child that she will want to pick up. Point to a puzzle piece that your child will want to pick up and put in the puzzle. Point to the place in the puzzle where the piece should go ("Jamie, it goes here!"). When your child follows your point to the object, help your child as needed to achieve her goal with the object (this is the reward for following your point). For an object your child wants, instead of giving it, put it down and point to it ("Here's the car!").

● If your child does not follow your point, reposition yourself, the child, or the object to help him complete the action. Point to something that is close by, between you and your child. Keep pointing while your child picks up the object, so that your child sees the relationship between your point and the object placement.

● Before using the give-to-me gesture (opening your hand while saying, "Give me"), point to the object you want your child to give you. Point, direct her attention to the object, and then turn your hand over into a "Give me" gesture and help your child give you the object. Give your child a lot of experience with following your points in all kinds of settings. Within a few days, you will probably see your child starting to follow your point and understanding what it means. When your child consistently follows your point, you know that she has learned its meaning.

● As your child learns to follow your point and touch, start to put more physical space between your point and the object you are pointing at, as you continue to say something like "Steffy, look! The baby!" Start by having 6 inches of space between your finger and the object. Later increase it to 12 inches, then 2 feet, then 3 feet (things on the floor, couch, or bed are appropriate for working on longer distances). Now you know that your child knows that pointing directs his attention to something important. Make sure your child gets the object after looking!

● Position objects or toys your child really likes out of reach and point to the objects, saying "Timmy, look! The jack-in-the-box," waiting until your child looks at the object before getting it down and giving it over.

There are many opportunities in your existing routines to help your child follow your point. During your turns, think about how you can vary the activity by pointing to different things your child might attend to.

Here are some ideas for different ways to demonstrate pointing:

- During toy play, use toys that have multiple pieces, so that during play you can point to where the next item might go—the place for a puzzle piece, the top of the tower for block stacking, the hole for the peg or shape that matches. Or hide the last piece on the floor nearby, and when your child is looking for the last piece needed to complete it, say, "[Name], look" while pointing at the needed piece.

- Point to button-activated toys, so that when the button is pushed, the fun effect will happen.

- Use picture books with large, clear pictures (but not too many on a page), because there is something on each page to point to and show your child.

- Try toys that might be a little difficult for your child to use on her own, so that your pointing to show how to operate them will help your child succeed.

- Point to things you know your child will likely want in all kinds of settings—to cereal on his high chair tray, to the next ring that goes on the ring stacker, to bath toys.

♟ Activity: *Teach Your Child to Point to Request Objects*

Now it's time to teach your child to point! To learn pointing, your child needs to be able to reach with her hand consistently toward distant objects to request them—to indicate choices and desires without having to touch the objects. You have started working on this in Chapter 8.

Here are suggestions for teaching your child to point:

- If your child can use a reach to communicate a request (rather than as a way to grab), hold the object slightly away from your child (e.g., "Do you want a drink?") to elicit your child's reach. Then very quickly mold your child's hand into a point ("Point; point to cup"), and bring the tip of your child's index finger over to touch the desired object. Then immediately give the object ("Here's the cup!"). It works a little better at first if you hold the object in your less dominant hand and shape your child's point with your dominant hand. Don't worry about molding a perfect point. Just work toward extending your child's index finger; with time and practice, you can help your child close the other fingers.

- Pointing is a challenge for children with ASD to learn, and you will want to help your child practice many times a day at times when your child really wants something (it's the getting it after pointing that rewards your child's point and builds the skill). Practice especially at meals, during object play, and during bath time. Try to practice it several times in each activity in which your child is "requesting" an object with her body. Once you give the object to your child, let her have it for a few minutes. You don't want to take it away and ask for another point; that would be very frustrating for your child!

● You should see, over time, that your child begins to extend the index finger without your having to shape it first. That's great! Don't expect a perfect point. It will evolve over time. A spontaneous approximation to a point, without your hand molding, is much more important than a perfect point.

● After your child is pointing spontaneously to objects within reach, you want to teach your child to point "through the air," without having to touch the object. This is called a **distal point**, while the closer one is a **proximal point**. To teach a distal point, hold the object a little out of your child's reach. As your child extends the point toward the object, give it to him without having your child's pointing finger touch it. Start with a 4- to 6-inch gap. Once your child is pointing easily to things just out of reach, hold it back more—12 inches. Then farther—18 to 24 inches. Now your child has a distal point. Now present things from the side or above. Help your child point to things in all directions.

● Once your child has mastered the distal point, provide a choice of two objects while naming the objects ("Andrew, car or truck?"), so your child can point to choose. This works well for larger things—cereal boxes, shirts,

> "Picture books were a wonderful resource for my son. We were able to find books with his favorite types of objects and then build more and more on the images. At first, we just used the books to encourage him to point. As he learned to point to things on request, he began to point to the things that interested him the most, to share his enjoyment of them. With time, we were able to ask more and more complicated questions. We initially asked him to point to objects, then to specific colors or shapes, then to parts of objects (for example, 'Where is the wheel?'), then to more abstract things (for instance, 'Which is your favorite car?'), and so on. I was able to find books that showed facial expressions as well, and that was a huge help in practicing recognition of expressions. Once he had the idea of pointing to things in the books, it opened up all sorts of possibilities for learning."

milk or water bottles, bath toys, and so on. Pointing to choose is a very functional skill. Be sure to name the choices; this is a great vocabulary builder.

As with the giving and showing gestures, we teach pointing first without expecting eye contact. But once your child is using pointing easily and consistently to request, start to expect eye contact after the point gesture before giving your child what she is requesting. This requires that you be in front of your child and offer things directly in front, so it is easy for your child to make eye contact. Once your child points, hold the object back and wait patiently for your child's eye contact before you release the object. If you need to, call your child's name or make a little sound to encourage her to look at you. Slowly increase expectations that eye contact will follow pointing to an object routinely.

Here are some specific ideas for teaching pointing to request objects:

- You can provide your child with lots of opportunities for practice by controlling multipiece materials, such as puzzle pieces, pieces for a shape sorter, pegs for a pegboard, or Legos, Tinkertoys. Have your child request several of them as you offer them by pointing.

- Putting little round dots or stickers on objects as "pointing targets" helps some children learn pointing more quickly. Each time, they will touch the dot with their point. After they learn to do this spontaneously and it is well established, you can peel off the dots, and they will continue to point.

♟ Activity: *Teach Your Child to Point to Show or Comment*

Children can use pointing to express several meanings. It can mean "I want this" (requesting). It may mean "Do this" (regulating another person's behavior). It may mean "Attend to this" or "I'm interested in this" (the showing or commenting function). The commenting function is really important for language and vocabulary, as well as social development. It is how typically developing children get parents to label objects of interest. We have already talked about teaching pointing for requesting and teaching giving to get help or to get someone to remove something. Now we shift to helping your child learn to use pointing and gaze as a way of showing or commenting.

Here are suggestions for teaching your child pointing to show or comment:

- Pointing to show is a more complex way of showing. Your child needs to have mastered showing on request before you start to work on pointing to show. One of the best ways to encourage pointing to show or comment involves developing commenting routines around books that have several very clear pictures on a page, or picture albums, or puzzles with pictures. In any of these routines, while facing your child, point to each picture in turn. When your child looks at the picture (short pause), name the picture (you have done this earlier, in teaching your child to follow a point). When you do this, you are modeling pointing to show/comment. When your child looks, make interesting sound effects to add to your child's engagement with the activity. Be sure your child is attending to each picture you point to. When your child's interest wanes, the activity is finished. Do the same books in the same way for a week or so; it builds up your child's learning about the routine, and your child's interest and attention will likely expand.

● Once your child enjoys and really understands this activity as a pointing and naming activity, you will begin the variation. Be sure to be in front of your child. Begin the activity, *point to the picture, but do not speak*. Don't name the picture. Just wait, ready to speak. Your child will likely look up to you to see why you are not naming. When your child looks at you, name the picture and make the sound effects. If your child doesn't look, refer back to the ideas in the preceding section. Do a few more pictures in the regular way to establish a pattern or theme, and then do this waiting variation again. Continue this way for a few days. You will probably see your child learn to use looking to cue your speech. You have taught the child to use eye contact as a way to get someone to produce a label—that is, as a way to initiate commenting.

● The next step involves teaching your child to use her own point to get you to comment. Position yourself in front of your child. Now, rather than your pointing to the pictures, let your child do the pointing. If she already does that spontaneously, great. Otherwise, take your child's hand and help your child point to each picture while you provide the word and sound effects right after the point, just as before. Once this becomes a set routine, provide less and less help with the point, until your child is leading the activity by pointing to each picture and you are responding to your child's point with a word.

● Once your child is initiating pointing to pictures for you to name, begin the activity, and when your child points to the picture, do not speak. Just wait, ready to speak. Your child will likely look up to you to see why you are not naming, and when your child looks at you, you name the picture and make the sound effects. Do a few more pictures for your child in response to pointing without requiring eye contact, and then do this waiting variation again. Continue this way for a few days. You will likely see your child learn to use pointing and looking to cue your speech. You have taught the child to use point and gaze as ways to get someone to produce a label—that is, as ways to initiate commenting. Your child is now combining pointing and gaze both to initiate and to comprehend commenting, just as it occurs in typical development.

- Generalize this skill by playing the point-and-name game in many situations. Bathtub toys allow for the point-and-name game. Crackers in the high chair work fine if you line them up and point and count. You can also do this with blocks in a line on the floor, with little cars, with objects on the coffee table, or with utensils at the table.

- Show your child objects outside by pointing and naming. Help your child show you interesting things outside—a flower, a dog, a bird, a sprinkler running—with the point-and-name game. (Remember, the showing routine is also a naming routine.) As you do pointing and showing in more and more situations, you will start to see your child spontaneously point to something, in order to show you something for you to name. This is a huge step and opens up a world of sharing thoughts, feelings, and words for your child.

Summary of Step 3

If you have followed along and carried out the preceding activities, you will have taught your child how to give, show, and now point to objects across different communicative functions (to request an object, to ask for help, to make a comment, to share an experience). See if you agree with most of the statements in the following checklist. If so, you are now armed with important skills for expanding your child's joint attention skills. If not, start experimenting during play and caregiving routines until you have found some methods that work for each statement.

Activity Checklist: Am I Teaching My Child to Follow My Point and to Point to Objects?

____ My child is able to follow my point to attend to, place, and pick up toys, food items, or other objects.

____ My child is able to make a point (with my help, if needed) when I offer an item or a choice between objects.

____ My child is able to follow my point to pictures during book routines.

____ When I point to a picture and pause, my child looks up at me during book routines.

____ My child points to pictures and looks at me during book routines.

_____ I feel confident that my child and I have the tools to share activities with each other.

What about Andrew? *Andrew loves balloons, so his parents think of several ways to work on pointing during this activity. First they start the usual routine or theme in which Andrew communicates to them (by blowing) to blow up the balloon and let it go flying around the room. After a few instances of this, his parents vary the game by kneeling next to Andrew so that he won't see where the balloon lands right away. Since his parents know where the balloon is, they are able to point to its location and help Andrew follow their gesture to pick up the balloon. They make sure he doesn't put it in his mouth (to prevent choking) by being right by his side. Instead, they point to the balloon in his hand and ask him to give it to them. Since his parents have been teaching Andrew to give objects, he doesn't need to see their outreached hand to understand their request and is able to give the balloon. His parents repeat the new game of Andrew asking them to blow up and let go of the balloon, waiting by his side for the balloon to land, and then pointing to its location. It works so well that Andrew starts looking at his parents before the balloon even lands for their cue.*

Next, his parents move on to teaching Andrew how to point. His mom blows a little air into the balloon and then points to the slightly inflated balloon, asking Andrew, "More blow?" Andrew makes a sound in response, so his mom blows a little more and then stops. This time she helps him point while making a sound, and then she blows two more times into the balloon before stopping. Again she points to the balloon, asking Andrew, "Blow?", and then takes his hand to point to the balloon before continuing to blow. She does this several more times until the balloon is large enough to let go. She releases the balloon, and Dad points once Andrew looks at him for where the balloon has landed. When Andrew gives her the balloon, Mom goes through the routine of blowing a little air into the balloon at one time before having Andrew request more by pointing to it. Although he doesn't point perfectly, Andrew does tap the balloon with his finger, and that's good enough for Mom and Dad!

What about Joshua? *Joshua has several train books that he and Mom usually look at when Mom is getting him ready for bed. Mom places the book between them on the bed and points to pictures that she notices Joshua looking at—"You see the caboose," or "Yeah, there's the smoke." After a few more pages of commenting on what Joshua sees, Mom points to a different picture on the page and says, "Joshua, look! There's the black train," and makes a train whistle noise to add effect. He looks up at her, so she points to the train on the next page and makes the whistle noise again. She continues pointing to the pictures Joshua sees, as well as those she wants to show him.*

Mom gradually starts to pause once she's pointed to the picture, because she wants Joshua to look at her. Once he does, she makes the whistle sound or names the picture. Over the next few nights, this is their new routine with train books, and it's not until the next week that Mom helps Joshua point to a picture before naming it or adding the sound effect. She continues pointing to pictures as well, so that Joshua doesn't have to point to a picture on every single page. This could be too much of a new skill to make him do in just one night. But each night during their bedtime routine, Mom helps Joshua do a little more—point to a few more pictures or wait for him to look at her before turning the page. The next 2 weeks are marked by definite improvement in Joshua's ability to share books with his mom. He eagerly chooses which books he wants to take to bed, and when Mom asks, "Where's the red train?" or "Do you see the conductor?", Joshua is excited to point to the picture and say "Train" or simply vocalize a sound. Recently he's started pointing to pictures on his own, in anticipation that Mom will acknowledge them or make the sound effect. Mom and Joshua can enjoy their special time even more, now that he has different behaviors to express and share his enjoyment.

Chapter Summary

Young children with autism face big barriers to understanding and using joint attention to coordinate and share their interests with others, and their lack of sharing often results in fewer and fewer opportunities to communicate and learn over time. Yet children with ASD are capable of making enormous gains in joint attention and other types of nonverbal (and verbal) communication. The crucial techniques involve creating many, many opportunities for your child to share attention with you, and for you to share with him or her, directing gestures to the child and prompting your child to make gestural responses. Remember that typical toddlers are communicating nonverbally with adults all day long. They have hundreds (maybe thousands) of learning opportunities in a day. You are creating these kinds of opportunities for your child. This is a necessary step for verbal language development. The work you are doing at this level is paving the way for speech. As we have discussed in Chapter 7, gestures and gaze are our first language—a language we use forever in social interaction. It is joint attention that allows your child to share likes and dislikes, desires, interests, thoughts, requests, and feelings about objects and events in the world. Gestures, eye contact, and facial expressions give direct access to other people's thoughts and feelings. Teaching your child how to use gestures and gaze in everyday activities to communicate preferences and interests helps your child learn what communication is all about: It is an intentional and powerful system that influences other people.

Learning how to communicate through gestures and gaze can prevent some of the problem behaviors that are often associated with autism, by giving children useful communication tools for expressing their needs, preferences, and wants. It provides your child with a strong base for further language learning with built-in, powerful, natural rewards.

Refrigerator List

Goal: To teach your child how to look at and share interest in an object or toy with you, by using the key joint attention behaviors: giving, showing, and pointing.

Steps:

✓ Giving is a powerful request for help!

✓ Teach your child to give to you and give it right back!

✓ Have your child "look" before you hand things over.

✓ Showing begins as giving without the "take."

✓ Pointing tells your child where to "look."

✓ A child's point commands language and action! Give your child this powerful tool.

✓ Add gaze to each step to finish it off!

11

It's Playtime!

Chapter goals: To help you (1) increase the number of learning opportunities in parent–child toy play, and (2) support constructive, varied, independent toy play.

Why Varied, Flexible Toy Play Is So Important to Learning

Young children spend most of their free time playing. If they are not in the middle of care routines or naps, they are playing with the people and objects around them. Playtime has a number of important functions:

1. **Young children use play to build new skills**—trying again and again to climb the stairs, to put things in and take them out of containers, to push the car, to fit the puzzle piece, or to arrange their toys just so.

2. **They also use play to practice skills they have already mastered.** It's easy to see how much pleasure young children receive from "exercising" their skills in play.

3. **They vary their play and try creative new ways to use their toys and other objects.** And they can turn almost anything into a plaything—plastic storage containers, rags, boxes, sticks, and sand work, just as well as the newest creative plaything from Grandma.

4. **Young children also use toy play to practice social skills.** We see this in the way they like to have others join in their toy play. They learn by watching what others do with toys, and they learn to share, take turns, and cooperate with others during toy play. In pretend play with others, they practice social routines from daily life in their play with dolls, toy dishes, doctor bags, and toy animals. They act out what they have seen people do in real life and what they

have experienced in their own lives. And, of course, when a partner is involved, playtime becomes language-learning time.

What's Happening in Autism?

Though all young children enjoy repetitive play (banging a spoon on the high chair, splashing water during bath time, playing with a pull toy), most young children vary their play routines. They do many different activities in a play hour, and they play with an object in several different ways. Young children with ASD usually enjoy toy play as well, and play with a range of objects. They often enjoy puzzles, blocks, cars, swings, and slides, like their peers, and play with them similarly. But their play may differ from that of their peers in these ways:

- They tend to **repeat an act or motion** more frequently than their age-mates.
- They **spend an unusually long time with their favorite toys**, doing the same thing over and over. They don't seem to become bored nearly as quickly as other children do.
- **Their play may be much simpler** than that of their age-mates. They may get much pleasure out of playing with simple toys, in simple ways, using skills they learned months or years ago, instead of using play to practice new skills.
- **They may play with unusual objects or in unusual ways.** They may prefer to carry their cars around, one in each hand, or to line them up rather than drive them. They may enjoy playing with objects like strings, shoes, or other materials and ignore their more typical toys.
- **They demonstrate less interest and skill with pretend play** than their age-mates do. Pretending with dishes, dolls or stuffed animals, doctor's kits, dress-up materials, and similar toys does not seem to interest them, and they may not appear to understand this kind of play.
- **They seem more content to play alone with their toys,** and for longer periods, than their age-mates do. They do not seem as motivated to include parents, siblings, or others in their play as their age-mates are.

Why Is It a Problem?

Of course, when children are playing alone, they don't have as many opportunities to learn language as they do when they are playing with parents, grandparents, and older siblings. But the differences in how they play limit their learning opportunities in two other ways as well:

1. Repetitive, simple play with few objects robs play of novelty, significantly reducing new learning opportunities.
2. Playing alone significantly limits children's opportunities to learn not

only new language from their partners, but also new play concepts and the social skills and scripts that usually accompany object play. Since children with autism have difficulty imitating others, they actually need more time playing with others, not less, to get the same benefit from social play as typically developing kids do.

The play that you've been encouraging with your child as you've read Chapters 4–10 of this book has been aimed at building specific other skills: language skills, social and cognitive skills, and communication. In this chapter, which is centered on constructive play, and the next one, which addresses pretend or symbolic play, we focus on play in its own right. Young children with autism will learn more through their play when they can learn to play with lots of different materials and lots of different people, in lots of different ways, in a social and reciprocal fashion. Increase your child's enjoyment in play, and you'll increase the breadth of learning opportunities that your child gains from play.

⟫⟫⟫ What You Can Do to Increase Variety, Flexibility, and Learning Opportunities in Parent–Child Toy Play

Caution! Teaching new and more varied ways to play requires using objects to imitate actions. If your child is not doing this very frequently yet, spend a little more time with the activities in Chapter 8 before focusing on the strategies described in this chapter. Imitating others' actions with objects is a building block for developing more mature and varied play.

Building Play Skills from Imitation

Good news! You already know how to teach your child to expand his play! That's because teaching play skills is just like teaching imitation with objects. You will use imitation as your main tool for teaching play skills, and you will teach play by using the same four-part joint activity framework that you have been using to build other skills:

1. You will **set up** object play opportunities that follow your child's interests. You will provide attractive materials and interesting activities that motivate your child to play with you, and you and your child will begin to play, following your child's interest into the materials.
2. You will develop a play routine, which involves joining in toy play with your child, taking turns, and establishing a main **theme.**
3. You will use **variation**, in which you show your child how to play in new ways and hand over materials to your child and help her imitate you and practice the new ways to play.
4. For the **closing/transition**, you will finish the activity when your child's

interest starts to wane; the two of you will then put the materials away and make a transition to another activity.

Deciding What Kinds of Play to Teach

How do you decide what play skills to teach your child? You already know more about the answer to this question than you might think. You know what toys your child has, what toys your child likes, and how your child plays with those toys. What you may need are some ideas for new play skills to teach.

You can expand your child's toy play skills in two main ways: (1) by increasing the number of toys your child knows how to play with and (2) by helping your child increase the complexity of his or her play. Let's start with the topic of increasing the number of toys your child knows how to play with. First, you will need to select toys (and household objects that support play, like nesting measuring cups, pan lids that bang, rolling pins and dough) that "fit" your child's current skills. All children have a wide range of play skills in their repertoire, and your child likely does too. Some of his skills may involve very simple play, play skills he has been carrying out for a long time (like shaking, banging, dropping, watching things move, and mouthing). Others are more mature play skills and involve handling objects in some type of cause-and-effect play, like putting blocks in a shape sorter, putting pieces in a puzzle, or driving small cars around on the floor. (Save the pretend play toys for the next chapter. In this chapter you will be focusing on toys that are interesting because of their cause-and-effect qualities.)

Start by making a list of all the toys your child has that seem to fit your child's more mature play skills. Once you have done that, circle the toys that your child currently knows how to play with without any physical prompts from you. These circled toys are your *maintenance* toys, the familiar toys that your child knows and likely enjoys. You will want to be sure to use some of these every day for play. Put an M for maintenance beside those. Now look at the remainder of the list; there are probably a lot of toys that your child has but does not play with. Circle the five that seem like toys your child could learn easily and would enjoy; these are likely very good choices for the toys you want to teach. Put a G beside those five—those are your *goal* toys. Gather them up, organize their pieces, put them in an easy-to-reach spot where you can pull them down for daily play. These are the five toys that you will focus on first. The next section will help you develop

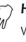

> **Helpful Tip**
>
> We'll say it again—electronic toys seem to stimulate repetitive and isolated play for young children with autism. So while you are working on expanding play, we suggest you put them away, and also turn off the TV and movies. Focus on simple constructive toys, household objects, and pretend play toys.

a teaching strategy. Once your child has learned those five, go back through this process, marking those with an M as well, because your child has now learned them, and choosing five more as goal toys. It is safe to assume that your child could learn to play with one or two new toys every week in a simple way if you play with them daily and help her learn them. In this way, week by week, you will be increasing your child's repertoire of toy play skills.

Playing with Cause-and-Effect Action Toys

Now that you have identified a number of goal toys or household objects to teach that involve cause-and-effect actions, you will begin by helping your child learn how to use each of these objects according to its *main theme*, the most typical way that other children would use it. You will use the joint activity framework to be sure your child learns both the main theme of each object and one or more variations. You have already begun this work by helping your child learn to imitate actions on objects (see Chapter 8). Here we are focusing on using the same techniques to build up your child's skill set with toys.

Helping Your Child Learn the Main Theme of a Number of Toys or Objects

Most young children's toys have at least one main theme. For books, it is looking at the pictures and words. For shape sorters and puzzles, it is matching the shapes and putting things in. For pegs, it is putting them in the holes. For blocks, it is stacking and building with them. You want to be sure that your child learns how to do the main action that goes with each object. If your child does not know how to play with one or more of his toys, start with that one main object and its main theme. You need only one action to create a theme for the play. If you're not sure what that is, observe your child's actions with the objects or think about the intended function of the object. Is it meant to roll, stack, bounce, push, pull, go in–out, or go up–down? Pick a name for the action, and take turns doing it with your child.

Here is the sequence:

- Bring out the toy. Get into a good face-to-face position with your child, either on the floor or standing or sitting at a little table or the coffee table.

- Put the toy between the two of you. Take one or two pieces, and show your child how it works by doing it—quickly, and with fun sound effects or simple words.

- Is your child interested? Is he looking at the toy, reaching for a piece, sitting down, or watching your actions? If so, then hand your child a piece and see if he copies what you did. If he does, give him a cheer and do a piece yourself, followed by handing your child another piece. He is playing with the toy appropriately! If he doesn't imitate what you did, help him do it, by physically guiding him through the action. You may have to repeat the action, exaggerating the effect and/or slowing down the motion, so your child can observe and process the steps. Or you might have to start the action and then let your child finish it. If this does not work, then again physically help your child complete the action. Give a cheer and hand over another piece, helping your child again.

- Is your child still interested? Terrific! Take a quick turn yourself, and give your child another piece. See if she starts to do it correctly. If so, wait for her to finish, give a cheer, and give another piece if she is still interested. If not, give enough help so that she is successful.

- Try to give your child three to five opportunities to carry out the single action involved in the activity, or more opportunities if he seems interested (staying seated, reaching, watching). Take turns, hand the pieces over, and help your child as needed. Have fun, label, cheer, and enjoy your child's efforts to learn.

- Bring this goal toy out for some playtime daily if you can while your child is learning it. It will probably be more fun for your child with repeated experiences.

- Remember to bring out several maintenance toys each day as well—different ones from day to day—so your child continues to practice and enjoy those familiar toys.

- Once your child is using a piece of the goal toy correctly, you can start expanding on his play by encouraging him to put in more than once piece. Set up the toy as you did before, but instead of handing the pieces over one

Helpful Tip

Many typical toys for young children have many pieces. If your child does not yet know how to carry out the main theme of the toy on her own with one piece, start with just one or two pieces, *not all the pieces*, so your child does not get distracted by the number of pieces. Similarly, having just one toy in front of her to play with may help your child focus on the skills being taught (the toy will be in your child's "spotlight of attention") and avoid becoming confused or distracted by having too many play materials available at once.

at a time, put two or three pieces down on the floor or table. Pick up one and do it yourself and then wait for your child to get the other. When your child can pick up two pieces, one at a time, and complete the action with both, you can put more pieces out. Remember to take some turns, label the objects, label the actions, show your pleasure at your child's efforts, and shift toys as your child's interest wanes.

In the Appendix at the end of this book is a list of toys to pick from that work well for teaching varied play with young children of various ages.

Here are some ideas for goal toys involving various types of toys that your child might not be playing with yet:

- Books

- Art materials

- Ball play

- Puzzles, shape sorters, color sorters, pegboards

- Building toys and nesting toys

- Stringing and lacing

- Musical toys (especially rhythm instruments, xylophones, and keyboards)

> "I found First Words, My Little Animal Book, My Big Train Book, First 100 Words, First 100 Machines, *and especially* My Little Word Book *from the [Roger] Priddy book series to be invaluable.* My Little Word Book *was one of the very most useful, and I can't recommend it highly enough.*"

Helpful Tips for Choosing Books
  - Look for minimal words and pictures on a page.
  - Look for simple stories that are repetitive and/or that rhyme.
- Board books (with mirrors, sturdy flaps, etc.), are a great way to involve your child.
- Look for common children's interests (baby faces, emotions, animals, actions, children's routines, etc.).
- As your child embarks on new adventures, such as potty training, washing hands, and so forth, it is helpful to incorporate books discussing these topics into your daily routine.
- And most important . . . follow your child's lead! Involve the child in the book-choosing process whenever possible. A great way to allow your child to choose books and to supplement your book collection is to visit your local library.

- Outdoor play—sand, water

- Bath play

- Pretend play sets like a farm set or dollhouse (see Chapter 12)

 Helpful Tip

The lists of toys and children's books in the Appendix at the end of the book are great sources of suggestions if relatives ask for gift ideas for your child.

Teaching Your Child a Variation on the Main Theme; Variations Add Complexity

Flexible play is very important for learning. You see flexibility when you see your child do more than one thing with a toy. So once your child learns to play with her toys in the main way for which the toy was intended (the main theme), you should introduce a variation. Blocks can be stacked, but also lined up as a road to drive with cars or trains. Connecting blocks (e.g., Legos or Tinkertoys) can be assembled and turned into a helicopter, ice cream cone, or rollers. Children can color with markers, but also with crayons, chalk, and with paintbrushes, and they can make marks, lines, and dots or can trace and color shapes.

Another way to add variation and complexity is to increase the number of actions your child is doing with each toy, both the goal toys and the maintenance toys. There are three ways to add complexity to a toy: (1) adding more pieces, (2) adding more actions, and (3) adding more "phases," or stages, to the play. Building play complexity encourages your child's thinking, memory, organization, and planning. It also holds your child's attention on a toy for longer and longer periods, so building complexity is building your child's thinking ability!

Adding more pieces is an easy way to build complexity, and it was mentioned in the steps above. Children begin with a new cause-and-effect toy by learning how one piece goes in or out or around. However, when your child works with multiple pieces, the whole play becomes more complex. If the toy is a puzzle or a small pegboard or the like, adding all the pieces introduces the idea of "completion": all of the pieces being placed, not just one. The goal has become much more complex, and your child has to maintain the goal of "completing" until all the pieces are placed. Build up the number of pieces as slowly as you need to to help your child sustain attention and motivation to "finish." The number of pieces remaining will define the "finish point" for a while. After your child learns the toy, the number of holes to be filled, if visible, also defines the finish point.

In addition to adding more pieces, you can start to think about adding more actions. What actions are involved in a five-hole pegboard? If you lay out the board, place one peg first, and then hand your child a peg, your child has one action to complete: put in. If you hand your child the five pieces one at a time, and she puts each in, then she has completed five actions, all involving putting in. If the five pieces are lying on the table and your child takes each in turn and places it, she has completed 10 actions, each involving a two-action sequence—pick up and put in. If after completing the pegboard you encourage your child to take each one out and put it on the table, you have added another 10 actions: 5 take outs and 5 put downs. So, as you are teaching the toys, you can build complexity by adding related actions to the play and encouraging your child to develop simple sequences of actions involving each toy, which builds independence in play as well as planning and sustained attention. For each toy you and your child play with, whether goal or maintenance toys, think about how to add these simple action sequences so your child is carrying out more related actions with each piece and each toy.

The final way to build complexity is to add more phases, or stages, to the toy play. Your setup and closing/transition routines are two such phases. In setup, selecting a toy from a shelf, carrying it to the floor or a table, opening it up, and getting the pieces out is a whole set of actions in itself for your child to learn. Picking up, carrying, placing on a table, and laying the pieces out for play is another series, or sequence, of related actions involved in preparing to play. These may involve 10 different actions for your child to carry out before the play even begins, adding more complexity to the play, mental stimulation for your child, language learning opportunities, and sustained attention toward the goal of the toy play.

Your closing/transition phase is similar. When you and your child decide you are done with a certain toy, and your child helps put the pieces back into the container, closes it, stands up, picks up the materials, and puts them away, your child has completed another series of actions and has benefited from the thinking, planning, attending, and communication that accompany it.

Each of your variations in play is also a phase, or stage, that allows for additional complexity. For example, let's say you are using play dough together, and the first theme after the setup is rolling the dough into snakes and then joining the ends to make O's. This involves multiple repeated actions for your child: (1) squeezing a lump of dough in her hand, (2) putting it on the table, (3) flattening her hand and rolling the dough back and forth until the dough is now a "snake," and then (4) using both hands to grasp the ends and pinch them together—four actions for every snake. For the variation, you demonstrate cutting the snakes into little pieces with a child's scissors (it helps your child learn to cut). Now your child has to take the first three actions to make a snake and then (4) pick up the scissors, (5) pick up a snake, (6) cut the snake, and (7) cut the snake again. These seven actions occur in an action sequence for each of the snakes.

So, if your child has had a setup phase, a closing/transition phase, the theme, and a variation phase, he may well have completed 100 actions, with your help, in this 15-minute activity—a very complex chain of actions with multiple goals, plans, language and communication opportunities, and sustained attention. This is where you are headed, over much time and practice with your child, into complex toy play that your child understands, carries out independently, and enjoys. See how well this prepares your child for both independent play and play in preschool with other children.

In this section we have been discussing how to teach your child to play with an increasing number of typical toddler–preschooler cause-and-effect toys, with increasing play complexity. For these kinds of toys, the theme of the play is in the *cause-and-effect actions* that the object presents, and the variations stay with that cause-and-effect theme. However, there is another type of play that children do with objects, which involves learning the conventional social use of objects—such as using a play phone, stove, cash register, and so on. This is often called *functional play* or *conventional play*. It's discussed in connection with pretend play in Chapter 12.

⟫⟫⟫ What You Can Do to Help Your Child Play Independently

Besides playing with others, your child needs to be able to play alone constructively with toys once or twice a day so that you can do something else—laundry, cooking, making beds, taking a shower, answering email, talking to a friend, and so on. Although most children will readily watch a video independently, constructive independent play does *not* mean watching videos repeatedly. Independent play that is appropriate and varied allows your child to continue to learn during these periods and to play as others do. To do that, your child needs to come up with appropriate play on his own, without imitating you. A reasonable goal is 10–15 minutes of independent play.

A good time to start to target this is once your child can easily and frequently imitate the actions you are modeling, has built up a number of play routines with different toys, and can sequence a number of actions with each toy, including setup and closing/transition with your support. To work on spontaneous and independent play, you will change strategies. Your new strategy will be to support your child to choose a toy, set it up, and begin to play without your taking any role as a model. How can you foster this? Here are five steps:

Step 1. Organize for independence.

Step 2. Ease out of the play partner role.

Step 3. Decrease support for the setup and closing/transition phases.

Step 4. Change toys frequently.

Step 5. Move farther away from your child.

Step 1. Organize for Independence

How you organize your child's toys can make a big difference in your child's independent play.

Here are some ideas:

- Limit the number of toys that are accessible. Too many choices leads to disorganized play and makes it harder for your child to focus on one toy at a time. Store extra toys in a closet or on a high shelf somewhere. Having six toys available to choose from is plenty.

- Organize the toys on a low shelf that your child can reach; try to get them off the floor. Don't stack toys; separate them so your child can easily pick one and put it back.

- Put out a few different cause-and-effect toys that your child likes and that have a number of different actions, all of which your child can carry out alone. Here are some examples: a puzzle, a shape sorter, beads for stringing, plastic bricks for building, and pegs and a pegboard. Avoid using electronic toys when you are beginning to teach independent play.

- Place the pieces in containers, bins, or baskets so your child can easily select a toy and put it away. Put multiple pieces in baggies; use clear shoeboxes to contain all the parts. Your child should be able to get the toy from shelf to floor alone in one trip. If the pieces fall out, or he has to make several trips, chances are that he will lose focus toward his goal. Watch what happens when your child tries to choose a toy and set it up for play; if it is hard for him, consider how you can make it easier. Does it need to be easier to reach? Fewer parts? Less difficult to make work properly?

- Make sure your child can open and close the containers independently.

- Be sure there is a little table and chair for your child nearby, or a rug or blanket or mat on the floor a little distance away (4–6 feet is a good distance from play area to toys). This is the setup for independent play.

- Do not have the TV on, and do not have food available. These are big distractions. Try to situate the play area so that other people do not need to walk through it as they do their activities at home.

If you need some ideas for activities, look at what other children your child's age are playing with. Objects that involve multiple steps are the right kinds of toys for expanding children's constructive play skills. Good choices include some of the ones listed in the Appendix at the end of this book, including board books with large pictures, blocks, multishape block sets, nesting toys, cups, simple shape sorters, Legos/Duplos, Magna Doodle, pegboards with multicolor pegs, and puzzles. If you need more ideas, check out websites for parents. Begin by reading the ideas for children your child's age. If those ideas seem too mature for your child, drop back an age level until you find something that fits with your knowledge about what your child can do and enjoys doing. When your child knows how to play as other children do, and with the same materials, your child has the skills needed to join other children in play and to learn from them by imitating them—and the other children can learn from your child as well, because you will have developed your child's play skills over many toys and many actions.

Step 2. Ease Out of the Play Partner Role

Your new strategy will be to support your child to choose a toy, set it up, and begin to play without your taking any role as a model or partner.

Here are some ideas:

- Try this when you and your child are playing with a favorite toy that your child can use easily. Once she starts playing, scoot back a little and turn your body a little to the side, so that you are not so available. Watch quietly and see what your child does. Does your child continue to play with the object for a few minutes without your help? If so, your child has succeeded in playing spontaneously! Hold back a little longer, and then comment approvingly about what your child has done ("Yes, ball in the bucket!" or "You shook it! Shake, shake, shake!"). This attention and narration should provide reinforcement for your child's independent behavior.

- If your child does not continue to play independently when you stop taking turns, no problem. You can build up this skill. Start again as you did before. If your child does not continue to play after you pull back, then prompt your child to continue, taking a turn if you need to. In your child's next turn, be more active as an observer: Narrate, show interest, smile, and nod approval, but don't take a turn until your child stops playing. Try to keep your child playing for a few minutes, giving as few prompts as your child needs to play in an appropriate and varied way. Then support your child through the closing and a transition to a new toy.

- Pay attention to how many times you need to help your child continue playing for 3–5 minutes of play. Over time, you want to see this number shrink as your child gets used to playing without your turn-taking support.

- As your child's interest wanes, encourage your child to clean up the toy and take it to the shelf himself. Help him if he needs it, but help from the side or from behind. If your child does not put the box on the shelf, prompt him to do so and then to choose another toy. Congratulations! Your child has just shown you some appropriate, motivated independent play!

Step 3. Decrease Support for the Setup and Closing/Transition Phases

Once your child can play out the theme and variation phases with a toy nicely and independently, and can sustain this for a few minutes, she needs to learn to carry out the setup and closing/transition steps independently to sustain independent play.

Here are some suggestions for all four steps:

- **Setup:** Have your child come over to look at the boxes, and physically choose one by picking it up. Support your child as needed, from behind, to carry the toy to the play space. See where your child is headed (table or floor), and then support your child as needed to put the box on the table or floor, sit down, get out all the pieces, and lay them out in front of him. Sit with your child, but not right in front and not too close. Beside is a good place for now, but eventually you will want to be behind your child.

- **Theme:** Wait for your child to begin and watch your child build the theme, narrating occasionally.

- **Variation:** Encourage a variation through language, prompts, and gestures. Try to go through these types of prompts before taking a direct turn:

  → Say or verbalize an action for your child to do: "Can the car drive fast?"

  → Offer, show, give, or point to what the child might do: "Look [point], the car can drive there," or "Can the car crash into the block [hand block]?"

  → Model or gesture as you need to so your child adds a variation, but don't then take turns. Continue to observe and comment.

- **Closing/transition:** As your child's interest wanes, encourage her to put the materials back in the box to clean up. Then have your child stand up, pick up the box, take it over and put it where it was, and pick another box. Notice that the closing leads into a transition to a new setup. By prompting as needed from behind or beside your child, rather than in front, you are teaching your child how to carry out this transition on her own. This is the key to independent play—your child's ability to sustain play across multiple toys.

> *"I didn't think there was any hope my son would learn to neatly take out toys, play with them, and put them away until he was much older. As a result, I didn't push him to do these things without help (I would always encourage him to put toys away). As soon as he started preschool, he was able to do all of the steps without encouragement. It made me realize I had held him back by underestimating what he could do."*

Step 4. Change Toys Frequently

Change one or two of the toy choices every day or two, but don't change them all. Do make sure to rotate all the toys, even your child's absolute favorites, so your child develops a wider and wider range of toys he plays with independently. When your child gets a new toy, join your child in turn-taking play until your child knows how to do all the steps. Then it can also become a choice for independent play.

Step 5. Move Farther Away from Your Child

Here are some suggestions:

- Gradually move farther away once your child starts with a toy, and make yourself less readily available (read a magazine page or two, put something away, move something to another room). Do not provide more support than your child needs; actually, try to provide a little less. It is okay for your child to struggle a little once the routine is very well established, so she can solve problems that arise in independent play. Helping your child learn to make transitions between toys independently is the key here, and soon it may be the only time you need to support your child in this.

- Remember that the goal here is child independence. Don't expect your child to play as creatively alone as he does with you, though he may. The goal here is playing alone constructively, not practicing every skill you have taught.

- After your child is playing well independently, choosing several different toys, and managing the transitions well alone, you can add an electronic toy to the set of choices if you want, to see what happens. If your child starts to choose it preferentially and "gets stuck," put it away again. This is true for any toy that your child uses in a highly repetitive fashion and cannot move away from. Repetitive play doesn't give your child many learning opportunities. That is why you are rotating choices frequently: to prevent repetitive play, to increase your child's play repertoire and flexibility, and to prevent boredom.

Summary of Steps 1–5

If you have followed along and carried out the preceding activities, you are establishing joint activity routines and teaching your child to play with toys flexibly and independently. See if you agree with most of the statements in the following checklist. If so, you are now armed with important skills for expanding your child's play–knowledge you will use in the next chapter. If not, start experimenting during play and caregiving routines until you have found some methods that work for each statement.

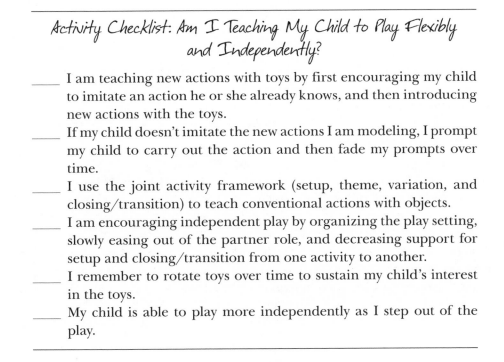

Activity Checklist: Am I Teaching My Child to Play Flexibly and Independently?

____ I am teaching new actions with toys by first encouraging my child to imitate an action he or she already knows, and then introducing new actions with the toys.

____ If my child doesn't imitate the new actions I am modeling, I prompt my child to carry out the action and then fade my prompts over time.

____ I use the joint activity framework (setup, theme, variation, and closing/transition) to teach conventional actions with objects.

____ I am encouraging independent play by organizing the play setting, slowly easing out of the partner role, and decreasing support for setup and closing/transition from one activity to another.

____ I remember to rotate toys over time to sustain my child's interest in the toys.

____ My child is able to play more independently as I step out of the play.

Questions You May Have

What about siblings? Your child with ASD will probably learn independent play more quickly if you can focus on teaching this when siblings aren't demanding your attention—such as when siblings are napping or off on their own activities. If you can't, however, you can teach both children to carry out the independent play routine, coaching the sibling with language while you prompt your child with ASD from a closer position. This will also provide opportunities to teach each child to respect the other child's materials—to wait until the other has finished if they both want the same toy.

What if my child does not add new actions to the play? First, make sure your child is interested in the play. Is he reaching for the materials, taking turns doing things with the materials, and watching your actions? Your child needs to be interested in the materials and enjoying the activity to learn how to do new actions. Second, be sure to model new actions when your child is watching; otherwise, he won't see the new skills you're trying to teach. Third, resist physically teaching your child to do things. Instead, model the action several times with your toy, add fun effects to increase motivation, and encourage your child with words and gestures. If you have to help physically, be sure to use it as the last resort, and continue to practice the new action so your child can strengthen his skills.

Chapter Summary

In this chapter we have focused on expanding your child's play abilities with a wide range of objects, using a wide range of actions. There are two main purposes for focusing so much on toy play: (1) to build your child's thinking, language, and social skills, and (2) to prepare your child well for participating in typical early childhood settings. Building your child's play skills with a typical range of toys found in any early childhood setting is crucial for both these purposes. In doing so, you are also building your child's curiosity, awareness of others, and sense of competence.

We have also focused on building children's independent play skills. The ability to play alone constructively for periods of time is an important skill for every child. Preschools expect that children will have independent play skills. We have provided steps for building up both your child's independence in play and your child's range of play skills. Constructive play is only one type of play that we want to encourage in young children with ASD. The other type is pretend play, also referred to as symbolic play. The next chapter will focus on this.

Refrigerator List

Goal: To increase constructive, varied, independent toy play

Steps:

✓ Teach your child to play with his toys! Go from easy to harder slowly.

✓ Model first, then prompt if needed. Fade prompts fast!

✓ Use the four-step joint activity framework (setup, theme, variation, and closing/transition) to teach your child more play skills.

✓ Encourage independent play by organizing well, sitting behind, and easing out.

✓ Rotate toys to prevent boredom.

12

Let's Pretend!

> **Chapter goal:** To give you strategies for helping your child develop pretend play that is spontaneous, creative, and flexible.

Why Pretend Play Is So Important

Pretend play (or *symbolic play*, as many people refer to it) helps expand children's thinking abilities, because it involves play ideas that come from a child's imagination rather than from the physical environment. When a child picks up a toy animal and makes it walk, growl, or eat, those ideas are coming from the child's mind, in contrast to picking up a puzzle piece and putting it in the puzzle—actions for which the goals are built into the physical materials. The mental aspect of pretend play is deeply connected to language and other kinds of thought, and it is thus a very important part of young children's mental or cognitive development.

What's Happening in Autism?

Young children with autism have difficulty learning and using pretend play. Although they typically have many object interests, the world of pretending does not seem to come naturally to them. Young children with ASD may be very adept at playing with puzzles, blocks, shape sorters, and even letters and numbers, and yet when faced with a doll, a toy bottle, a spoon, and a plate, they may seem to have no idea what to do with the objects. Pretend play goes beyond using an object as it was intended (such as picking up a fork and putting it in your mouth), though that is an important beginning point; it involves using ideas that come from the imagination, rather than from the objects themselves (such as pretending there

260

is ice cream in a bowl and scooping up the ice cream, eating it, and then getting another "scoop of ice cream" and saying, "Want some ice cream?").

By about 2 years of age, children typically start to use pretend play. You will see them treating a block as if it were a piece of cake, "combing" a doll's hair by using a rectangular block, and so on. However, this development of pretend play doesn't emerge naturally in most young children with autism; it needs to be taught. One theory regarding why it does not develop naturally is that parts of the brain that are important for abstract thinking, such as the frontal lobe, develop more slowly and aren't as well connected to other parts of the brain in autism. The parts of the brain that are responsible for perceiving and remembering the concrete world and for understanding concrete information and facts appear to be functioning well—in fact, more strongly than in other children in some cases. This helps us understand why many people with autism have excellent memories for concrete details but some difficulty with pretend play and, later, abstract thought.

Imaginary play skills are closely linked to language skills. In fact, studies have shown that when a child with autism develops pretend play, his language abilities also increase, even if therapy has focused only on improving pretend play skills and not on language directly.[1] Why? Pretend play activities teach a child skills that allow him to develop a "shared experience" with another person, a joint focus of attention. This provides a context for developing, using, and practicing language.

Why Is It a Problem?

As just explained, the close relationships among symbolic play, language development, and abstract thought highlight an important area of relative weakness in autism. The themes of pretend play are about people and their lives; developing pretend play skills helps young children with autism expand their knowledge about the social world. Pretend play abilities also help young children with ASD join in such play with their typically developing peers and expand the learning opportunities available through such interactions. It allows them to learn what others are thinking and feeling by pretending to experience what others are experiencing. And finally, in pretend play, the world of ideas overpowers the physical world. This capacity for thought to overrule the physical world is quite important for children with ASD, for whom the physical world seems to speak very strongly. When a block becomes a key for a car engine, a bar of soap for a baby's bath, or a handful of food for a toy horse, the child's ideas are molding and shaping the physical world into the child's mental world.

---

[1]Kasari, C., et al. Language outcome in autism: Randomized comparison of joint attention and play interventions. *Journal of Consulting and Clinical Psychology*, 76(1), 125–137, 2008.

➤➤➤ What You Can Do to Increase Your Child's Symbolic Play Skills

Young children with autism can learn to produce and enjoy symbolic play, just as they can learn to use and become proficient with language. They need exposure, practice, and guidance to develop these skills, but parent–child daily toy play is a powerful tool for developing pretend play. You can teach symbolic play in just the same way that you have taught the other play skills in Chapter 11—through joint activity routines. The time to start introducing symbolic play is after your child is playing with many different toys, combining objects in play, and combining several different actions in his play with individual toys. Your child needs to know how to imitate, how to engage in joint attention, and how to use many objects in functional play spontaneously and reciprocally before it is time to move forward and build more imaginative, make-believe play.

Symbolic play involves three types of play skills:

1. The first is called *animate play* and involves using dolls and animals as if they were alive and could act on objects themselves, such as having a doll pick up a cup and drink from it, or having an animal brush its own hair or fur with a comb.
2. The second is called *symbolic substitution* and involves using objects as if they were something else, as when a child uses a Popsicle stick to stir in a cup as if it were a spoon, or flies a block in the air as if it were a helicopter.
3. The third type involves *symbolic combinations*—putting together several different pretend play acts to create a more complicated scene. An example would be stirring pretend water in a teapot, putting the lid on, pouring the water into cups, and then taking a drink, making sipping noises, and maybe using a spoon to stir the cup. This sequence involves six different symbolic actions that together make a logical flow, the way the scene really happens—a symbolic combination.

There are five specific steps you can carry out to facilitate these three different types of pretend play skills:

Step 1. Teach conventional, or functional, play skills.

Step 2. Animate dolls and animals.

Step 3. Move from imitation to spontaneous symbolic play.

Step 4. Teach symbolic substitutions.

Step 5. Develop symbolic combinations.

In the following pages, we describe how to carry out each of these steps, give you some ideas for activities to try, and suggest what you can do to solve problems that may come up. Be aware that this sequence takes a long time for young children to develop. Toddlers typically develop these skills beginning at age 12 months and continuing to 36 months and beyond. Think of this as a long-term activity that may take a year or two to complete, but one that you can start immediately.

Step 1. Teach Conventional, or Functional, Play Skills

Rationale. *Conventional (functional) play* involves playing with objects whose meanings are defined socially—that is, by how people use them. Conventional play teaches children the social meaning of people's actions: Objects carry significance beyond their physical attributes or cause-and-effect relation. In other words, an object has a meaning defined by society rather than by its sensory characteristics. Let's use a comb as an example. A comb's meaning, or identity, is defined by how people use it—in contrast to, say, a jack-in-the-box, whose meaning is defined by its physical causality (the relationship between turning the lever and the clown popping out of the box). The cause-and-effect relationship defines the jack-in-the-box, but the meaning of a comb, a toothbrush, a tissue, or a spoon is defined by how people functionally use each object. Conventional or functional play is being used when a child picks up a play tea set and stirs a spoon in the empty cup or pretends to drink by putting cup to mouth, or picks up a hairbrush and briefly touches it to his hair, or puts a hat on Dad's head, or tries to put on Mommy's sunglasses. It is as if the child is saying, "I know what people do with this; it's for your nose," or "This is for drinking." The child is "naming" and giving a social meaning to the toy with his gestures in his play.

♟ Activity: *Teach Your Child to Use Realistic Objects during Conventional Play*

Conventional play is an important step in play development, because it means that the child has learned certain actions from watching other people. This demonstrates social learning—attending to what other people are doing and imitating what they do. You can help your child develop conventional play skills through adapting the steps of your regular joint activity framework, as follows:

1. Introduce the object(s) during setup (e.g., a toy phone).
2. Model and prompt the main theme (e.g., putting the phone to your ear and saying, "Hello?").
3. Use imitation to help your child coordinate actions on her body and on yours (e.g., give the phone to your child and encourage her to answer it and put the phone to her ear).

4. Vary and expand the play to include other "characters" (e.g., putting the phone up to a doll's or another family member's ear).

5. Expand the play into other activities, especially self-care and household tasks (e.g., have Dad call on the real phone and let your child answer it).

Here are ideas for adapting the steps:

● **Setup:** Offer functional play objects like toy animals, comb, brush, cup, fork, tissue, hat, beads, mirror, toy food, dolls, tea sets, doctor kits, sunglasses, phones, and toothbrushes in a box to your child. If she shows some interest, let your child choose an object and explore it, just as in any other object play routine.

● **Theme:** For your turn, model the "conventional" (social) action with the object, using relevant action words ("Brush hair" while briefly brushing your hair or your child's; "Zoom, zoom" while rolling a car fast; making drinking noises with a cup and saying, "Yum, good juice"; etc.). After your demonstration, hand the object back to your child and encourage him to imitate, prompting, shaping, and fading your prompts just as you have done in teaching any other kind of object imitation.

● **Role reversal:** As you model conventional play acts, model them on both yourself and your child. As your child takes the object, prompt her to act on you with the object, as well as on herself. When you do this, the two of you are reversing roles! Encourage role reversal games (e.g., you put a hat on the child and the child puts the hat on you). Hats, beads, brush, cup, sunglasses, spoon, and many other toys/objects work very well for role reversal. Experimenting with double toy sets (two of each object) can turn into lovely, imitative, role reversal games. As you practice the role reversal in these games, use your name and your child's name to mark turns ("Mama's hair, Jerrod's hair," "Emily's turn, my turn").

● **Variation: Using dolls, toy animals, hand puppets, and other people.** After your child is both imitating and spontaneously producing conventional actions on you and on himself, it's time to bring other "characters" into the play. Large dolls with clearly defined facial features; stuffed animals; hand puppets like Elmo or Cookie Monster; other family members—including these characters in your role reversal games will expand your child's play and move your child closer and closer to symbolic play. To introduce these new characters, first model a conventional play act on yourself while labeling it (and making sound effects). Then do the same action on the doll or animal, using the same simple descriptive language, and follow that by encouraging and prompting your child to "feed Pooh," "brush Teddy," "hat for baby."

- **Expansion:** Finally, you can expand the number of conventional objects and actions that you model and the situations in which you use them. You can model conventional actions on objects during bath time, by modeling rubbing your face or arm with a washcloth and then handing it to your child. When it's time to brush teeth, first model toothbrushing with your own toothbrush on your own teeth. During mealtimes, model eating a bite of fruit with a fork, and encourage your child to do the same. When your child needs a messy face wiped, first model it by wiping your own mouth with a napkin, and then encourage your child to do so. If something spills, model wiping up the spill with a paper towel, and then encourage and prompt your child to imitate you. If you are mixing pancake batter or eggs and milk for scrambled eggs, model stirring for your child, and encourage her to take a turn. Help your child learn the social meanings of the many conventional objects that you handle in your child's presence during the day. Including your child in these kinds of activities for a few minutes gives your child many more opportunities to learn from you about what people do and the words that go with objects and actions in life's daily routines. Conventional play is the stepping stone to symbolic play.

Here are some more activity ideas:

- Use themes your child knows: bathing, eating, dressing, going to bed, familiar songs and finger plays, playing on swings and slides. Use a washcloth to pretend that you're washing a bear's hands, face, and tummy. Add the "soap" to make sure the bear gets really clean. Or dress your child and his favorite stuffed animal together, taking turns to put a shirt, shorts, and socks on each one. Maybe your routine for putting your child to bed is to get a drink of milk or water, sing a song, and then kiss her goodnight. Help your child carry out these actions with her doll. Carry them out on the doll yourself as you put your child to bed, and encourage your child to do likewise.

- A community outing—especially a new experience, like going to the zoo or going to the doctor's office—opens up a new set of experiences to act out in pretend play. During play, act out the steps involved in the recent experience: buying an admission ticket to the zoo, walking around the house to look at the different animals, and pretending to feed the nice ones; or using a doctor's play kit to take an animal's temperature/blood pressure, give it a shot, put on a bandage, and give the animal a lollipop.

- Sensory social routines can be acted out with animals and dolls too. If your child has a favorite song sequence, like "Ring-around-the-Rosy," you can incorporate a doll into the routine as if it were another person. You can also hold two small action figures as if they are holding hands and have the dolls act out "Ring-around-the-Rosy." Or if you and your child are each holding the doll or animal's hand, you can swing it back and forth to the tune of "London Bridge."

- Self-care activities are great ways to incorporate this theme. When bathing your child, putting her to bed, having dinner, or brushing teeth, incorporate the same actions on yourself or on a large doll or favorite animal. Encourage your child to act on you or on the doll, just as you are acting on your child.

- During book routines, have the doll or animal sit beside your child. Show pictures and label them for your child, then for the animal.

- Household chores can also be used as character play opportunities. Your child's dolls, animals, or characters can help water the garden, feed the dog, and participate in other activities, just as you have your child join in.

What if my child is not interested in conventional play? Initially your play might need to focus more on the objects involved in conventional play than on the social meaning. For example, mealtime is associated with plates, bowls, and feeding utensils. Encourage your child to feed you a bite off her spoon or to share her sippy cup. Show her with your fork how to feed a doll or stuffed animal seated on the table. Add fun effects, sounds, and lots of enthusiasm and praise to each attempt your child makes to participate (even watching what you're doing counts), to increase the social appeal of the play activity. Try extending the number of play actions or length of time your child can continue before transitioning to the next activity. This idea can also work during other daily routines, like dressing or bathing. You could take turns dressing the doll, animal, or each other, or using a washcloth to give mini-baths to each other and play objects. The goal is to keep it creative, so your child will become more interested in what you're showing her with the materials.

Summary of Step 1

If you have followed along and carried out the preceding activities, you now have ideas for using real objects to teach this first step of symbolic play—functional play—during daily joint activities with your child. You have also introduced a doll or other figures into functional play. See if you agree with most of the statements in the following checklist. If so, you are now armed with important skills for expanding your child's play—knowledge you will use in **Step 2**. If not, start experimenting during play and caregiving routines until you have found some methods that work for each statement.

Note: This is a good time to move on to the next chapter. Continue to read this chapter and to focus on building pretend play skills with your child, but start

Chapter 13 as well. Chapter 13 focuses on developing speech, and the kinds of play you are doing here will help your child make progress in speech as well.

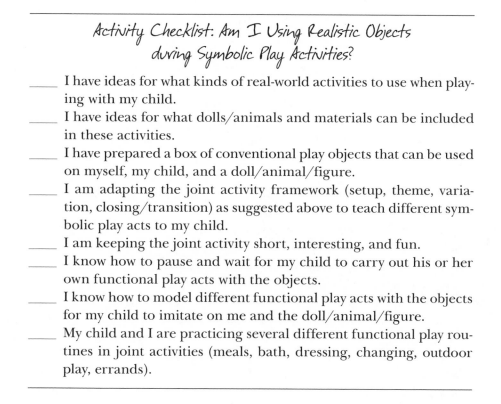

Activity Checklist: Am I Using Realistic Objects during Symbolic Play Activities?

_____ I have ideas for what kinds of real-world activities to use when playing with my child.

_____ I have ideas for what dolls/animals and materials can be included in these activities.

_____ I have prepared a box of conventional play objects that can be used on myself, my child, and a doll/animal/figure.

_____ I am adapting the joint activity framework (setup, theme, variation, closing/transition) as suggested above to teach different symbolic play acts to my child.

_____ I am keeping the joint activity short, interesting, and fun.

_____ I know how to pause and wait for my child to carry out his or her own functional play acts with the objects.

_____ I know how to model different functional play acts with the objects for my child to imitate on me and the doll/animal/figure.

_____ My child and I are practicing several different functional play routines in joint activities (meals, bath, dressing, changing, outdoor play, errands).

Gracie is 28 months old and has recently started using single words to communicate greetings, protests, and some needs and wants. Gracie's mother wants to expand her functional play skills to help usher in pretend play. Gracie loves her Yo Gabba Gabba! *dolls, and she often carries one or two in her arms when walking around the house. When it's time for a snack, Gracie's mom starts to include the dolls in the routine. Gracie seats herself in her chair; Mom sits kitty-corner from Gracie; and two of the dolls are seated on the table between Mom and Gracie. Gracie selects juice from her mother's choice of crackers or a drink, and Mom responds by pouring juice into the cup, followed by pretending to pour some into the dolls' cups (she adds a "sssh" sound for effect). Gracie watches her mom intently as she gives the doll a drink from the cup. Mom makes slurping sounds as the doll drinks, which Gracie finds funny. Gracie takes a drink from her cup, which Mom has the doll imitate. When Gracie finishes, Mom encourages her to give a sip to the doll, modeling with her own cup. Gracie watches and then imitates her mother's action, extending the cup to the doll. Her mother makes the slurping sound, and Gracie laughs. Gracie holds out her cup again and looks right at her mother, as if signaling her mother to make the slurping sound. Her mother responds immediately with the sound again, letting Gracie know that she has understood her gesture. Next, Gracie's mom shows Gracie how to feed a cracker to the doll, and she adds chewing sounds while the doll eats the cracker. Her mom holds up the juice container or bowl of crackers for Gracie to choose what to give the doll. Gracie says "ca" for cracker, and Mom gives her two pieces—one for Gracie to eat herself, which she does immediately, and the second to feed to the doll with Mom's help. Mom accompanies the doll's bite with chewing sounds ("yum yum yum"), which makes Gracie smile. Mom gives the doll a drink and intentionally spills a little juice on its face. She points out to Gracie that the doll's face is dirty, and hands Gracie a napkin to wipe its face. Gracie wipes her own face first, but after Mom points to the doll and explains again, Gracie helps to wipe the doll's face. Mom and Gracie continue with these three actions—drink, eat, and wipe—for a few more minutes, until Gracie indicates that she is finished and snack time is all done.*

Ben's mother often finds that it's difficult to keep Ben, her 4-year-old, occupied when she is grocery shopping. He often whines and wants to get out of the grocery cart seat. She decides to use pretend play to teach him some appropriate actions. At home, she writes out a list with some food items, and then she places the items (bananas, carrots, toy pizza, ketchup bottle, and a box of animal crackers) in various locations throughout their family room. After she gets Ben's little sister's grocery cart, she tells Ben that they're going to the grocery store at home! She reads the list and says they need to find bananas somewhere in the family room. They stomp around the room looking until Ben vocalizes and points to the bananas on top of the couch. Ben and his mother run over to the bananas and put them in the cart. Next, his mother asks whether they should look for the bottle of ketchup or the pizza. Ben chooses the pizza, and the search is under way. Ben finds the pizza next to the television. Mom chooses the next item from the list to look for and gives Ben a clue to its location. The game continues until all five items from the grocery list have been found. The last item is a box of animal crackers—a favorite of Ben's. They roll the cart into the kitchen, and Mom puts the items away and has Ben put the animal crackers on the table. They then sit down at the table together with the animal crackers and a drink, ready to celebrate their shopping trip.

Step 2. Animate Dolls and Animals

Rationale. Step 2 helps your child understand that dolls can represent people and their actions. Agents of action—people and animals—act spontaneously on the world. They cause actions to happen; this is what defines them as agents, or animate beings. Toys and other inanimate objects cannot act spontaneously, but living things—people and animals—can. Very early on, children understand the difference between animate and inanimate objects. They act it out when they manipulate dolls and animals so that the figures are acting on things—walking, growling, waving, eating, drinking, dancing, and so on. The strategies described above have taught your child how to easily incorporate dolls and animals into lots of pretend play actions. The next step is to help your child learn about how figures can also "act" as independent agents.

You will continue to use joint activity routines, offering objects and following your child's interest, taking turns, both participating, both adding ideas, and following your child's cues about when it is time to be finished.

♟ Activity: *Have Dolls Take on Human Actions*

Here are ideas for adapting the joint activity routine to your child to use dolls or stuffed animals as if they were "alive" and able to act on their own:

- **Setup:** Begin by bringing out a box of conventional toys or objects that people use on their bodies (brush, comb, sunglasses, hat, necklaces, bracelets, cup, feeding utensils, plate, plastic food, washcloth, soap, telephone, napkin, tissue, and so on). Have your child choose one of the toys, and either show your child an action that she already knows, or let your child show you a functional action with that object. The action will be directed to either your child's body or yours.

- **Theme:** As the two of you act this out, name both the action and the person ("Feed Mommy," "Joshua drink," "Comb hair").

- **Variation:** As you have done before, bring out a doll or an animal, demonstrate doing the action to the animal or doll while naming the action and animal/doll ("Feed Oscar," "Brush kitty"); then hand the object to your child, and encourage your child to carry out the same action on the figure ("Joshua, feed kitty," "Joshua, give baby a drink"). Provide physical prompts if your child needs them to succeed. Then take a turn yourself and perform the action on the toy. Go back and forth a few times, you and your child acting on the toy, the child, yourself, while labeling the action and the recipient each time (e.g., "Feed Mama," "Feed baby," "Feed Joshua").

- **Variation:** Now have the doll do the action on itself. Hold the object in the doll's hand, and move the doll's arm through the action. Narrate for your child ("See, Elmo is eating," "Baby brushes hair"). Have the doll carry out the act on your child's body ("Elmo brushes Caitlin's hair"). In this step, the doll is acting as if it were alive, or animate; it is an independent agent of action.

- **Closing/transition:** As you run out of ideas, or as your child's interest starts to wane, offer the box and ask, "All done?" while putting your object into the box. If your child also puts his objects in the box, you can say, "All done with Oscar" (or "kitty," etc.), and have your child help you put the box away and make a different choice.

You have just shown your child how the doll can carry out an independent action. Now, as you play out the themes that you have developed in Step 1 with functional play, add this step to each of your routines: Have the doll or character use the objects on itself, on you, and on your child. As this becomes familiar to your child, give your child a turn and help your child "animate" the figure by making it act. In addition to having the figure use the objects, the figure can also jump, run, and go to sleep. Toy animals can "drink" out of water bowls, "eat" their food in their food dishes, and walk on all fours. They can lie down on their sides and go to sleep. Help your child learn to imitate these kinds of actions, in which the characters themselves are doing the actions that are part of the scenes from life you have been playing out with your child. Once your child easily produces acts in which he directs actions to other people and dolls and animals in play (feeds them, gives them drinks, etc.), you will begin to model how the doll or animal can also direct actions inside the play scene.

Now, in your daily pretend play activities with your child, have the animals or dolls routinely participate in the actions as actors once the theme gets going, and help your child carry out these actions. After you have had your child imitate this successfully many times, wait to see if your child will make a figure act independently, either spontaneously or after your suggestion. If your child helps the character produce an action without a physical prompt, imitate the action on your own body right away, and respond with enthusiasm! If not, keep trying. As your child builds up more ideas, more skill, and more enjoyment from pretend play, he will begin to have characters create actions.

Here are more ideas for animate play:

● You can incorporate animate play actions into all kinds of daily routines. Having a big doll in the bathtub allows you and your child to wash the baby's belly, hair, face, and feet, just as you wash your child's belly, hair, face, and feet. Baby or Elmo can be at the table during a meal, sitting beside your child, getting a bib, getting some "bites" and "drinks," and having his face wiped with the napkin. Lion can sit on the potty after your child sits on the potty. The baby doll can have a diaper changed after you change Madison's diaper. Your child can take Curious George on a walk in the stroller after you come back from a walk with your child in a stroller. Thomas the Tank Engine can take turns in the swing with your child, can be on the swing next to your child, or can take turns on the slide. Cookie Monster can go to the doctor's with your child and have his ears checked, his height measured, his chest listened to. He can go get his hair cut right along with your child. Dora the Explorer can draw her own picture with crayons. Incorporating figures into your child's daily routines emphasizes the "human" qualities of animate toys and helps your child develop the ideas behind pretend play.

● Physical actions can also be used to illustrate animate characteristics. Have the characters kick balls to your child, jump on the trampoline with your child or off the bottom step, bounce on the bed, and act out song routines that your child knows and loves. Characters can splash water, blow bubbles, drive cars and trucks, and be part of "Ring-around-the-Rosy." Encourage your child to include the characters and act out these actions, prompting if you need to and then continuing the action with your child so there is a fun reason to continue.

Summary of Step 2

If you have followed along and carried out the preceding activities, you will have found object routines that you can make dolls and other figures act out on themselves, on you, and on your child during your joint activity routines. You have also shown your child how to do this, and your child is imitating you in "animating" the figures. See if you agree with most of the statements in the following checklist. If so, you are now armed with important skills for facilitating spontaneous symbolic play—knowledge you will use in **Step 3**. If not, start experimenting during play and caregiving routines until you have found some methods that work for each statement.

Activity Checklist: Am I Using Dolls/Animals as "Action Agents"?

_____ My child likes the dolls, animals, or figures being used in play.

_____ I know how to offer choices among objects to keep my child motivated to continue a joint activity.

_____ My child and I are able to carry out conventional play acts with objects on each other and the doll/animal/figure.

_____ My child can imitate my actions with the figures in several different scenes, including making the figure act independently.

_____ My child and I clean up the objects together and choose the next joint activity to do.

What about Gracie? *Gracie and her mother have been following the joint activity script to take turns giving crackers and juice to Gracie's dolls. After reading the suggestions in this part of the chapter, Gracie's mother sets up snack time a little differently just by adding a variation to the usual routine. She takes Gracie to her room to have a pretend snack, and together they set out the cups, saucers, spoons, plates, and* *napkins and take a seat along with Gracie's doll on the floor. Gracie's mom takes out a bib and asks Gracie to help her put it on the doll (just to vary the play); this is followed by pouring "juice" into each of their cups, including the doll's. Gracie's mom now models having one or the other of the dolls carry out one of the different play actions that she has planned with the objects, by manipulating the doll's hands with an object so that it feeds itself from the plate. (Other actions could be pouring drinks, stirring with the spoon in a cup, placing items on its plate, wiping its mouth.) After she models, it's Gracie's turn, and Gracie carries out the action on herself. She is imitating the doll! In Mom's next turn, she has the doll give Gracie a bite of real cookie. Gracie eats it and then offers a piece to the doll. The doll then gives it to Mom. They continue to carry out actions from snack time with each other, so that there's a round robin of turn taking among the three play partners—Mom, Gracie, and the doll. When Gracie's interest in the activity fades, Mom has her help place the materials and dolls in a container, and they move on to the next play activity. In this routine, the doll has acted as an independent agent, and Gracie has treated it as such.*

What about Ben? *Ben likes his toy cars more than any doll or stuffed animal, so his mother decides to use these in the play. She tells Ben that his cars need a bath, and they go to the bathroom sink and get a washcloth, soap, lotion, and a towel (all the items she would use for giving Ben a bath). She also includes an Ernie doll as a character. Since this is a new routine for Ben, she models each step with the first car (pouring water into the sink, putting soap on the washcloth, rubbing the car with the washcloth, rinsing the soap off, drying the car off with the towel, and putting lotion on the car), helping Ben participate with each action. With the next couple of cars, Ben is able to do more of the routine, with her prompts. Mom now has Ernie join in the car washing, and Ernie gives props to Ben and also helps with the steps. Mom now uses Ernie instead of herself as the participating partner. Ben likes this new activity and starts to imitate Ernie; he also gives Ernie a car and a towel when Mom suggests it. When all the cars have had their bath, Ben and Ernie empty the water, put away the props, and take the clean cars back to their garage. Mom is pleased that she has figured out a routine that 4-year-old boys might do together. It is the first time Ben has related to a doll as if it were a person.*

Step 3. Move from Imitation to Spontaneous Symbolic Play

Rationale. As you and your child play out more and more actions with various props and various action figures (dolls, animals, etc.), your child is building up more and more ideas about pretend actions. The more ideas your child has, the better prepared she will be for suggesting some of these ideas to you. As you play out more themes, you will use more props, and the boxes of objects and action figures will probably be getting fuller and fuller. As your child picks out some toys, add enough so that there are several different actions that you and she could do in these "scenes."

♟ Activity: *Follow Your Child's Lead in Spontaneous Play Actions*

Set up the materials in some kind of orderly way (e.g., cups on saucers, eating utensils laid out by the plate; cup and napkin; pitcher or bowl of pretend food; two different action figures available). Then, instead of modeling an action, just wait, looking expectantly at your child, to see what she will do first. When your child produces a spontaneous play action, first comment on it ("Kitty is eating") and then join in the play by imitating your child and using a related action, following your child's lead (make another animal eat the food with the kitty). If your child waits for you to start, offer a choice of two objects, and see if your child then begins an action rather than doing the action yourself. Give as little help as is needed to help your child produce the first action directed either to the figure, you, or herself. (This is called a *least-to-most prompting hierarchy*. You are giving as little help as your child needs to be successful.) Following your child's lead by imitating her actions with enthusiasm and fun provides your child with reinforcement for her spontaneous play. This is the key to increasing your child's spontaneous play: Provide familiar and interesting materials, wait, and then follow your child into the play, adding fun and interest to your child's themes. When you are focusing on spontaneity, you want to follow your child's lead and be less active than you have been in starting all these routines. It's fine to add new ideas here and there to keep the play lively and interesting, but you want your additions to be responses to your child's ideas, rather than leading and directing, so your child's initiations are being strongly supported.

Summary of Step 3

If you have followed along and carried out the preceding activities, your child will be initiating pretend play routines and may also initiate using figures (dolls, animals, figurines) as animate beings. See if you agree with most of the statements in the following checklist. If so, you are now armed with important skills for teaching other kinds of symbolic play—knowledge you will use in **Step 4**. If not, start experimenting during play and caregiving routines until you have found some methods that work for each statement.

Activity Checklist: Can My Child Carry Out Spontaneous Play Actions with Props and Action Figures?

____ My child is able to choose different objects and props from the box for character play.

____ I know how to set out the materials in an orderly way to help my child start to play.

____ I know how to wait and follow the least-to-most prompting hierarchy to encourage my child's spontaneous play actions with the character.

_____ I know how to follow my child's lead when he or she chooses a play action to do on the doll/animal/figure.

_____ My child is able to use different objects or props and initiate different play actions among the doll/animal/figure, my child, and me.

_____ I know how to model and help my child use the doll/animal/figure to act out different play actions.

_____ My child, the doll/animal/figure, and I can act out different play scenarios during daily routines.

What about Ben? *As you have read earlier, Ben doesn't care much for dolls or animals. Mom has introduced the idea of animate toys by teaching Ben how to carry out different play actions with objects and props on his cars and having a character help him. However, he engages the characters only for car play. Mom tries to come up with other ideas for character play. She thinks about how much Ben loves his Lightning McQueen pillowcase, which shows a race car from the Disney movie* Cars. *She wonders whether the pillow might work as a "doll" to bring to life. Since Ben can easily feed his toy cars, she decides to seat the pillow in a chair next to Ben during lunch and tells him it's hungry. When Ben doesn't respond, she asks him whether McQueen would want a bite of his peanut butter and jelly sandwich or his apple. She's glad that she has offered Ben a choice rather than taking the first turn to feed something to the pillow, because Ben picks up an apple slice and touches the pillow. Mom does her best imitation of McQueen's voice and thanks Ben for sharing. Next McQueen asks for a bite of Ben's sandwich, and Ben obliges. Then McQueen says he's thirsty and asks if Ben could get him a cup. Mom gets up to retrieve an empty cup and hands it to Ben. When he doesn't place the cup in front of the pillow, McQueen says, "Hey, buddy, don't forget that I'm thirsty. Give me a drink, please." Ben smiles as he raises the cup to the pillow. McQueen and Ben continue their lunch together and make sure that Mom doesn't feel left out.*

Step 4. Teach Symbolic Substitutions

Rationale. The next type of pretend play that your child will develop is the ability to treat objects as if they were something else. You have probably seen a child invent objects "out of thin air," such as handing you a pretend cookie to eat, putting a cereal bowl on her head as if it were a hat, or sitting in a cardboard box as if it were a car. Just like play with action figures, this is an important step in children's pretend play and thinking skills. It shows that thoughts and ideas can guide their actions—that they are no longer bound to the world of objects.

Instead, their mental world is becoming stronger and more abstract, and they can impose their ideas on the world of objects. This is a huge step for little children with autism, and a very important one to develop for thinking skills, for language skills, and for social development. It will help them understand the play of their age-mates and participate with other children as competent play partners.

Activity: *Help Your Child Learn to Create Pretend Objects in Play*

You will use the same joint activity format that you have used to teach all the other play skills. In this type of play, you will model using ***ambiguous*** materials— materials that do not have a clear function in and of themselves—as if they were the familiar props your child is using in your pretend play routines.

Here are ideas for adapting the joint activity routine for this purpose:

- **Setup:** Using the set of props you have been using for pretend play, include some ambiguous objects that can easily represent objects your child likes to use. These are objects that do not have a strong identity of their own. For example, instead of using a play cookie, use a round piece of cardboard: It is shaped like a cookie, but doesn't have a strong identity as anything on its own. The ambiguous object should resemble the realistic object that it will be a substitute for in some key physical features. For example, a Popsicle stick is a good ambiguous object to represent a spoon, fork, or knife. It is not a good substitute for a towel, however. A small piece of cloth is a good substitute object for a towel, or a hat, or a diaper, but it is not a good substitute for a spoon. However, they are both ambiguous; neither has a strong identity of its own. Blocks are particularly good ambiguous items. A cylinder-shaped block is a good substitute for a baby bottle or drinking glass. A square block is a good substitute for a cookie or a bar of soap. Small pieces of cloth, Popsicle sticks, small pieces of paper, baby blankets, shoeboxes, and other random household materials work well as ambiguous objects. Try to find two ambiguous objects to substitute for two key objects in each of your play scenes with your child. Add them to your box of objects for pretend play.

   Now that you have these props in your box, let your child pick out some familiar objects and choose the theme, or suggest it yourself and follow your child's lead into the pretend scene. Action figures will be present, of course, and multiple props related to theme, all realistic except for the one or two ambiguous objects that you have chosen for this scene. They will be substitutes for the realistic objects in the play.

- **Theme:** Use the realistic (not ambiguous) objects to start off the pretend play scene with your child, as you two typically do, doing the actions on each other and on the doll, animal, or other figure. Have an ambiguous object that will be used next to represent the realistic object nearby.

● **Variation:** After you have played out a theme involving the realistic object for which you have a substitute available, immediately repeat the action using the ambiguous object, while narrating and modeling the action as you typically do. Label the ambiguous object with the name of the real object it is representing: "Look, here's my [comb, shoe, cookie, etc.]!" For example, if the goal is for the child to pretend that a triangular block is a baby bottle, then have the block, bottle, and baby present. First set up, model, and have your child imitate feeding the baby with the bottle, with you and your child each taking a turn. Then immediately model feeding the baby with the block, calling it a bottle, and encourage your child to imitate this. Play this back and forth a few times, and also include the other realistic props in your typical actions involving feeding. This might be a good time to have two figures available, so when your child feeds one figure with the bottle, you can feed the other figure with the block, and vice versa. Imitating your child while using the equivalent object will make the idea of the substitute stronger.

● **Closing/transition:** As usual, begin an organized closing and transition to a new activity as interest or ideas wane.

● If this is not becoming clear to your child, back up and go back to pretend play themes with dolls or other figures and realistic, miniature props for a while. Continue to expand the number of themes your child can play out with realistic props. As we have said earlier, children generally prefer

---

⟲ Helpful Tip

Other ambiguous objects include the following:

- *Popsicles stick, Lincoln Logs, Tinkertoys.* These can be good substitutes for feeding utensils, ice cream cones, rocket ships, pencils/pens, thermometers, brushes/combs, keys.
- *Blocks and shoeboxes.* These can be substitutes for cars, trucks, planes, food, pillows, beds, roads, houses, garages.
- *Yogurt and cottage cheese containers, orange juice boxes cut in half vertically.* These can be substitutes for drinking glasses, bowls, plates, bathtubs, pools, hats, spaceships.
- *Necklaces, artificial leis, and beads.* These can be substitutes for snakes, crowns, belts.
- *Pieces of cloth.* These can be substitutes for towels, washcloths, scarves, diapers, bibs, tissue.

to use realistic props rather than ambiguous ones, and building up pretend play themes with realistic props is setting the stage for your child to learn to use an ambiguous prop as a substitute. After you have a very well-established theme that your child enjoys and can play out with all the objects without your prompts, try the substitute object again. Remove the key realistic item from a favorite theme, and have only an ambiguous substitute object available for that key part. As you play along, request the needed object. Feign ignorance and ask for it, such as "I need a spoon" when there are only tongue depressors there, along with a real bowl and cup. Point to a tongue depressor, say, "Here is a spoon," help your child give you the tongue depressor, label it as a spoon, and immediately use it to eat "cereal" from the bowl. Ham it up with sound effects ("Yum, yum, delicious!"), and then offer a bite of cereal to your child with the spoon. Encourage the pretending, and then give your child a tongue depressor to use as a spoon. Help him if needed. Then produce a real spoon and imitate your child eating the cereal. These are the steps for teaching symbolic substitutes.

● Build up your child's knowledge of many ambiguous objects representing many different props. In each of your play theme boxes, have multiple ambiguous objects available that can be substituted for the object necessary for that theme; be sure your child has learned to use the ambiguous objects and can use them in more than one way. For example, a Popsicle stick can be used several ways: as a spoon for feeding, a crayon for writing, and a thermometer for doctor scenes. As the play evolves, your child may well begin to use the ambiguous objects spontaneously. If so, label the object with its pretend identity with enthusiasm! If your child does not do this spontaneously, continue to hand the ambiguous object to the child, label it with its pretend identity, and ask the child to use it (e.g., to feed the baby, comb the baby's hair, etc.).

Activity: *Help Your Child Learn about Invisible "Objects"*

The next activity in this sequence is the use of invisible "objects," represented by gestures and pantomime. Don't start this activity until well after your child spontaneously uses a number of ambiguous objects to represent realistic objects during play. Be sure your child really understands the use of substitute objects before you move to this skill. You will help your child develop an understanding of invisible "objects" exactly as you have helped her develop the use of substitute objects. However, now you will completely leave out a key prop in a set of pretend play objects. For example, you might leave the bottle out of the prop set for feeding the baby. In this case, you will play out the familiar and well-loved baby-feeding scene—but when it is time for the bottle, and you and your child see no bottle, you will pretend by holding the invisible "bottle" in your hand, saying, "Here is a pretend bottle." Take your turn to feed the baby, using the same language you always use. Then pass the turn to your child, saying "Here's the bottle. You feed the baby," while you hand the invisible "bottle" to your child. Help your child do the same thing, pretending that her hand is holding a bottle. You will go back and forth a couple of times this way—asking her to give you the "bottle," pantomiming the routine again, taking turns back and forth. At the end, produce the real bottle and let your child use it on one figure while you demonstrate the pantomime gesture once again on another.

After your child can act out a key prop using an invisible "object" by gesturing to represent it, do the same thing in another prop set. Leave out the main object—the cookie, the cup, the comb, the steering wheel—in a favorite play scene and represent the invisible "object" with your own pantomimed gesture, playing out the routine just as you usually do. Be sure to use the same language and actions you typically use, so your child will really understand what you are doing. Then help your child imitate the invisible "object" as you do. As your child catches on to a new one, slowly add invisible "objects" through pantomimed gestures to your other pretend play themes with your child, and help your child understand them. Go slowly from one routine to the next, and use the real objects intermixed with the invisible "objects" if your child seems confused. If this seems very difficult for your child, go back and spend some more time using substitute objects and then try this again. There's no hurry; this is an advanced level of pretend play for young children.

> ### Helpful Tip
>
> In each theme or scene you are playing out, don't use more than one invisible "object" as a substitute for a key object. Children much prefer realistic objects, or ambiguous objects, over invisible "objects." However, it is quite important that your child learn about invisible or pantomimed "objects," for two reasons: because it allows play to become more creative and less limited by props; and because other children will do this at times, and your child needs to understand it to play along. Many children will think this is funny and will enjoy pretending to feed you or to drink from "nothing." Persist gently, and your child will come to understand this.

Summary of Step 4

Congratulations! You have now taken your child through this whole sequence of learning about symbolic substitutes. This process of learning about pretend play and substitutions takes a long time for all young children. It is a gradual process of learning about more and more scenes from life, more and more ways of playing them out, and more and more props and language. Your child can learn this too! And it opens up your child's ability to understand pretend play, to participate with peers and siblings, and to use pretend play to learn about the social world. See if you agree with most of the statements in the following checklist. If so, you are now armed with important skills for teaching the final type of symbolic play—knowledge you will use in **Step 5**. If not, start experimenting during play and caregiving routines until you have found some methods that work for each statement.

Activity Checklist: Can My Child Substitute Objects during Play Activities?

____ I have ideas of what kinds of ambiguous objects or invisible "objects" can be used in play with my child.

____ I know how to set up and use real objects and dolls/animals/figures to develop the first play theme with my child.

____ I know how to model the action with ambiguous objects for my child to imitate.

____ My child is able to play with ambiguous objects to represent realistic objects in different ways.

____ I know how to model actions using invisible "props" for my child to imitate.

____ My child can carry out play actions with several invisible "objects" when I set them up.

What about Ben? *Ben and his mother pretend that Ben's cars need to be fixed by the mechanic. They drive the cars to the "garage," using pillows to build the structure and a stuffed bear to act as the mechanic. Ben and his mom hand the bear straws, plastic forks and spoons, and pieces of tape to use as the tools to repair the cars. They take turns helping the bear talk about what he's doing to fix each car. Since Ben is very knowledgeable about cars and their parts, he is able to provide a lot of the dialogue. Mom then takes over the role of mechanic and models actions using pantomimed "tools" with her hands as Ben explains procedures for fixing specific car parts. She then reverses roles and has Ben become the mechanic, suggesting that he fix something. Ben likes this idea and pantomimes filling up the "tank" and pumping up the "tire" while Mom makes suggestions, just as he did earlier. Mom makes sure he narrates what he is doing.*

Step 5. Develop Symbolic Combinations

Rationale. The last category of pretend play to help your child develop involves combining various pretend play actions so that your child is able to play out a whole scene from life, rather than just one or two related actions. Think about a scene from your child's life, like bedtime, and how many different actions are involved. For some children, bedtime begins with taking a bath, changing into pajamas, and brushing teeth. Then parent and child may head to the bedroom and sit in the bed together to read a book. Then the parent tucks the child in, covers her up and gives her a kiss, sings a song, provides a favorite toy or blanket, turns out the light, and closes the door. Each of these activities involves a number of actions in and of themselves, and when you consider all of them together, there could be as many as 50 separate actions involved in this whole string of events. Right now your child may play out a going-to-bed sequence that involves putting a doll onto a toy bed and covering it up, which involves two actions. Even adding the book, the story, the kiss, and the lights out makes this a much more elaborate scene, with many actions combined. Once your child can combine one or two actions into a pretend play scene easily, you can help your child expand the number of actions involved, so the play becomes richer and more elaborate.

 Activity: *Combine Symbolic Play Actions into "Scenes from Life"*

The time to start focusing on combining actions is the point at which your child can easily play out several different themes with you (eating, bath, and bedtime are each a theme), and can imitate *and* spontaneously produce several different pretend actions on objects in each theme.

Here are ideas for adapting the joint activity routine for this purpose:

- **Setup:** Have your child choose a theme for pretend play from some choices of objects. Have your child choose a figure or two to add as characters in the play, sit down with you, and label and organize the props. You will want at least four or five props.

- **Theme:** Wait for your child to begin a pretend act; if he doesn't begin, then encourage and help him begin. There is the theme. Imitate it in parallel play so that you have joined in the theme.

- **Variation:** In your next turn, play out and narrate the theme action, and then follow it with an additional action that in real life follows those your child has already produced, narrating as you go. By doing this, you are demonstrating a sequence of actions that occur together in the scene from life that you are acting out (e.g., pour from pitcher to cup, stir the drink, and drink from the cup; then put down the cup on the saucer and wipe your mouth with the napkin), while narrating your actions ("Pour the juice. Stir it up. Drink my juice. Um, good juice. Uh-oh, I dripped some juice"). Then share the props with your child and encourage your child to "have some juice too," using whatever prompts you need to have your child combine multiple actions as well. Having a double set of toys may help, so that you can model multiple acts and prompt your child through imitation. Your goal is to build a sequence that is one or two steps more than your child is already doing easily.

- **Closing/transition:** As your child's interest begins to wane, or the play is feeling too repetitive, suggest that it is time to finish and offer the cleanup box. If your child does not want to clean up, offer another choice of theme in the box, and see if your child will make another choice. If so, then put the new materials down and encourage your child to help clean up the pretend play set so she can move to something else.

Here is a list of pretend themes and related actions, in case you need some ideas:

- **Having characters go to bed:** Take off clothes, put clothes in hamper, put on PJs, brush teeth, pick out book, sing lullaby, kiss/hug good night, turn off the light.

- **Having characters wake up:** Get dressed (take off PJs, put PJs in hamper, put on clean clothes), wash face, brush teeth, comb hair.

- **Mealtime:** Set table, pour juice, put food into plate/bowl, eat, drink, wipe face, clean up.

- **Running errands:** Pretend to get in the car and go to a post office, grocery store, toy store, or restaurant. Go through some steps, then go home (cardboard boxes make good "cars").

- **Going on an outing:** Go to preschool, church, doctor/dentist appointment, play date, birthday party, Grandma's house, zoo.

- **Playing at park:** Go on swings or slide, climb up–down, build sand castle.

- **Giving/taking a bath:** Fill up tub, pour bubbles, wash body parts, rinse off soap, dry body parts.

- **Playing out stories**: Act out the themes from your child's favorite books, movies, and classic fairy tales after your child knows the stories well.

- **Going to the doctor's office:** Go in the door, sign in, get weighed and measured, go into the exam room, sit on the table, have the doctor listen to heart and chest, look in ears and mouth, check reflexes in feet.

- **Going to the dentist:** Go in and sign in, go to the exam room, sit in the chair, put on the bib, tip back a little, open mouth, look in with a mirror, tap some teeth, rub the gums, squirt water in, sit back up, take bib off, get new toothbrush.

Note: Not only can you and your child play out these themes yourself with props from home, but as your child becomes a more advanced player, you can play these themes out with small doll figures, houses, cars, and props. Now the little figures can go to the zoo, the doctor, camping, to the park, to the farm, and so on, using commercial toy sets for props. You and your child can act out themes from favorite books or movies this way. Helping your child learn to create these stories with doll figures is great preparation for thematic play with other children.

Activity: *Use Pretend Play to Help Your Child in Real-Life Experiences*

Amazingly, this process of playing out scenes from life will also help your child understand more aspects of real-life experiences. As you play these out, you may find that daily routines that are difficult for your child (toothbrushing, bedtime, haircuts, etc.) become easier as your child learns and practices the steps and narration in play. Pretend play offers a way to prepare your child for a new experience that has the potential for being difficult or scary! Creating a "script" for what your child can expect in a new experience is called ***priming*** and is a research-based strategy for familiarizing a child with the skills and behaviors to use inside a sequence of events.

Here are suggestions for priming your child for a first trip to the dentist, using pretend play:

- Two weeks before a dentist visit, start to play out a dentist visit with Winnie-the-Pooh, Mickey Mouse, or another favorite figure of your child's—preferably one that has teeth or at least a mouth that opens. Play out with your child on the character the main simple steps—the chair, the bib, opening the mouth, the dentist looking at teeth with a mirror and touching them with a stick, and getting down. Start very simply, with the chair, the light, a bib, and a tongue depressor. Call it "playing dentist." Play it out several days in a row with the figure, having your child take a turn acting as the dentist with the doll or animal, and also with you.

- As this play theme becomes familiar, add a couple more steps, and also play it out with another person if possible. If Mom has been playing this out, Mom can recruit Dad or Grandma to be the patient. Be sure to cheer for the "patient" when the "exam" is finished. As the theme gets to be familiar, use turn taking to have your child be the "patient" sometimes—to sit, put his head back, put on the cloth, open his mouth, and let you touch a couple of teeth with the tongue depressor. Then take off the bib and cheer. Your child now has a "script" for the dentist's office and is prepared for what will happen.

- A few days before your scheduled visit, ask the office if you can come in for a "preview visit," with an assistant playing out the steps you have practiced on you and then on your child, so your child sees the familiar script in the new place and knows what to expect. Take your camera and your child's favorite doll or other figure with you! When you go there, have the receptionist greet your child and your child's toy, and take a picture of the receptionist. Then walk into a dental suite, look at the chair, and perhaps put the toy figure in the chair. Take a picture of the chair. Have the assistant show your child how the chair goes up and down with the figure in the chair; then take a ride on the chair yourself, holding your child and the toy if she is relaxed about it, or just with the toy if your child seems anxious. Then sit in the chair holding your child and the toy, lean back, and have the assistant look in the mouth of the figure with an instrument and then in your mouth. Get a picture of the assistant looking into the mouth of the toy. If your child is relaxed, you can encourage your child to let the assistant look in her mouth. Try to get a picture of this. Then be finished and cheer the child and the toy. Get a picture! If it is possible, get a picture of the dentist who will see your child. Then have the celebration that you have practiced in play. Take a picture!

- Print out the pictures that you have taken, and make a little book with the pictures in order. Read it with your child to your child daily before the real visit. Be sure to end the book with the celebration picture and story.

- After the event is over, continue to play it out in pretend play, that day and here and there in the days after that. You can add more and more props (mask, cup, light, etc.), and it can be a theme for your child to choose from for pretend playtime.

As your child has new life experiences, they all become possible themes for pretend play, both for preparation and for review play afterward. Critical social events are important themes for pretend play: birthday parties; doctor and dentist visits; getting "owies" and having them washed and bandaged; playing circle games with others; sitting in restaurants; going to the library for story hour; family and holiday routines; going to religious services—whatever repeated events you do with your child or events that cause your child anxiety. As you expand the number of props, figures, and actions, you will also naturally expand your language, and your child will be learning both the actions to anticipate and the language that goes with each event.

Summary of Step 5

This step has focused on helping your child learn to create scenes from life by combining pretend play actions into logical sequences. You have been building up the number of combined acts in your child's pretend play themes. At some point your child will know the whole "script" for each of these themes, from beginning to end, and will be able to participate in playing them out with you, with brothers and sisters, and with other children at preschool and at home. See if you agree with most of the statements in the following checklist. If so, you are now armed with all of the necessary skills for teaching different kinds of symbolic play to your child. If not, start experimenting during play and caregiving routines until you have found some methods that work for each statement.

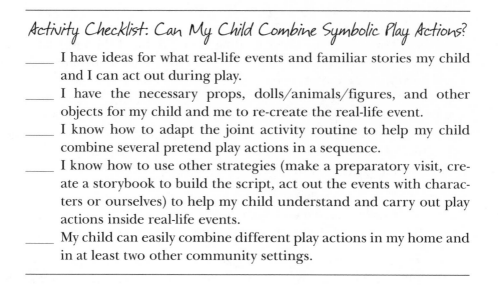

Activity Checklist: Can My Child Combine Symbolic Play Actions?

_____ I have ideas for what real-life events and familiar stories my child and I can act out during play.

_____ I have the necessary props, dolls/animals/figures, and other objects for my child and me to re-create the real-life event.

_____ I know how to adapt the joint activity routine to help my child combine several pretend play actions in a sequence.

_____ I know how to use other strategies (make a preparatory visit, create a storybook to build the script, act out the events with characters or ourselves) to help my child understand and carry out play actions inside real-life events.

_____ My child can easily combine different play actions in my home and in at least two other community settings.

What about Gracie? _Gracie's mom likes the idea of including dolls and animals inside other daily routines. Right now Mom is working on potty training with Gracie and thinks that having her_ Yo Gabba Gabba! _dolls also use the potty might motivate her daughter to do the same. Since Gracie can already carry out the actions with the objects on her mother, herself, and her dolls, Mom moves straight to having a doll act as its own agent. She speaks for the doll as it walks into the bathroom ("I have to go potty") and completes each step that's part of the potty-training routine ("Pants off," "Underwear down," "Help me sit on potty, please," "Go pee-pee," "Wipe-wipe," "Panties up," "Flush toilet," "Wash hands"). Mom congratulates and praises the doll for doing each step while Gracie watches. Mom even hands a little reward to the doll for cooperating—a ribbon to put in its hair (Gracie loves ribbons and barrettes in her hair). Next Mom has the doll say to Gracie, "Your turn," and through Mom the doll helps Gracie move through the potty-training steps. The doll then offers Gracie a choice of which ribbon to put in her hair. Gracie is very excited to have a pretty new ribbon to wear, and happily gathers up her dolls at the end of the routine._

"*Learning good pretend play skills has been extremely valuable for my son. Because he was very interested in playing with cars, we helped him develop complex adventures for his cars (taking turns with his sister to fill cars with gas in a toy garage, racing down the ramps, becoming stuck on a ramp). He can now develop complex stories by himself and can spend long periods of time playing independently or with his sister. I think this has also been extremely helpful in teaching him empathy and understanding of other people, because we can talk about why a car might be happy or sad, or why his sister might be happy or sad with a particular development. Coincidentally or not, he has simultaneously developed a much better ability to look at a picture and describe how a person is feeling (e.g., 'She is sad because she fell off her bicycle').*"

Chapter Summary

Pretend play is a crucial developmental skill for all young children. It fosters thinking skills, language skills, and social skills. In particular, pretend play helps all children understand social expectations and social roles; it helps them learn the "rules" that underlie social events. Pretend play can also be used to prepare children for real-life events. Once your child understands pretend play, has some language, and can spontaneously come up with pretend play actions, you can help your child use pretend play to practice upcoming events. Pretend play routines, including storyboards and storybooks, can be used to practice novel situations—a first airplane ride, a trip to the hospital, the first day of a new group program, a birthday party, going to church, a new baby in the family, adjusting to a new pet. They can help your child become less afraid of certain triggers: the wind, hair washing or haircuts, the vacuum cleaner, the lawn mower, the shower. Symbolic play can also be used to help your child practice the rules for group games and activities. Learning the rules for "Duck, Duck, Goose," circle time at preschool, "Musical Chairs," "Stop and Go," and so on can be fun and extremely helpful for your child when you play these out with your child and also play them out with dolls. Practice birthday parties, dentist visits, greetings, and other routines between dolls, so your child can learn the social scripts that go with these routines. Practice what a child should do when a friend gets hurt while playing: what to say, what to do. This is how your child will learn how to respond appropriately to others. Your child will learn these from your using the imitation and language skills you are teaching (which is how all children—and adults!—learn social scripts). Thus pretend play is as useful for young children with autism as it is for children without autism: It helps them make sense of real life and play with other children.

Refrigerator List

Goal: To help your child develop pretend play that is spontaneous, creative, and flexible.

Steps:

✓ **Use everyday objects during play.**

✓ **Bring dolls/animals/figures to life.**

✓ **Substitute objects for other things.**

✓ **Combine multiple actions to make scenes from life.**

✓ **Everyday life events are the right themes for play.**

✓ **Playing out social interactions and other new experiences helps your child understand them.**

✓ **Playing out scenes from favorite movies and books is great for advanced pretend play.**

13

Moving into Speech

> **Chapter goal:** To help you support your child to use and understand speech through active social interaction with people, their facial expressions, and their gestures.

Why Speech Development Is So Important

Speech is our main mode of self-expression and of social interaction. It is the skill that parents of young children with ASD are typically most worried about. You may very well have turned to this chapter before reading the rest of the book. Or you may wonder why we've waited so long to discuss this critical topic. It's because everything else we have discussed so far is part of the foundation for speech development in young children. Just as children have to sit up and stand before they can walk, they have to be able to attend to parents, imitate their sounds, communicate with gestures, and shift their attention from objects to people and back again before they can learn the meaning and use of speech. So if you have not yet read Chapters 4–12, please do so before trying to apply the strategies in this chapter.

Learning to talk involves two skills: using words to convey desires, experiences, feelings, and thoughts to other people, which is called *expressive language*; and understanding what others are saying, which is called *receptive language*. Young children with ASD often have much difficulty learning to understand and use speech, but most are quite capable of learning to communicate with words, with the help of their parents and professionals.[1]

---

[1]A small minority of children with autism do not learn to use spoken language. These children, however, can learn to communicate by using pictures and other visual devices. All children need to learn to communicate by using either speech or other communication methods.

What's Happening in Autism?

Although not all children with ASD are delayed in developing language, most are. Many children struggle with learning to use speech, but all are helped by the strategies we discuss in this chapter. Many children with autism have overall slower rates of development in all areas (cognitive, social, communication), and this means that they will also learn language at a slower rate. In addition, as discussed in Chapter 4, autism is associated with a very specific difficulty in paying attention to other people. Finally, some children with autism have a specific difficulty with speech above and beyond their other problems. However, most children with autism can learn to use speech, provided they have enough support and the right kind of support.

Why Is It a Problem?

Autism's effect on children's social attention to others—their decreased social initiative, social responsiveness, and social engagement—results in fewer opportunities for these children to listen, learn, and respond to language. Therefore, we need to increase their opportunities for social interaction, as this will help promote language development. We have spent most of this book discussing ways to decrease the amount of time your child spends playing alone, wandering about the house, watching movies, and spending time relatively unengaged with others. You have already put many changes in place to help your child learn to talk by increasing the amount of time the child participates in meaningful social activities with others throughout the day.

You already know that helping your child learn language means helping your child interact face to face with you and others in the family whenever possible. Watching movies or playing with electronic "educational" toys or computer games may be entertaining, but children learn to communicate by interacting with other people. Words they may pick up by imitating a movie script or an electronic program are often not used to communicate with others. Children learn *communicative* language from their *interactions* with other *people.*

Given the demands of running a household, working outside the home in some instances, and caring for other family members, it simply isn't possible to spend most of your day on the floor playing with your child. However, during the moments you are naturally with your child—such as during meals, bath time, or at the playground—you can drastically increase the number of language-learning opportunities you provide for your child by using the strategies discussed in this chapter. By including your child with autism in more household activities, and by making the care and play routines you already have with your child more interactive and language-focused, you can help your child's language abilities grow. So let's discuss the specific strategies for promoting speech and language development. We discuss expressive language first, followed by receptive language.

➤➤➤➤ What You Can Do to Build Your Child's Expressive Speech and Language

Does your child make many sounds? Does your child use his voice as a way of communicating, even though he has not yet learned to talk? Can your child imitate any simple sounds you make, like animal sounds, or car sounds during car play? Can you and your child make noises back and forth to each other? Developing these skills paves the road to speech. Here are the steps to building expressive speech and language:

> **Step 1.** Build up your child's vocabulary of sounds.
>
> **Step 2.** Develop vocal games with your child's sounds.
>
> **Step 3.** Increase opportunities for listening and responding to sounds made by others.
>
> **Step 4.** Talk to your child in a way that promotes language development.
>
> **Step 5.** Add sounds to gestures.

In the following pages, we describe how to carry out each of these steps, give you some ideas for activities to try, and suggest what you can do to solve problems that may come up. *We have had an extremely high rate of success in teaching young children with autism to speak by using these techniques. Most develop first words within a year.*

Step 1. Build Up Your Child's Vocabulary of Sounds

To develop speech, your child needs to be able to make a lot of sounds, and to make them frequently and in response to you.

Rationale. Often very young children with autism produce very few sounds, especially consonants. Vowel sounds, like "ah," "ee," and "oh," are easier for children than consonant–vowel combinations, like "ba," "da," and "ta." The first step is for your child to make a lot of simple vowel sounds and to make them frequently, in response to your making similar or other sounds. If your child does not yet do this, this is where you will start to focus—on increasing the frequency with which your child makes sounds, and also the number of different sounds your child can make.

♟ Activity: *Treat Sounds Like Words and Repeat Your Child's Sounds*

One of the most effective strategies you can use is to respond to your child's sounds *as if* they were words: by answering your child, by imitating your child's sounds, or by saying something that sounds like what your child said. If your child is vocalizing to himself, go up to him and imitate the sounds. Get in a good position for attention (see Chapter 4), repeat the sounds your child is making, and then pause. Your child may vocalize again. If so, respond again. Then, see how many times you and your child can go back and forth. This is a little conversation, and it shows that your child can control his voice, can choose to turn it on and off, and is aware of taking turns with voice. If your child stops vocalizing, that's okay! It doesn't mean that you've done anything wrong or that your child doesn't like it. Maybe it's really hard for your child to choose to turn on his voice right now. Maybe it is a new experience and your child has to think about it a little. Maybe he is surprised! You've done the right thing; keep doing it. With enough experience, your child will probably start to vocalize back when you repeat his sounds. Persistence will pay off.

Step 2. Develop Vocal Games with Your Child's Sounds

Once you and your child can vocalize back and forth easily when your child starts to vocalize, try starting the vocal game yourself, before your child makes a sound.

♟ Activity: *Use an Everyday Activity as an Opportunity to Make One of the Sounds Your Child Typically Makes*

Try this activity while you are face to face and you have good attention—in the high chair, at the changing table, on your lap, on the bed. Look at your child, make a sound you know your child can repeat back and forth, and wait expectantly for your child to "answer" you. If she does, answer back and carry out your mini-conversation. Practice starting these with the various sounds you and your child use to play turn-taking sound games.

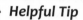 **Helpful Tip**

Some families like to keep a list of sounds their child makes on the refrigerator or a kitchen cabinet. Watching the list grow over time lets you know that your work is paying off.

When your child can sustain the back-and-forth interaction with you when *she* starts it, and when she can "answer" you with the various sounds she has when *you* start the "conversation," you and your child have taken a giant step toward speech.

> ### ✋ Helpful Tip
>
> Toy microphones that echo or carry sounds may encourage "quiet" talkers to experiment with their voices. Try voicing (or singing) an extended vowel sound into the mike while your child watches—something like "oh-oo-oh-oo-oh" or "la-la-la-la-la." When you are finished, hand the mike to your child. He may look at it, mouth it, hold it to the mouth, or put it to your mouth for more. Take it back after a short time, vocalize again, and hand it over again. You can also pat your child's mouth with your fingers to encourage mouth movement and emerging sounds. Try it on yourself while chanting and then again with your child. Do this several times in a row, and play either or both games daily. In a few days, you may see your child begin to vocalize into the mike or pat your mouth to start a vocal game as well.

If your child does not answer you when you start the vocal play, don't worry. At some point, she probably will. Continue to imitate your child and build these little back-and-forth exchanges from your child's vocalizations, and continue to try to start them several times a day. Your child will very likely follow your lead in the near future.

Twenty-month-old Sabrina was a quiet little girl who rarely sat still and had little interest in objects. Her vocalizations were infrequent and occurred when she was moving around the room. Her mother, Christie, consistently imitated her, but Sabrina was not yet responding. Christie also sang to Sabrina many times a day, with animated face, voice, and gestures, and she found that Sabrina particularly liked "Twinkle, Twinkle, Little Star." When Christie started to sing it, Sabrina would stop, turn, and come close to her to watch and listen.

A few weeks after Christie started to use the techniques in this book, she heard Sabrina making song-like vocalizations. These sounded a bit like "Twinkle," so Christie sang back what she had heard. Sabrina turned and approached her mother. Then Christie stopped the song, and Sabrina started to "sing" again. They went back and forth several times in a row.

Christie took this as a cue to augment the song repertoire and started to sing during many of her dressing and changing routines—just little made-up songs as she went along. Within a week or two she started to hear "words" inside Sabrina's songs; her daughter was learning speech sounds inside the music. When Sabrina started a song, Christie continued it. She found that if she started a favorite song and then stopped at the end of the line without finishing it, Sabrina would fill in the missing word. Sabrina's consonants and vowels, and her word-like utterances, were increasing steadily inside the song bits, and Christie started to hear these new sounds when Sabrina was vocalizing to herself as well.

They had had so much practice going back and forth in songs that Sabrina now began to respond when Christie imitated her vocalizations. She repeated them, and the two could go back and forth with sounds as well as songs. Sabrina now had enough sounds that Christie could begin to embed them into their play routines. Sabrina loved feeding one of her baby dolls and watching bubbles. Christie could use Sabrina's "ba-ba" sound inside both of these routines, for bottles and for bubbles. And when she got one of these routines going, Sabrina did imitate the "ba-ba" sound, several times a day. In a few weeks, Sabrina had moved from no consonants or imitation to many episodes every day of back-and-forth vocalizing and singing, and Sabrina was now ready and able to start to imitate some word approximations inside the routines that Christie chose, using the sounds Sabrina had already mastered.

Step 3. Increase Opportunities for Listening and Responding to Sounds Made by Others

Another technique to use with a child who is just beginning to develop control over her sounds is to increase the range of sounds you provide by using non-speech sounds, songs, and chants.

Rationale. Animal noises, car noises, and other types of sound effects made during play routines are important steps toward speech, even though they are not speech sounds. Activities involving songs and sensory social routines generally involve words used in ritualized, playful ways that will engage your child.

Activity: *Increase the Number of Times Your Child Hears Nonspeech Sounds*

When you are playing with toys with your child, weave sound effects into your social exchanges with the toys.

Here are some activity ideas:

- Say "Ringggg" dramatically when you put the phone up to your ear.

- Make engine noises ("vroom-vroom") when you play with trains, cars, and planes, and also when you do books or puzzles about vehicles.

- Make animal noises for toy animals and pictures of animals in books and puzzles.

- Make silly noises like tongue clicks, raspberries, lip pops, and other crazy fun sounds you can think of during diaper changes, mealtimes, toy play, and sensory social routines.

Watch your child's reactions, and repeat those effects that catch your child's interest and attention. Make each sound and patiently wait for your child's turn to imitate or make a sound back. Whether or not your child responds, take another turn. The predictability of your sounds will help your child learn to make them.

♟ Activity: *Increase the Number of Times Your Child Hears Words*

These kinds of activities generally involve words or sounds used in playful ways that are built into chants, play routines, or songs. Here you can use all those "baby games" that combine words and gestures, like peekaboo, chase/"I'm gonna get you," bumblebee, "Round and Round the Garden," and "This Little Piggy." We also include songs with action, like nursery rhymes—"This Is the Way the Ladies Ride," "The Noble Duke of York/Grand Old Duke of York," "London Bridge," and "Ring-around-the-Rosy." Bubble routines that involve "pop and poke," as well as routines with balls, jumping, swings, and slides that involve "Ready, set, go!" and "One, two, three!", provide opportunities for words to enter your child's ears in rhythmic and predictable ways. When your child is involved in any rhythmic activity like jumping, swinging, or banging, add the words "jump, jump, jump" (or "up and back" for swinging, or "whee" when the swing comes toward you) in rhythm with your child's activity.

Children seem particularly attracted to these kinds of rhythmic social sound and action routines, and these are often the first words they say. Try to build up lots of fun sensory social routines every day with these kinds of sounds, words, and songs. Hearing all these sounds will help your child build up more and more sounds and learn much more about the social aspects of sounds and the meanings of some words.

Summary of Steps 1–3

Thus far in this chapter we have been talking about helping your child develop the sounds that she will need for speech production, and helping your child use those sounds in back-and-forth imitation games. See if you agree with most of the statements in the following checklist. If so, you are now armed with important skills for helping your child learn to speak and use language. These are skills you will use throughout your child's first language-learning stage—building on the sounds your child can already produce, offering new sounds and words in interesting contexts, and helping your child expand sounds in meaningful activities. If you don't feel secure in these skills, turn back to the start of the chapter and ask your child's speech–language therapist to observe your interactions and give you some feedback or coaching with these techniques. Eventually this style of talking with your child will become so natural that you will not even think about it. Maybe it already is!

Activity Checklist: Am I Helping My Child Develop New Sounds?

_____ I know the sounds my child makes regularly, both vowels and consonants.

_____ I typically imitate my child when he or she is vocalizing, and I try to be positioned for eye contact.

_____ I know how to pause and wait for my child to take a turn after I make a sound.

_____ I know how to develop some back-and-forth sound games with my child.

_____ I use lots of sound effects, single words, song routines, and "baby games" that combine action and simple words or sounds with my child.

_____ I routinely pause when I am playing games with sounds or words, and wait for my child to look, gesture, or vocalize (take a turn) before I continue.

Step 4. Talk to Your Child in a Way That Promotes Language Development

Rationale. How parents talk to their children has a big influence on their children's language development, and this is also true for children with autism. Parents who talk frequently to their children (face to face, using simple language) about what the children are doing, seeing, and experiencing; who label their children's actions and objects; and who narrate activities as they are carried out help their children talk more and develop larger vocabularies. Parents who use speech mostly to give their children instructions or corrections limit their children's opportunities for language learning. You want to be sure you are talking to your child throughout the day during both play and nonplay activities, and that whenever possible, you have your child's attention when you are talking.

> "So important to talk to your child! So many parents talk about the child, around the child, but since the child is not verbally communicating back, they slow down or stop communicating to the child."

Talk about what? The easiest thing to do is simply to talk about what your child is doing. "You want the ball?" "Here's the ball." "That's right—roll on the ball!" Follow your child's focus of attention. You know that what your child is attending to is what your child is thinking about. Put words to it: "There's the bed." "You want on the bed?" "Up on the bed!" "Time to sleep." *Put the words in your child's ear that* *you want to come out of your child's mouth.* Name the object your child is looking at. Name the action your child is using with the object. If your child is looking at what you are doing, describe it. If your child is looking at you, say something. Act as your child's narrator or translator; name what your child is looking at, playing with, touching, or using.

Helpful Tip

If you have any doubts about how many words to use, think of yourself as your child's translator, and stick to what is most important to conveying the meaning of the action: Name what your child is looking at, playing with, touching, or using. Limit your language to simple words and short phrases to capture the key nouns and actions of your child's movements.

How complex should your language be? For children who are not talking yet, you want to keep your sentences really short and to the point. Limit your language to simple words and short phrases to capture the key nouns and actions of your child's movements.

Activity: *Make Your Language Just a Little More Complex Than Your Child's*

In general, you want your language to be just a little more complex than your child's. If your child doesn't talk yet, or if your child is just beginning to use words, then these one- to three-word phrases are just about right.

Here are some ideas:

- Name people:
  - → "There's Mama!"
  - → "Hi, Daddy!"
  - → "Grandma's here. Hi, Grandma!"
- Label objects:
  - → "It's a ball. See the ball."
  - → "That's a doggie."
  - → "That's the light."
- Label actions:
  - → "Bang, bang, bang the drum."
  - → "Jump, jump, jump" (on the bed).

> ### ✍ Helpful Tip
>
> You want your language to be just a little more complex than your child's. This is what we call the **one-up rule**: make your sentence one word longer than your child's. If your child doesn't talk yet, or if your child is just beginning to use words, then these one- to three-word phrases are just about right. If your child is combining a couple of words (e.g., if your child says, "Bang drum," or "Big car"), then use slightly longer phrases ("Yes, bang the drum fast," or "It's a big red truck").

→ "Splash, splash" (water in the bathtub).

→ "Pour the water" (from cup to cup in the kitchen sink).

→ "Water on" (as your child turns the faucet on). "Water off" (as she turns it off).

You can think of a simple vocabulary of the words you want your child to learn, and then use those words frequently (many times a day) until your child learns them. Provide words for the objects and actions your child encounters in daily life. Everything needs a name—sensory social routines, foods, toys, people, and pets—and actions are important to highlight as well as names of things. There is no need to focus on colors, counting, or letters for children who are just beginning to talk. Those will come later. In the beginning, focus on names, labels for objects, and actions of the objects and activities that engage your child.

> *"Just labeling the environment for the child is huge, even if your child can't engage in a reciprocal conversation with you."*

> *"I think parents gets so worried about the developmental level of typical peers that they feel their children need to know things like colors, letters, and numbers, but do not realize they do not have the foundation for it yet."*

Sixteen-month-old Manuel's parents do an excellent job of narrating his activities. They use a mixture of Spanish and English, just as they speak with others in their family. It is quite important to their family to raise bilingual children, since the grandparents speak only Spanish. Manuel's brother also has autism and speaks both languages well, so the parents are confident that Manuel will also learn both. Here is what Manuel's father says as Manuel is playing with a ball maze on the coffee table.

Manuel goes to the coffee table and begins to put a ball in one of the holes that is part of the toy on the table. His father, Ramon, goes over to the coffee table and sits on the floor across from Manuel (he is now at eye level and close). Ramon places a ball—"Pelota aqui [Ball here]"—as he points. Manuel hammers the ball; Ramon accompanies with him "Boom, boom, boom." Then he asks for the ball—"Dammi a Papa? Pelota? Gracias [Give to Papa? Ball? Thank you]"—as he reaches out his hand and Manuel gives it. Manuel pushes several balls into their holes. "Push, push," says Ramon.

Then Ramon picks up the hammer and a ball. He offers both to Manuel, while saying, "Te quieres, Manuel? Quieres pello or pelota?" Manuel reaches for the ball. "Pelota? Si? [Ball? Yes?]" As Manuel takes it, Ramon says, "Si, la pelota. [Yes, the ball.]" Manuel reaches for the hammer, and Ramon says, "Quieres pello. Aqui e pello." Then, as Manuel hammers the ball, "Bang, bang la pelota." Then he asks for it: "Dammi a Papa" [Give to Papa], aqui [here]," as he points to his hand. He says, "Thank you," as Manuel gives it to him. "Papa's turn," Ramon says as he hammers: "One, two, three!" Then he says, "Manuel's turn," as he hands it over to Manuel. Manuel bangs the hammer: "Bang, bang, bang." Ramon offers a ball—"Manuel, pelota?" He gives Manuel all three balls, and as Manuel puts them in the holes he counts: "Uno, dos, tres; tres pelotas [three balls]."

In this narration, we see all the features we have discussed. Ramon, the father, uses simple words and phrases to describe all of Manuel's actions and the objects that he is looking at. He takes turns with his son and uses simple language to accompany his own actions. His language is repetitive, and his sentences are generally one or two words long, just right for a child who is not yet speaking. He uses sound effects (such as "Bang, bang"), ritualized phrases ("One, two, three"), and simple gestures (such as extending his hand) when he makes a request of his son. He helps Manuel follows his simple verbal instructions, and he uses a happy, positive voice throughout.

Ramon also joins Manuel in an activity that Manuel has chosen, and he positions himself so that he can easily follow Manuel's actions and gaze so he can label just what Manuel is focused on at that moment. This is what we mean by "narrating your child's activity" at just the right level for this child. In this episode Manuel vocalizes only three times (we have not described these here). However, within 1 month, Manuel is imitating many of these words and is initiating some of them as well: "One, two, three," "thank you," "ball," "please," "*mas* [more]," "*agua* [water]," and several other words in both languages. At 18 months he is well on his way to becoming a verbal child, and at 22 months he speaks in short Spanish and English phrases, has well over 50 words, and understands his parents' simple speech in both languages.

Step 5. Add Sounds to Gestures

Rationale. We have been talking about how to help your child do three things: (1) develop more sounds and words; (2) develop the ability to "turn on" his voice;

and (3) make words or sounds back and forth with you and others in vocal play—
"mini-conversations." For children who can do these three things, the next step
is adding gestures to their sounds, to increase their nonverbal communications.
We talked about how to build up your child's gestures and body language in
Chapter 7. Now it's time to put sounds to those gestures.

To help your child learn to put word approximations or sounds to gestures,
you will need to model the skill very consistently. The procedure should follow
these steps:

1. Choose a gesture and a word or word-like sound that your child uses frequently, and model them together.
2. Add sounds or simple words to accompany all your child's gestures.
3. If your child is making sounds but not words with her gestures, add word
   approximations—nouns or verbs—to the simple sounds.

Here are some ideas for carrying out this sequence:

● **Choose a gesture and word or word-like sound to target.** Pick a sound
  your child can already produce. Now choose a gesture your child already
  uses frequently that the sound could easily be paired with. Let's say, for
  example, that your child has learned to consistently reach or point to an
  object to request it, and that your child makes many requests by pointing
  every day (because you are offering many choices every day—good for
  you!). Now think about what sound or word your child uses that could be
  paired with a point. Does your child say "da"? Is "da" something your child
  can repeat after you? If so, it's a great choice for pairing with a point—it's
  close to the word "that." What about "ah"? Can your child repeat "ah"? It
  also sounds a little like "that."

  After deciding on the gesture and word you plan to use, ask your
  child to hand you things during a game by pointing and saying, "that, give
  me that." You have just modeled what you want your child to learn. And
  when your child points to or reaches for something, before you give it, imitate your child by pointing to the object and say, "That? You want that?"
  Wait and see if your child will try to imitate the word "that" by saying
  "ah" or "da" before you give it. If she says anything at all, give the object.
  If she looks at the object but doesn't say anything, give the object. Model
  this when your child makes requests every day. Pretty soon your child will
  probably begin to add a sound to the requesting gesture.

● **Add sounds or simple words to all your child's gestures in the same way.**
  In the gesture games you play, try to add a sound consistently—"boo" when
  your child uncovers his face during peekaboo, "bye" when your child waves
  bye-bye, "no no" when your child protests and pushes away an unwanted

food or object. Follow the suggestions we have just laid out above to find a simple "word"—a sound to pair with your child's gesture. Start modeling it and trying to get your child to imitate it. Your animal sound games and books, and your sound effects in your toy play routines, are other places to encourage your child to imitate your sounds with gestures.

Remember! The first time your child imitates your word and gesture, imitate your child's word and gesture right back, give the toy to your child as quickly as possible, and keep the game going. Don't ask your child to imitate you again right away. It's really tempting, but it's a brand-new skill, and it may be really hard for your child to do it twice in a row. Instead, go ahead and take your turn, and just model it again a couple of times. Then give your child another turn. She may model the sound as well as the gesture; she may not. But try it again the next day or the next time you do the routine. As it becomes easier for your child, you will expect more of these, and you can expect more imitations in a row. But baby steps are the way you will get there.

- **Add nouns or verbs to the simple sounds.** Now, at this point, your child is vocalizing with his gestures and in your baby games and sound games, but he may be saying only an "ah" or a "da." You are still playing your vocal games, right? So your child is likely increasing the number of sounds he is making, and can now imitate back and forth with you. So now, after your child gestures and vocalizes with his "ah" or "da" or other sound, imitate back and then model the correct word. For instance, if your child points to a cereal box and says "da," you say, "That? Cereal! [emphasizing the "s"]. Cereal!" And hand it over. Add a real word to all your child's gesture-plus-sound routines—ideally, a word that contains some sounds your child can already make and imitate in games with you. After you have done this for a few days, if your child is not starting to imitate the new word, get closer, look at him, say "Cereal? Cereal? Sss-cereal?", and look expectantly, waiting for your child to imitate. Give the cereal regardless of what your child says or doesn't say.

> **Helpful Tip**
>
> As you begin to use the correct words for your child's sounds, try not to use the word "more" or "please" as a general term for requesting, and instead use the object or action name as the target. This will expand your child's vocabulary and prevent overuse of "more." This way your child can understand and start to use the names of objects and actions to communicate.

If you and your child have a number of vocal imitation games going, and if you have a number of sounds in them that your child can imitate, her ability to start imitating and adding sounds should come along. Accept any sound match your child makes. It's a long way from "Sss" to "cereal," but this is the way that all little children learn to speak. They say what they can, and over time—as their speech muscles and skills develop through practice, and as they learn to hear the sound differences more precisely—they come closer to saying the real word.

Summary of Steps 4–5

If you agree with most of the statements in the following checklist, you are now armed with important skills for helping your child build an initial vocabulary. These are skills you will use throughout your child's language learning—building on what your child can already produce, offering new words in interesting contexts, and helping your child expand her utterances in meaningful activities. If you don't feel secure in these skills, turn back to the start of this section and review. Consider asking your child's speech–language therapist to observe your interactions and give you some feedback or coaching with these techniques.

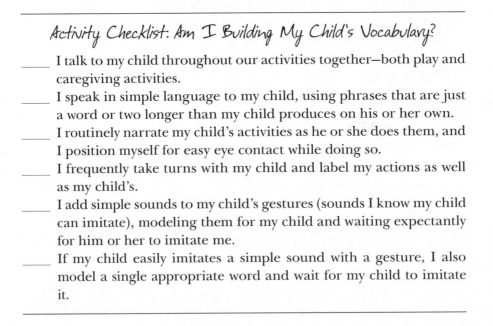

Activity Checklist: Am I Building My Child's Vocabulary?

_____ I talk to my child throughout our activities together—both play and caregiving activities.

_____ I speak in simple language to my child, using phrases that are just a word or two longer than my child produces on his or her own.

_____ I routinely narrate my child's activities as he or she does them, and I position myself for easy eye contact while doing so.

_____ I frequently take turns with my child and label my actions as well as my child's.

_____ I add simple sounds to my child's gestures (sounds I know my child can imitate), modeling them for my child and waiting expectantly for him or her to imitate me.

_____ If my child easily imitates a simple sound with a gesture, I also model a single appropriate word and wait for my child to imitate it.

Caution! Does your child imitate, or echo, easily? If so, you may find it very tempting to provide the child with phrases and encourage him to echo every word, hoping that he will learn multiword speech more quickly. *Don't do this!* It doesn't help; we think it actually fosters more echoing. Instead, base your own word length on the length of your child's spontaneous, meaningful, nonechoed utterances. Your child may be able to echo a whole sentence, but may produce only single words spontaneously. If this is the case, then base your sentence length on

Summary: Building Expressive Speech and Language

Steps	Activities	Techniques
Step 1. Build up your child's vocabulary of sounds.	**Activity:** Respond as if your child's sounds are words: Repeat them, answer them, or say a word that is similar to the sound and that makes sense in context.	**Techniques:** Position yourself face to face. Repeat or otherwise respond to your child's sounds, and then pause, waiting for your child to make another sound. When your child makes another sound, respond again in a similar manner.
Step 2. Develop vocal games with your child's sounds.	**Activity:** Carry on a "mini-conversation" by making one of the sounds your child makes, waiting for your child to respond, and answer back with the same or different sound.	**Techniques:** Gain the child's attention first by initiating the game while you are face to face. Look at your child, make the sound, and wait expectantly. Sustain the back-and-forth interchange as long as your child is interested.
Step 3. Increase opportunities for listening and responding to sounds made by others.	**Activities with nonspeech sounds:** Make noises such as animal sounds, car noises, phone rings, and so on while playing with your child. Make noises such as tongue clicks, raspberries, and lip pops while interacting with your child. If your child shows an interest, repeat and pause, waiting for your child to imitate.	**Techniques:** Watch for your child's reaction to the sounds. Repeat the sounds to increase your child's interest and attention. Wait for your child to respond. Have fun!
	Activities involving words and sounds in songs and sensory social routines: Make sounds and use words while playing familiar games involving songs or other routines (e.g., peekaboo, chase/"I'm gonna get you," bumblebee, "This Little Piggy").	**Techniques:** Use songs or routines that involve anticipation and a sound, such as "Ready, set, go!" Songs or routines that have a predictable rhythm are especially effective.

(cont.)

Summary *(cont.)*

Steps	Activities	Techniques
Step 4. Talk to your child in a way that promotes language development.	**Activities:** Talk to your child throughout your shared activities: while you are playing, riding in the car, making dinner, and so on. Label objects and actions, describe in simple words what your child is seeing and doing. Narrate your own activities, and narrate your child's activities.	**Techniques:** Follow the focus of your child's attention and actions by describing what your child is seeing and doing. Narrate whatever your child is doing with simple language. Use short and simple phrases or single words. In general, your language should be just a little more complex than your child's language. (If your child uses only sounds, use single words that expand on those sounds; if your child uses single words, use simple phrases using those words.) Decide on the words you want your child to learn, and use those words frequently in different situations.
Step 5. Add sounds to gestures.	1. Choose a gesture and word or word-like sound, and model them together. 2. Add sounds or simple words to your child's gestures. 3. Add word approximations to your child's gestures. **Note:** Skip #2 if your child is already using words.	**Techniques:** During a game or other interaction, model the gesture and word you wish your child to learn. When your child uses a gesture such as reaching or pointing, use a sound or word to indicate what your child wants before giving it to your child. When making sounds or using words with your child during play or other types of interaction, add a gesture to that sound.

your child's one-word *spontaneous* utterances. Hold your sentence length to two or three words (the one-up rule), and follow all our guidance above. For example, if your child spontaneously says "milk" to request it, don't tell your child, "Say, 'I want milk.'" Instead, just say something like "Here's your milk," or "Want more milk?" or "Yummy milk" as you hand over the milk. Focus on slowly building up your child's spontaneous speech, and all should progress well.

►►►► What You Can Do to Help Your Child Understand Speech

At the time they are diagnosed with autism, young children typically understand very few words that the people around them use. Some children might seem to understand more than they actually do, because they may learn to "read" the whole situation and make good guesses about what will happen next, based on their past experiences. For instance, you may say, "It's time to go to preschool. Let's get in the car," and your child may head to the door. It looks as if your child has understood your words. But you have also picked up your keys and your jacket, as well as your child's backpack and jacket, and these may be the nonverbal cues your child is using to interpret what is going on.

Sometimes young children with autism seem to ignore the speech that is being directed at them. You may be doing a terrific job of narrating play, using simple language, and providing language models, but the words may not "penetrate" your child's attention. Your child may not have learned the importance of listening, or the need to follow through by responding to your words. But you can teach your child to listen and respond to words. It will come.

> ### 🖐 *Helpful Tip*
>
> To know whether your child really understands the meaning of a word or phrase, speak it without any gestures and see what happens. If your child follows the meaning—reaches for the object, follows the instruction, carries out the action—then it is clear that she understands your words. If not, then your child may understand the situation well, but not the words alone yet.

"One thing I found helpful was to realize when my son was following other cues rather than words, so that I could fade out the other cues gradually. My son loves to go on walks outside, so one of the earliest commands he would follow was 'Let's go outside.' By initially giving lots of cues (pointing toward the door, etc.) and then reducing them, I was able to encourage him to rely on the words more, and then could see when he was responding to the words alone. One of our biggest breakthroughs occurred when I asked him to get his shoes and take them to the door, and he actually did! At the time, he rarely responded to verbal commands. However, the fact that he'd picked up on the nonverbal cues showed us that this was a highly motivating phrase to learn."

The best news about receptive language learning is that when you follow the guidelines we have given you for expressive language development, receptive language understanding will develop right alongside it. The techniques actually develop both sets of skills. Over time, as you follow the techniques we have already covered, your child will learn that speech is important, that she needs to listen and attend to what is being said, and that she is expected to respond when spoken to. If you've been helping your child make sounds with her gestures, you've already been expecting your child to listen to the word or sound you've modeled and imitate it back. You've waited to give your child the cereal until she responds with a sound. In this situation, you expect your child to listen to you and to respond. You make it clear that a response is required, and your child has learned this. This is how your child will learn to respond to other spoken requests you make or spoken instructions you give to your child.

In the previous chapters, you added labels to objects and actions throughout the day during your child's activities. These techniques are powerful for building receptive language. Now we will address a different topic: understanding other's instructions.

Continue using the previous steps and add these other steps, which focus precisely on understanding and responding to others' speech:

Step 1. Expect a response, then get it.

Step 2. Be clear about the natural reinforcers of your child's speech, and be sure to use them for responding to speech.

Step 3. Instruct less and follow through more.

Step 4. Teach your child to understand brand-new words and instructions.

Step 1. Expect a Response, Then Get It

Part of teaching your child to understand is raising your expectations for your child's response.

Rationale. When a young child with autism does not speak or understand speech, over time you may stop expecting the child to respond. But a child who isn't expected to respond won't learn the importance of speech. So it's critical to start requiring a response.

Activity: *Follow Through on What You Say to Ensure a Response*

When you are focused on teaching your child to understand speech, your expectations and follow-through are crucial. For this step, you need to get your child's attention, give your child a simple instruction, and wait briefly for the child's response. If there is none, quickly physically cue or prompt your child to follow through, and then follow with the reinforcer, whatever it may be. The turn-taking routines discussed in Chapter 6 are great examples. When it's your turn, you can extend your hand, say, "Give me," wait briefly for the child to give, and prompt your child to place the object in your hand if the child needs help completing this step. Then you take a very fast turn and give the object right back, so that the child ends up with the object he wanted in the first place. Making gentle and easy but frequent requests or instructions and requiring follow-through is a crucial teaching technique for developing children's understanding of words and their attention and responsiveness to adult speech.

Step 2. Remember the Natural Reinforcers of Your Child's Speech, and Be Sure to Use Them for Responding to Speech

Step 2 may sound simple enough, but it's important to choose the right reinforcers—the rewards for cooperating. You need to work with your child's own goals and motivations. So the time to teach your child the instruction "Sit down" is when your child wants something that you have. Have your child sit down on a small chair or the floor before you hand over the glass of juice she is requesting, or "Come here" to go outside to play, or "Stand up" to transition from a sitting activity to a fun physical game. In all these examples, the instructions are followed by a powerful reinforcer. They are also physical skills your child already has—sitting, standing, walking to you. If you provide an instruction right before doing something that your child wants, your child will get used to hearing your instruction and the rewarding activity and words that follow. Inserting simple demands before delivering what your child wants is a very powerful part of teaching the child to follow simple instructions.

> Two-year-old Alex plays happily alone, and he pretty much ignores his parents' efforts to engage him. As he puts pegs into a little car, his mom says, "Put it here," and points to a hole. He ignores her and puts it elsewhere. He reaches for a pompom, and Dad sees his goal, picks it up, and offers it to him. "Want the pompom?" says Dad, but Alex turns away from Dad and picks up the other pompom lying within reach. Dad hands him the other pompom, and he drops it on the floor. He turns back to the car, and Mom models driving it while making "vroom-vroom" noises. He blocks her and starts to put pegs in again.
>
> Alex's lack of response discourages his parents, and they don't know how to motivate him to engage with them. They decide to use identical cars in play activity and to imitate his actions with one of the cars with an identical one they are holding. As they begin to imitate his actions and narrate, he begins to look at what they are doing. After about 10 minutes, his father holds back for a minute, and Alex looks at him and makes a little emphatic noise, as if to say, "Come on, Dad, do it!" Dad does, and Alex smiles and looks up at Dad briefly. As they continue to imitate him, they now begin to add a piece to his car. He does not reject this, but rather looks up

at Mom and then continues. After a couple more minutes, Mom hands him a peg and he puts it in his car. Then, as he reaches for the pompom, Dad hands it to him, saying "Here, Alex, pompom," and he takes it. Dad picks up the other pompom, says "Alex, pompom," and hands it to him. Alex takes it. He turns back to the car and puts another peg in, which Mom imitates. She then drives her car, making a "vroom-vroom" sound, but he places another peg. She picks up a peg and offers it: "Alex, peg." He says "peg" and puts it in.

Mom and Dad have developed a very effective strategy in this play. They imitate him, narrating and helping him for several turns, and then they place an instruction (e.g., "Alex, peg") inside the flow of activities. They make sure to follow through (either by handing it over or by placing the piece), but their play interactions with him are so rewarding that he follows through with the instructions, and this keeps the game going. After another few minutes, his father offers a choice: "Alex, peg or pompom?" as he holds both out. Alex says "peg" and selects the peg, which Dad then labels ("You chose peg"). Lo and behold, he is communicating, with gestures, gaze, and even a word imitation!

Alex is harder to engage than some young children with ASD, but his parents are persistent. They do not give up, and they find a way to join him in play. Like most children, he enjoys being imitated, quickly experiences the contingency, and comes to expect it—and that becomes the reward for this shared activity. His parents choose their words and actions carefully, fitting them into his preferred activity and being careful to space their instructions out so they follow several minutes of Alex-led activity. Their persistence, their ability to establish a powerfully reinforcing joint activity, and their wisdom at putting simple instructions into the play, directing him to do things he already wants to do—these techniques allow them to begin to work on receptive language, the names of the objects. Within 12 weeks, Alex is playing cooperatively in toddler-type toy activities with both parents, imitates single words easily, and uses about 25 words spontaneously.

But what if there is no built-in reinforcer in the play activity? In the example above, Alex's parents find a reinforcer inside the activity—pegs and pompoms—and focus their language and expectations for Alex's responses on these items. However, if there is no intrinsic reinforcer (a reward that relates to the child's behavior) in a routine, you can create one. As you know from Chapter 9, learning happens only when behaviors are followed by reinforcers. How can you create reinforcers where there don't seem to be any?

Sometimes you can use activities your child really likes and rearrange the order of household routines to capitalize on the reward power of the favorite activity. For instance, it is a struggle for many parents to motivate their children to get dressed for school in the morning, even when the children are perfectly capable of self-dressing. Think about the reward structure for getting dressed. Is there any? For children who are hungry in the morning and are motivated to eat breakfast, parents can establish a new rule—that the children have to be dressed

> **Helpful Tip**
>
> Follow **Grandma's rule**, or **Premack's principle**. Grandma's rule is "First work, then play." Premack's principle (coined by David Premack, a professor of psychology) is that when a more preferred activity follows a less preferred activity, the more preferred activity can act as a reinforcer for the less preferred activity.

before breakfast. Now breakfast, which would have happened anyway, gets repositioned to follow self-dressing and can reinforce the activity.

There has to be some reward for a child for following an instruction. This doesn't mean you are spoiling or bribing your child, regardless of what others say. This is how children learn. You wouldn't go to work if you were not receiving a paycheck, would you? It's the same for your child. You need to find something your child is motivated to have: a favorite activity, an object that your child really loves to handle, an electronic toy, or even a little piece of a favorite cereal or a sip of juice. Some desired event must follow your child's cooperation with the instruction, no matter how much you had to help, for your child to learn. If your child has a runny nose and you provide a tissue and help him wipe it, the natural thing to do then is "throw it away." Say it and help your child do it. Once it is thrown way, clap and cheer for your child, pick him up and play a favorite game in the air, or go back to the very fun activity that was interrupted by the runny nose. All of these will provide rewards for throwing the tissue away.

> **Helpful Tip**
>
> Think about what rewarding event can follow your child's response. Sometimes the reward might be more logical than naturally related to your child's behavior. Here are some examples:
>
> - First dress, then eat breakfast.
> - First wash hands, then have a snack.
> - First go potty, then play outside.
> - First put jacket on, then go for a ride.
> - At bedtime, first brush teeth, then read a book.

Step 3. Instruct Less and Follow Through More

To teach your child that your words have meaning, you must follow through—happily, playfully, but consistently. So be careful what you say! Be ready to act. Giving instructions without following through actually teaches children to ignore their parents' instructions. If you are not in a position to assure that your child follows through on an instruction by helping your child through it, don't give the instruction in the first place. Fewer instructions, with more follow-through, often aids children's learning of others' speech.

Step 4. Teach Your Child to Understand Brand-New Words and Instructions

So far, we've been talking about giving children instructions involving things they can actually do. They are capable of sitting, standing, giving, approaching you, and throwing things in a trash container. You give them the instruction and walk them through it, fading your supports as quickly as possible. Through this process, they learn what the instruction means. However, most of the instructions you will give your child a little later on will involve skills your child does not yet have. Now you will be teaching the skill and the language for it, all together. Putting on a coat, taking off shoes, bringing you her pajamas, sharing his toy with his brother—these all involve new skills your child will need to learn from you.

The process will be the same: (1) You will figure out the reward—fun bath time follows undressing; taking off a coat or jacket and hanging it up on the hook is necessary before entering the preschool room; bringing you the pajamas is followed by a favorite storybook; sharing a toy involves getting it back very quickly and getting another one to play with. (2) Then you will give your child the instruction and help her follow it. (3) Finally, you will reward her for following the instruction.

Over repeated practice opportunities (daily or several times a day), you will slowly decrease the amount of help you give (fade your prompts) to ensure that your child follows through. That is, you will be giving less and less help once you give the instruction, until you are just gesturing that your child should follow through. Then you will fade your gestures, and your child will follow your verbal instruction and use the skill independently.

What about skills that have lots of steps? For multistep tasks like bathing, your child may need quite a while to learn them all. In this situation, it is often useful to begin to work toward independence by having your child learn the very last step independently, then the last two, then the last three. This is called *backward chaining*. For instance, you would help your child take off his clothes up until the very last step (shirt off head), which your child would do alone. Once that is mastered, you would focus on the next-to-last step as well (shirt off neck and head). This is the process we have discussed in Chapter 7, in which you are breaking down the skill into its various steps and teaching each step as its own skill—even while you have your child participate in all the steps, so he learns the chain.

Caution! We recommend that you *not* use verbal instructions in the various steps of a chain. The instruction to "Wash hands" needs to mean all the steps of washing hands. Teach your child the intermediate steps through physical prompts and gestural prompts, but don't use verbal instructions to prompt your child to do the individual steps; otherwise, you are in danger of having a child who waits to be told each step. You want each *action* to become the antecedent for the next action. So use physical prompts or gestures to keep the chain of steps going, and physical arrangement of materials if you need to, to help your child through a complex set of actions involving objects (e.g., laying out the clothes to be put on in order on the bed, or putting all the pieces for table setting on the table).

Summary of Steps 1–4

Your child's intervention team will be able to help you figure out how to help your child learn all kinds of instructions. We are really just trying to give you a beginning point here (a place to start after diagnosis while you are waiting for your child's services to get organized and get going) and a follow-through point (a way to work with your child at home and in daily life that augments other interventions your child will receive). To monitor your own learning, see if you agree with most of the statements in the following checklist. If so, you are now armed with important skills for helping your child build her understanding of speech. These are skills you will use throughout your child's language learning—building on what your child can already do, offering new vocabulary words in their appropriate contexts, and helping your child follow through with instructions in meaningful, enjoyable activities. If you don't feel secure in these skills, turn back to the start of this section and review. Consider asking your child's speech–language therapist to observe your interactions and give you some feedback or coaching with these techniques.

Activity Checklist: Am I Building Up My Child's Understanding of Speech?

_____ I routinely put simple words and instructions into our play and caregiving routines.

_____ I monitor myself and consistently help my child follow through with instructions.

_____ I make sure there are rewarding consequences that follow my child's successful cooperation with instructions.

_____ I foster my child's independence at following instructions by fading my help rapidly.

_____ When teaching my child a new skill, I use simple, direct language to introduce the activity.

_____ When working with my child, my instructions or directions are balanced by the many opportunities my child has to make choices and have fun with me; we are partners in the process.

Summary: Building Receptive Language

Steps	Activities	Techniques
Step 1. Expect a response, then get it.	**Activities:** During turn-taking routines, use gestures and words and expect a response in return. Make gentle requests or commands and require a response from your child. Reinforce every response.	**Techniques:** Get your child's attention, give your child a simple instruction, and wait briefly for a child response. If there is none, quickly physically cue or prompt your child to follow through, and then follow with the reinforcer.
Step 2. Be clear about the natural reinforcers of your child's speech, and be sure to use them for responding to speech.	**Activities:** Notice your child's goals and motivations, and use these as reinforcers for following instructions, requests, or commands. During everyday activities, insert simple demands before delivering what your child wants.	**Techniques:** When your child wants an object, ask your child to follow a command, such as "Sit down" or "Come here," before giving your child the desired object. Provide an instruction right before doing something your child wants and that you would have given anyway; your child will get used to hearing your instruction and the praise or other reward that follows.
Step 3. Instruct less and follow through more.	**Activities:** During your typical daily routines or during playtimes, teach your child that your words have meaning by consistently following through with whatever you request and comment on.	**Techniques:** Use fewer instructions throughout the day, but always follow through by expecting your child to respond to your instructions, even if this requires that you walk your child through the response, fading your gestures, prompts, and supports over time.

Summary *(cont.)*

Steps	Activities	Techniques
Step 4. Teach your child to understand brand-new words and instructions.	**Activities for teaching simple one- or two-step skills:** During everyday activities, when you wish to teach a new skill, figure out the reward (fun bath time follows undressing; taking off a coat or jacket and hanging it up on the hook is necessary before entering the preschool room; bringing you the pajamas is followed by a favorite storybook; sharing a toy involves getting it back very quickly and getting another one to play with). Then you will give your child the instruction, help your child do it, and then give the reward.	**Techniques:** Over repeated practice opportunities (daily, or several times a day), you will slowly decrease the amount of help you give, to ensure that your child follows through (fade your prompts). That is, you will be giving less and less help once you give the instruction, until you are just gesturing that your child should follow through. Then you will fade your gestures, and your child will follow your instruction and do the skill independently.
	Activities for teaching multistep skills: During activities (such as getting dressed) that require multiple steps, use the same teaching methods as for single-step skills, but start by teaching the last step, then add the next-to-last step, and so on.	**Techniques:** Break down a complex skill into a series of single steps. Teach each step as its own skill, starting with the last step. Chain all of these steps together to teach the complex skill. Avoid using a different verbal instruction for each step. Instead, use one verbal instruction for the entire sequence of steps that make up the complex skill. Use physical prompts and cues (e.g., laying out materials needed in a sequence) to help your child chain the different steps together.

Chapter Summary

Young children with autism often have significant difficulties using and understanding speech. However, they are capable of making enormous gains in these areas. We believe, and have demonstrated in our studies and clinical work, that the majority of young children with autism can learn functional, spontaneous, phrase speech. To promote their language development, children need to receive high-quality language experiences and intervention throughout the preschool years. Parents are in the best position by far to provide the greatest number of language-learning opportunities, regardless of the intensity of "outside" therapies.

Speech builds on gestures, imitation, shared attention, and vocal and object play. Functional communicative speech begins with these skills. The fundamental techniques that you as a parent can use involve simplifying your language; creating many, many opportunities for the child to engage with you and communicate throughout the day; using gestures, words, and sound effects in all your activities with your child; building up your child's repertoire of speech sounds through vocal games involving imitation, sound effects, animal sounds, and song patterns in play; increasing your expectations for your child to vocalize along with his gestures; and increasing your expectations and follow-through to show your child how to listen and respond to your simple instructions. Let communication routines become part of all your caregiving routines and play routines with your child. Include your child in as many of your household activities as possible. Interacting with others who are speaking to them and doing shared activities is how children learn functional language skills. This is how every child learns to use and understand spoken language.

Refrigerator List

Goal: To help your child use language and understand speech.

Steps:

✓ **Raise your expectations!**

✓ **Continue imitating your child's sounds to develop vocal games.**

✓ **Everything, and every action, and quality, needs a name.**

✓ **Use simple language; follow the one-up rule.**

✓ **Put in your child's ear the words you want to come from your child's mouth.**

✓ **Instruct less; follow through more.**

14

Putting It All Together

We are coming to the end of a long time spent together. You've accumulated a lot of strategies for directly addressing the learning challenges of early autism. All of these are based on the success we've had with the Early Start Denver Model, which helps young children learn naturally by building learning into everyday routines, and particularly by incorporating it into play. Children with autism need to discover the rewards of social interaction, because being engaged in activities with others and communicating with them are the routes to all learning, including learning to speak.

We hope that by now, with practice, use of the strategies we've described comes naturally to you too. And we hope, as a result, that you've seen your child turn a corner toward becoming engaged, communicating, and learning, which will lead to success in the years to come.

In this final chapter we'll review the building blocks you've accumulated, to give you a picture of how they all fit together in your daily interactions with your child and propel your child along a typical developmental path at this crucial early stage of life. We'll also show you how these parent-delivered strategies can intersect with the early intervention efforts of the professionals who are assisting you and your child. Finally, we'll help you keep the most important principles in mind as you continue to teach your child in the months and years ahead, and we'll steer you to the appropriate chapters to review if you run into any problems with using the strategies you've learned in this book.

But first, here are two important bits of advice if you've just gotten started and are worried that weaving these strategies into your already busy life will be too difficult:

- **Carve out moments to interact and play with your child.** It's a challenge to use teaching strategies, set up play activities, and arrange everyday activities so they can provide teaching moments. Things go slower; less gets done. It takes young children with autism time to learn new routines. Working them into these new routines takes time, and your child may protest changes in his or her routines. However, this will become more and more automatic, both for you and for your child. As you practice these routines, they will become like second nature to you. You will no longer have to think or plan or monitor yourself—it will be natural. The same will be true for your child. Young children are flexible and can learn new routines, and they enjoy interacting with parents (and the younger they are, the more flexible they are!). Whether it is dressing, mealtime, playtime on the floor, or reading books at bedtime, the important thing is to find interactive time throughout the day to engage your child face to face with you as you narrate your shared activities and elicit your child's participation. That is how your child will learn.

• **Take baby steps.** Go one little step at a time, making sure there are fun activities, things your child enjoys—rewards for participation—built into each activity. You will be rewarded by seeing your child become much more of a participant in family life, learning much more about language and about how the world of your family works. Remember, "slow and steady wins the race." Take your time to adopt new routines. The routines are always going to be there. The strategies described in this book should offer pleasurable parenting experiences for you, as well as your child.

Please share these techniques with your child's circle of concerned others: your partner or spouse, grandparents, siblings, babysitters, preschool teacher, and other caregivers. That way, your child's learning opportunities will increase; others will have more satisfying experiences with him or her; and you can share the responsibility for helping your child learn among the many people who care about your child. You will be able to talk to others about what is working well and what is not. Your child will learn how to use his or her new skills with many different people, not just one. And each person will bring to the learning situation his or her own style and ideas, which will enrich the learning experience.

Your Foundation for Giving Your Child an Early Start

At this point you are undoubtedly very aware of how many learning opportunities you can create for your little one in every one of your play and care routines. If you've started incorporating our suggestions into your day, you're applying many critical principles for teaching a child with ASD.

You are likely quite skilled now at gaining and holding your child's attention. You know that learning cannot occur without attention, and if you have followed the guidelines for positioning yourself with your child, for rewarding attention, and for making sure you have your child's attention before trying to teach anything new or reinforce anything already taught, your child probably pays much more attention to you now than when you started with this book. **If you take**

away only one thing away from this book, take away this principle: the importance of gaining and holding your child's attention for learning from you.

You understand the structure of a joint activity and its importance as the framework for teaching and engaging your child. In joint activities partners share control of the activity, at times leading and at other times following each other. They play together, building on each other's actions by imitating, elaborating, or taking turns. It is through joint activities that young children learn in natural settings—at home and out, with you and the rest of your family—and ultimately with their friends and classmates too. Joint activities begin with your child's attention, motivation, and interest in an activity. In a joint activity you and your child are face to face, so that both of you are attentive and involved with the materials and with each other. Together you develop a theme, and then variations to expand the theme. Finally, the two of you close it down and transition smoothly to another activity; you sustain your child's attention through the transition and into the next activity, so there is no break in attention and learning.

You have probably experimented a lot with the joint activity structure, using it at meals and in care interactions like bathing, dressing, changing, and bedtime, as well as in play routines. You and your child probably have a wide range of joint activity routines at this point. Some of your routines use toys and other objects. These object-oriented routines highlight cognitive, play, motor, and language growth. Other play routines occur without toys. These sensory social routines create emotional exchanges and shared attention, and especially foster language, imitation, and social learning. You are probably seeing some very big differences now in your child's willingness to engage in joint activities with you and others—better attention, more motivation to engage, many more skills, more mature and sustained play with toys, much more communication. Take a deep breath, to remember and appreciate what you and your child have accomplished.

You have learned a lot about how children learn. Now you understand that you've been applying the ABC's of learning in all your routines with your child. The terms *antecedent*, *behavior*, *consequence*, and *reinforcement* have come alive for you. You know that your child's behaviors occur in response to some stimulus or another (the antecedent), and that the teaching–learning process ties antecedent and behavior together by following them with a desirable consequence for your child—one that occurs right after the child uses the skill you are trying to develop. Understanding this ABC relationship will allow you not only to teach your child new skills, but also to replace unwanted behaviors that may crop up with more acceptable and more communicative ways for your child to achieve his or her goals. It will also help you develop plans to teach your child new skills and behaviors, by thinking through the ABC's for yourself.

If you have completed this book, you now know a great deal about the development of communication skills. The developmental skills young children use to learn from others—imitation, joint attention, gestural and verbal communication, speech, practice in play, and practice during daily activities—are part of your moment-to-moment awareness. You have learned how to embed imitation into all kinds of joint activities. Imitating actions on objects is particularly easy to target in open-ended joint activities with objects. Gestural imitation is particularly salient in sensory social routines, especially songs and finger plays. And verbal imitation to learn new language structures occurs during language-learning activities in all kinds of joint activities.

You now know much more about how language develops—from meaningful gestures, from your child's use of his or her voice, and from the ongoing process of learning how speech and gesture influence others. You know the importance of functional communication: helping your child develop the gestures and words needed to indicate what is already in your child's mind. You are giving your child the gestures and words that label his or her desires, actions, interests, and feelings. You are putting the words in your child's ears that you want to come out of the child's mouth.

The purpose of language is to coordinate and share information and experiences with other people. Language is primarily a social behavior. You are emphasizing the functional and social aspects of communication when you respond to your child's gestures and speech by following through on their meaning—that is, by saying back what your child has said with the body or with speech (with a little elaboration), to let the child know that you have heard and understood it, and to provide a model for a slightly more mature way to say it. This is the one-up rule. You are responding to communication with meaningful communication rather than praise. And you know how to embed all this into playful routines, both during play and during caregiving. You are an expert in play! You are likely to be a very fun play partner and to have all kinds of play routines involving toys, social games, pretend, physical games, and outdoor activities in your repertoire.

Finally, you have learned how to make the most of the learning opportunities afforded by your everyday activities and routines with your child. Remember the big six types of activities introduced in Chapter 4: toy or other object play, social play, book activities, meals, caregiving (bathing/dressing/changing/bedtime), and household chores. Here is a review of the basic guidelines for making the most of these opportunities.

Meals

Does your child eat at the table, in either a booster seat or a high chair? If not, work to make that change and then sit down and eat with your child. Incorporate your child into family meals. Try to structure three meals and three snacks a day, all at the table and all involving others, while you decrease (or eliminate) eating on the run. Having a child sit down to eat or drink (even to sit down on the floor to drink from a cup) gives you the chance to work on many requesting skills, imitating skills, and communication skills centering around food and drink, which are usually very motivating for children.

As you read this, you may realize that you had once successfully established organized mealtimes and snack times, but that now your child has gone back to eating and drinking whenever and wherever he or she wants. These patterns have probably evolved slowly over time, and you can slowly undo them, step by step:

1. Begin by having your child sit down to eat. At the table is the best place, but if that is too far a stretch, begin by requiring the child to sit down wherever he or she is. Once seated, you can hand your child food or drink. If your child starts to get up while holding the food, consider taking the food away and encouraging your child to sit down again. Your child may well refuse to sit any longer after a few bites, at which time you will remove the food. However, if your child isn't yet full, he or she will be hungry or thirsty again soon, and you can practice again. If you are warmly and gently persistent, you will likely teach this skill quickly.

2. Once your child sits, switch to having the child sit in the kitchen, near the high chair. Try to give your child as much as he or she can eat and drink at one time, and then put off the next snack or meal for an hour or two.

3. Once your child is sitting in the kitchen for all food and drink, move the eating place to the high chair or booster seat, where you can sit right across from your child at a corner and provide the food there.

4. Be sure to eat or drink a little something yourself—a cup of coffee, piece of fruit, something to make it a social time. If you typically have a TV or video running during meals, turn it off, either quickly (if your child tolerates it) or slowly if needed, by first muting the sound for a few meals, then dimming the picture for a few meals, then keeping it off. Instead, sit with your child; have your child's food on the table (ideally, with you and the other family members); offer your child food and name the food; and wait for eyes, voice, or gesture to request. Don't give very much in a portion, so that your child needs to request many times to end up full. Shifting your child to eating three meals and three snacks a day at the table will result in better nutrition, better eating habits, and much more communication. If you can't do this for three meals, do it for one or two.

Caregiving Routines

Build social play routines into changing, bathing, dressing, washing hands, brushing teeth, and getting ready for bed. Add songs, social games, and object play routines to all your caregiving routines. Help your child do many of the steps of each routine him- or herself, instead of being passive (or resistant!) while you do it all. When you help your child participate in washing and drying, brushing teeth, washing hands, handing you a diaper, or giving you a sock or shoe, you will also be adding language and increasing communication during these activities—the building blocks of speech and language. You already spend time doing these things, and adding communication games and child expectations to those routines makes them richer learning experiences for your child. For example, if your child is watching a video while being dressed, little learning about dressing can take place. If the TV is off, you and your child are face to face, and you are helping your child complete each step of the routine (pull on each piece of clothing; hand you shoes, socks, or diaper; help pull zippers or button buttons), as you talk to your child in simple language about each step, narrating the activity, your child is learning language, self-care, social, and motor skills.

Bedtime is an especially important time for language learning. Does your child have a set bedtime routine? If not, can you begin one? Bathing your child and playing with bath toys nightly provide a very rich setting for language learning and social exchange. Following the bathing and drying routine with lotion and pajama-dressing routines that are language-rich and full of social exchanges provides two more learning-rich activities. Brushing teeth can be another language- and learning-rich activity. So, finally, are putting your child into bed and reading a book together (which for young children means naming and talking about the pictures and creating sound effects, not reading the script).

We have just walked you through close to an hour of a bedtime routine. It takes time, and parents with multiple small children and other demands will have many limitations on their time. However, this is a whole hour filled with language and social learning activities, and it is a routine that will also build better sleep habits. Even picking out one or two of these routines nightly will be very helpful for your child. Their consistency and repetition are what make these routines such powerful learning experiences.

Toy and Social Play

You have probably already increased your toy play routines and sensory social routines with your child, since we have been focusing on these so strongly throughout the book. Finding 15–30 minutes two or three times a day (morning, afternoon, and evening?), indoors and out, will help you continue to build the communication and learning value of these routines. The critical factor in play is the joint activity routine structure, with partners face to face, actively engaged with each other and the toys or social games, and communicating back and forth throughout. Try to help others who play with your child—parents, older siblings, grandparents, babysitters, and others—use these techniques as well.

Household Chores

Don't forget about household chores! There are many ways young children can participate with you in chores. They can help you feed the dog, water the plants, pull the clothes out of the dryer, wash the tires on the car. They can play in the kitchen sink with water, scrubbers, and vegetables while you prepare a salad. They can play beside you in bubbles while you wash dishes. They can participate in making cookies or putting cut-up vegetables in a cooking pot or salad. They can help unload the dishwasher and put the silverware into the correct slots in the silverware drawer. In the grocery store, they can put objects into the cart. When you include your child in your everyday routines, you are automatically talking to your child about the task and helping your child do it. Your child is having new experiences, learning new skills, learning how the world works, learning new words, learning from you! Just participating with you in your chores increases your child's learning opportunities enormously during daily life.

Partnering with Your Professional Team

By this point you have likely enrolled your child in early intervention services (or are trying very hard to do so) and are working with professionals to continue to help your child progress. Your child's therapists and educators have likely identified a number of developmental gains that your child is ready to make, written as a set of learning objectives. Everything we have covered so far will help you teach these skills to your child through your ongoing play, caregiving, and daily routines, at home and out and about. You will be working very closely with the professionals on your team, and you should never hesitate to ask for information, clarification, or advice when in doubt about anything involved with your child's treatment.

- If you need your therapists to break down the learning goals they have developed into smaller steps so you can work them into your routines more easily, ask them to do it for you, so you can figure out where to start on each skill.

- If you do not have a copy of each professional's treatment goals, ask each of your child's team members for them.

- If you need help in figuring out how to work on those goals at home in your natural routines, ask your professional team members to show you and to write out a home program for you.

Watch how the different professionals work with your child. Identify what works and what doesn't. Join in your child's treatment sessions, so you can learn from the therapists and carry out their goals at home. This is how your child will benefit from their knowledge. Help your team members identify what is helpful and what is not for your child. They are the experts in their disciplines, but you are the expert in your child. You know what your child likes and does not like, how he or she learns best, what your child can and cannot do yet at home, what is working and what is not. Help your team understand all this about your child. If you see your child not progressing in his or her treatment with others, speak up! Lack of progress signals a problem in the teaching plan, not a limit in your child's ability to learn. If your child is not progressing in one area, ask your team to come up with a different approach. You know your child can learn: Look at all the things you have taught your child over the past weeks as you have worked your way through this book.

Above All Else

- **Every interaction you have with your child is an opportunity for your child to learn and for you to teach.** Your child learns something in every one of these interactions, so ask yourself whether what is happening is what you want your child to learn. Maximize your child's learning by using the incidental (already existing) experiences you have with your child—family routines, outings, chores, caregiving, time in the car. When you use these times to engage your child in the activity, rather than moving your child through routines without engaging him or her in the step-by-step process, your child can be receiving hundreds of learning opportunities every day.

- **Try to teach your child the skill he or she needs in the setting in which your child will use it.** Practice eating communication skills at the table where your family eats. Practice taking off a coat and putting it on a hook when your child comes in from outside, both at home and at preschool. Teach your child to dress and undress when and where it's appropriate, and to name the objects used in each setting or activity in which the child encounters them in daily life. Children learn real-life skills more quickly and more deeply in real-life settings and situations, rather than through flash cards and computer games. Learning "sticks" when it occurs in daily life.

- **Work toward age-appropriate initiative and spontaneity.** Spontaneity and initiative indicate independence. You are not teaching your child simply to follow directions for everything your child needs to accomplish throughout the day. That's the reason behind strategies that involve following your child's attention, reading his or her cues to direct you to rewarding activities and materials that motivate your child to engage and participate. We've encouraged you to be alert for spontaneous performing of skills that you're trying to instill. When your son makes a sound on his own (not just one elicited by you during a game), or your daughter takes the initiative to lead you to the refrigerator when she's hungry instead of screaming, your quick response with a reward or reinforcer at the ready will solidify this skill. But be sure that demonstrations of independence are age-appropriate and are not substitutes for communication. Most 2-year-olds, for example, do not have unlimited access to the refrigerator, because it's not age-appropriate behavior. So if your 2-year-old with ASD opens the fridge to get a drink, it may very well be because he or she does not have a way to request it from others or is not motivated to use the communication skill of requesting it from others. You have likely taught your child ways to participate in many, many new activities, both regular household routines and play routines. All of these together foster your child's ability to initiate an activity and spontaneously begin communication, play, and social exchanges. Try to support your child's initiation of age-appropriate play skills, personal skills, and language.

• **Help your child regulate his or her arousal and activity levels to optimize availability for learning.** We have discussed this idea in terms of the choice of joint activities. There is a rhythm to interactive play that you have likely already discovered. You probably now know how to optimize your child's attention and energy for learning by alternating between quieter activities and livelier ones. As we've said before, it also helps to alternate between object-oriented joint activity routines and sensory social routines. Move from place to place as you create different joint activity routines. Children's body movements and positions can tell you something about what they need. Quieter, more passive children may need to be energized for learning through lively, physical, sensory social routines that involve fast, quick movements. An active, busy child who has trouble attending for more than a few seconds needs periods of lively, physical, social play (think playing chase, running outside, climbing stairs or slide ladders, or other types of backyard play) to alternate with quieter, slower, rhythmic, sensory social activities that focus attention for learning (such as being rocked on a ball, chair, or lap as you sing a song together; walking and moving to rhythmic music; or being rocked in a rocking chair while you go through an interactive book). Organize the physical space for a busy child by putting away things that are out, by limiting the number of materials available at any one time, by using boxes and containers and shelves or closets for toys, and by being ready to transition smoothly from one activity to another to extend and maintain your child's attention. Remember to use the structure of joint activity routines in the lively activities as well as the quiet ones, to take advantage of the learning opportunities that are already there. Helping your child stay in a well-regulated state for learning also helps markedly with behavior. It's a "two-for-one" deal!

• **Don't forget to take care of yourself emotionally.** When you feel emotionally spent or discouraged, don't forget to rely on your social support network, as we have talked about earlier in the book (see especially Chapter 2). Call a friend, touch base with other parents by email or on Facebook, or talk to your partner or other family member. Talk to your physician if you feel down or blue most days.

Get the help and support you need, so you can enjoy life and continue to help your child succeed and grow.

Reviewing When You Hit a Snag

Here are some questions to consider if you run into difficulties along the way. If you answer no to one or more of the questions, think about the strategies you are using by revisiting relevant chapters:

- ✓ Am I using simple words and phrases (the one-up rule) to communicate with my child? (If you might not be, review Chapter 13.)
- ✓ Am I waiting first to see if my child can do a new skill without my help? (If you're not sure you've been doing this, see Chapter 12.)
- ✓ If my child needs help, am I giving as little help as needed for my child to demonstrate the new behavior or skill? (If you think you might have gone astray here, review Chapter 12.)
- ✓ Do I have my child's attention before communicating with him or her? (If not, review Chapter 4.)
- ✓ Is the activity fun for my child? (If the child doesn't show signs of enjoying the activity, go back to Chapter 5.)
- ✓ Is the activity fun for me? (No? See Chapter 5.)
- ✓ Does my child experience the "reward" of the routine as soon as he or she tries to use the target skills I am trying to teach? (Not sure? Review Chapter 9.)
- ✓ Do I see and respond to my child's efforts to interact and communicate with me (even if they're not perfect)? (To be sure, see Chapter 7.)
- ✓ Is my child getting enough practice to master the new behavior or skill? (See whatever chapters address the skills you're working on. They all discuss practicing to cement the skills.)

In closing, we have written this book for you parents, your child's first and most important teachers. Parents are the most influential teachers children will ever have. We hope the tools we have passed on to you will help you and your child continue to learn from and teach each other for many years to come. We hope we have helped you experience the pleasure of watching your child master new skills, step by step. Know that all of those little steps are adding up to big gains as your child engages, communicates, and learns from others. As you watch your child develop and engage with others, we hope that your confidence in your child's future—in his or her ability to have a fulfilling, meaningful, joyful, and productive life—will also grow.

Appendix

Toys, Materials, and Books for Your Young Child with Autism

Age-Appropriate Toys for Children through Prekindergarten

Playthings in Your Cupboard

Tupperware; measuring cups; rolling pins and dough; clothespins; jelly jars; silverware tray; plastic cups, bowls, spoons, forks, and knives; child scissors; crayons and markers; shelf paper or printer paper; magazines and photos of people in the family; pictures of various objects, animals, and people that you take and store on your cell phone; empty cereal boxes; oatmeal containers; magazines; dishwashing soap (for bubbles); laundry basket; trowels from the yard; and many more.

Playthings You or Others Can Purchase

This list is meant just to give you a wealth of ideas to choose from; it is not a shopping list.

- Board books with large pictures, simple stories (see "Age-Appropriate Books for Young Children," below)
- Books with photographs of babies
- Blocks
  - 1-inch wooden blocks with letters or pictures
  - Multicolor, multishape block set
- Nesting toys
  - Cups, boxes
- Simple shape sorters
- Legos/Duplos
- Magna Doodle
- Pegboards with pegs
- Puzzles
  - Wooden inset puzzles with knobs
  - Wooden inset puzzles with matching pictures
  - Noninterlocking puzzles of up to five pieces
  - Simple interlocking puzzles of three to six pieces

- Toys that encourage make-believe play (toy lawn mower, kitchen sets, brooms, etc.)
- Digging toys (bucket, shovel, rake)
- Dolls of all sizes
- Cars, trucks, trains
- Unbreakable containers of all shapes and sizes
- Bath toys (boats, containers, floating squeak toys)
- Balls of all shapes and sizes
- Push and pull toys
- Outdoor toys (slides, swings, sandbox)
- Beginner's tricycle
- Connecting toys (links, large stringing beads, S shapes)
- Stuffed animals
- Farm set with barn and animals
- Little dollhouse set with small plastic people
- Zoo animals
- Child keyboard and other musical instruments
- Art supplies
  - Large crayons
  - Markers
  - Dot markers
  - Stamps
  - Play dough (Play-Doh or other brands) and accessories
  - Stickers
  - Child-safe scissors
- Toy telephone
- Unbreakable mirrors of all sizes
- Dress-up clothes
- Wooden spoons; old magazines; baskets; cardboard boxes and tubes; other similar safe, unbreakable items the child "finds" around the house (such as pots and pans)
- CD or MP3 player
- CDs or MP3s of popular songs
- Large wooden beads for stringing

Other Fun Items to Encourage Engagement and Communication

- Bubbles
- Balloons
- Play food

Age-Appropriate Books for Young Children

Books are a great way to share enjoyment and time with children. Books are also an important teaching material that can be used in your everyday life as well as in your child's early intervention program. Following are suggested children's books, many of which are available at your local library. This list is by no means exhaustive. We encourage you and your child to continue to discover great new books!

Great Books for Young Children with ASD

Quiet Loud, by Leslie Patricelli
Big Little, by Leslie Patricelli
Happy Baby Words, by Roger Priddy
My First Word Board Book, by DK Publishing Staff
My First Colors Board Book, by DK Publishing Staff

Animal Books

Brown Bear, Brown Bear, What Do You See? by Bill Martin (Eric Carle, illustrator)
Polar Bear, Polar Bear, What Do You Hear? by Bill Martin (Eric Carle, illustrator)
Panda Bear, Panda Bear, What Do You See? by Bill Martin (Eric Carle, illustrator)
Carl's Afternoon in the Park, by Alexandra Day
Good Dog, Carl (Classic Board Books Series), by Alexandra Day
Moo, Baa, La La La! by Sandra Boynton
Touch and Feel: Farm, by DK Publishing Staff
Baby Einstein: Baby MacDonald on the Farm, by Julie Aigner-Clark (Nadeem Zaidi, illustrator)
My First Farm Board Book, by DK Publishing Staff
My First Animal Board Book, by DK Publishing Staff
The Very Busy Spider, by Eric Carle

Counting Books

1, 2, 3 to the Zoo, by Eric Carle
Fish Eyes: A Book You Can Count On, by Lois Ehlert

Books about People, Faces, and Body Parts

Oh, Baby!: A Touch-and-Feel Book, by Elizabeth Hathon
Baby Faces, by DK Publishing Staff, Funfax
Where Is Baby's Belly Button? by Karen Katz
Baby Einstein: Mama and Me, by Julie Aigner-Clark (Nadeem Zaidi, illustrator)
My First Body Board Book, by DK Publishing Staff
Toes, Ears, and Nose! by Marion Dane Bauer (Karen Katz, illustrator)

Books about Actions

Baby Einstein: Mirror Me! by Julie Aigner-Clark (Nadeem Zaidi, illustrator)
Fuzzy Fuzzy Fuzzy!: A Touch, Skritch, and Tickle Book, by Sandra Boynton
That's Not My Teddy . . . : Its Paws Are Too Woolly, by Fiona Watt (Rachel Wells, illustrator)
That's Not My Puppy . . . : Its Coat Is Too Hairy, by Fiona Watt (Rachel Wells, illustrator)
That's Not My Dinosaur . . . : Its Body Is Too Squashy, by Fiona Watt (Rachel Wells, illustrator)
Snap! Button! Zip! by Abigail Tabby (Christopher Moroney, illustrator)

Resources

Associations, Organizations, and Independent Websites

Autism-Specific
United States

American Academy of Pediatrics (AAP)
http://www.healthychildren.org/English/Pages/default.aspx

The AAP is a nonprofit organization of pediatricians. This section of its website offers numerous parent resources about ASD, including checklists for early warning signs by age and informational brochures and booklets about typical developmental milestones, understanding ASD, and related medical information. It also includes "Sound Advice for Autism," a collection of interviews with pediatricians, researchers, and parents to answer diagnostic, treatment, and general care questions about ASD.

Association of University Centers on Disabilities
www.aucd.org/directory/directory.cfm?program=UCEDD

The University Centers for Excellence in Developmental Disabilities Education, Research, and Service (UCEDDs) are part of the Association of University Centers on Disabilities. The UCEDDs work with people with disabilities, families, government agencies, and community providers in projects that provide training, technical assistance, service, research, and information sharing, with a focus on building the capacity of communities to sustain all their citizens. The UCEDD section of the Association's website has a national directory for all 67 UCEDDs, listing technical assistance resources.

Autism-PDD.net
www.autism-pdd.net

This is an information and resource site for parents that provides an online support community forum and message board, as well as a place to post personal stories, photos, and local events. It also provides basic information about symptoms, diagnostic criteria, and treatment options. At *http://www.autism-pdd.net/autism-resources-by-state/*, you can search for ASD resources in your state, including legal, educational, and financial planning and assistance.

Autism Service Dogs of America

http://autismservicedogsofamerica.com

This nonprofit, community-based organization raises and trains service dogs specifically for children with ASD. The website includes information about what an Autism Service Dog can do for a child with ASD, how the dogs are trained, and how to submit an application.

Autism Society

www.autism-society.org

The Autism Society is the leading grassroots ASD organization in the United States. It is dedicated to increasing public awareness about the day-to-day issues faced by people on the autism spectrum; advocating for appropriate services for individuals; and providing the latest information on treatment, education, research, and advocacy. The website features links to nationwide ASD-related services and supports by location.

Autism Speaks

www.autismspeaks.org

Autism Speaks is the nation's largest ASD science and advocacy organization. It is dedicated to funding research into causes, prevention, treatments, and a cure; increasing awareness of ASD; and advocating for the needs of individuals with ASD and their families. Its website is one of the most comprehensive sites for families, providing links to the other major online resources. A resource link (*www.autismspeaks.org/community/fsdb/search.php*) offers specific services by geographic location to families of children with ASD. Click on your state for a list of diagnostic, intervention, educational, and community support resources. The 100 Day Kit (*http://www.autismspeaks.org/family-services/tool-kits/100-day-kit*) helps families navigate the first 100 days after diagnosis, providing critical information about autism and its effects on development, tips for assembling services for your child, various intervention approaches, a glossary of key terms, and week-by-week plans to help you stay organized. The Autism Speaks Official Blog (*www.autismspeaks.org/blog*), updated daily, provides up-to-date information on autism news, research, advocacy efforts, and family resources.

Centers for Disease Control and Prevention (CDC)

www.cdc.gov/ncbddd/autism/index.html

The CDC is a branch of the U.S. Department of Health and Human Services. This section of its website provides information about the prevalence of ASD, in addition to screening, treatment, and research resources.

Educating Children with Autism

www.nap.edu/openbook.php?isbn=0309072697

Here is the National Academy Press book *Educating Children with Autism* (2001), prepared by the National Research Council's Committee on Educational Interventions for Persons with Autism. Chapters on diagnosis and prevalence, family roles and planning, educational services, comprehensive and domain-specific treatment approaches, public policy and legal issues, and scientific recommendations can be downloaded for free via the links in the right-hand column.

Everyday Health

www.everydayhealth.com/info/v1ss/autism-basics.aspx

Everyday Health is a leading provider of online consumer health solutions and medical news that complies with the Health on the Net Foundation (HON) code standard for trustworthy health information to consumers. This section of the website shares basic information about ASD, caregiving information, treatment, and management of symptoms.

Families for Early Autism Treatment (FEAT)

www.feat.org

FEAT is a nonprofit organization of parents, family members, and treatment professionals, designed to help families with children who have ASD. It offers a network of support where families can discuss issues surrounding autism and treatment options. This website refers specifically to the FEAT in northern California, but it provides links to other FEAT programs around the United States, most of which have a directory of local resources.

First Signs

www.firstsigns.org

First Signs is a national nonprofit organization dedicated to educating parents and professionals about the early warning signs of ASD and related disorders. The website offers information to help you identify possible developmental concerns, a resource directory for services by state, and the free "ASD Video Glossary," which contains over a hundred video clips to help you see the subtle differences between typical and delayed development in young children and to spot the early red flags for ASD.

Global Autism Collaboration (GAC)

www.autism.org

The GAC is a nonprofit organization created in response to a global need for networking and communication about ASD. The website gives information on the "Parents as Partners" research initiative. The GAC also offers free informational videos on ASD symptoms, community resources (e.g., going to dentist's office or getting a haircut), and other forms of support.

Healing Thresholds: Connecting Community and Science to Heal Autism

http://autism.healingthresholds.com

Healing thresholds is an organization dedicated to healing the lives of families touched by ASD. The website includes information to help families deal with their child's new diagnosis, as well as therapy fact sheets about the different treatment options and the science behind each approach's effectiveness. The list of therapy options on this website is comprehensive (from diet to speech–language therapy to behavioral interventions) and includes the percentage of parents that chose each option. The site also provides daily updates of ASD therapy research and coverage in the news. A global directory of ASD-related therapists and services by geographic location is available.

Interactive Autism Network (IAN)

www.ianproject.org

The IAN is a nationwide online project connecting researchers with individuals and families affected by ASD to recruit more information about causes, diagnosis, family background, home environment, child behavior, and services received. Families can complete online questionnaires.

Mayo Clinic Health Information

www.mayoclinic.com/health/autism/DS00348

The Mayo Clinic is the first and largest integrated, not-for-profit group practice, with physical locations in Arizona, Minnesota, and Florida. Its website is compliant with the Health on the Net Foundation (HON) code standard for trustworthy health information to consumers, and received the 2010 *Time* Magazine Top 50 Websites award. This section of the site offers health information specific to ASD, such as risk factors, treatment and drug information, and coping and support resources. It also provides information to assist parents in communicating with their child's pediatrician about possible ASD symptoms (e.g., it describes what to expect during the visit and what questions and information about their child's development to discuss). The 21 research articles that were referenced to create these web pages are listed for review.

National Dissemination Center for Children with Disabilities (NICHCY)

http://nichcy.org

NICHCY is a division of the Office of Special Education Programs of the U.S. Department of Education. Its website provides information on specific disabilities; early intervention services for infants and toddlers; special education and related services for children in school; research on effective educational practices; resources and connections in every state; parenting materials; disability organizations and professional associations; education rights and what the law requires; and transition to adult life. Of particular interest to parents of children with ASD are links to information about how to write an individualized family service plan or IFSP (for children from birth to 3 years) and an individualized education program or IEP (for children from 3 to 22 years of age). In addition, this website provides links to numerous additional resources; a toll-free number that connects you to an information specialist; and resources in Spanish.

Organization for Autism Research (OAR)

www.researchautism.org

OAR is an online source for applied research to answer questions that parents, families, individuals with ASD, teachers, and caregivers confront daily. The website includes downloadable volumes in Spanish and English on research and assessment for parents.

Pathfinders for Autism

www.pathfindersforautism.org

Pathfinders for Autism is a parent-sponsored nonprofit organization that guides parents to resources in Maryland, where it is based. However, it also offers a free copy of the Modified Checklist for Autism in Toddlers, an ASD screening tool, which can be completed by parents and shared with pediatricians to discuss possible symptoms. In addition, it provides a toll-free number for families to call to speak with a trained staff member, an email link to ask questions, and a sign-up to receive informational emails.

Schafer Autism Report

www.sarnet.org

The Schafer Autism Report is a nonprofit online newsletter produced entirely by volunteers to promote awareness and education toward finding the best treatments, preventions, and cures for the range of ASD. You can read the most recent issue free of charge and then subscribe to future issues.

University of California–Davis MIND Institute

www.ucdmc.ucdavis.edu/mindinstitute/resources

The University of California–Davis MIND Institute (MIND stands for Medical Investigation of Neurodevelopmental Disorders), a collaborative international research center, is committed to the awareness, understanding, prevention, care, and cure of neurodevelopmental disorders. This section of its website offers a comprehensive guide to medical and behavioral treatment approaches, disability information, state and federal resources, available print materials, and support group information. At *www.ucdmc.ucdavis.edu/mindinstitute/videos/video_autism.html*, the MIND Institute's Distinguished Lecture Series videos on autism (featuring internationally renowned researchers) can be accessed. Each video is approximately 1 hour long.

Zero to Three

www.zerotothree.org/about-us/areas-of-expertise/free-parent-brochures-and-guides

Zero to Three is a national nonprofit organization that informs, trains, and supports professionals, policy makers, and parents in their efforts to improve the lives of infants and toddlers. This section of its website includes many parenting resources, including developmental milestones and ways to support your child's development from birth to age 3 during everyday moments.

Canada

Autism Society Canada (ASC)

www.autismsocietycanada.ca

ASC is a national, incorporated, nonprofit charitable organization started by a group of parents committed to advocacy, public education, information and referral, and support for its regional societies.

Autism Speaks Canada

www.autismspeaks.ca

See U.S. Autism Speaks listing for details.

United Kingdom

National Autistic Society

www.autism.org.uk

Ireland

Irish Autism Action

www.autismireland.ie

Australia/New Zealand

Autism Spectrum Australia (Aspect)

www.autismspectrum.org.au

Child Care

Center for Inclusive Child Care

www.inclusivechildcare.org

The Center for Inclusive Child Care is a nonprofit organization that strives to create, promote, and support pathways to successful inclusive care for all children. Its website is a comprehensive resource network for inclusive early childhood programs, school-age programs, and providers. It also includes an online consultation service for child care providers to support retaining children with special needs or challenging behaviors in community child care programs.

Child Care Aware
http://childcareaware.org

Child Care Aware, a program of the National Association of Child Care Resource and Referral Agencies, is partly funded by the U.S. Department of Health and Human Services. The website provides articles titled "Learning about Inclusive Child Care" and "Is This the Right Place for My Child?", which help parents select high-quality child care. Videos about high-quality child care can also be viewed from the website, and the online publication "Choosing High-Quality Childcare for a Child with Special Needs" can be accessed.

National Association for the Education of Young Children (NAEYC)
http://families.naeyc.org/

NAEYC is dedicated to improving the well-being of all young children, with particular focus on the quality of educational and developmental services for all children from birth through age 8. NAEYC is committed to becoming an increasingly high-performing and inclusive organization. This section of its website provides information about high-quality child care, as well as inclusive care for children with disabilities.

National Child Care Information and Technical Assistance Center (NCCIC)
http://www.nifa.usda.gov/nea/family/part/childcare_part_nccic.html

The NCCIC, a division of the U.S. Department of Health and Human Services, provides comprehensive technical assistance and information services about early and school-age child care and education. This section of its website features links to information on quality in child care programs, including links to the quality rating systems in each state. These quality rating systems address best practices in early childhood education, above and beyond each state's licensing requirements. Resources for choosing high-quality child care and different child care options are available at *http://childcareaware. org/parents-and-guardians*, as well as answers to frequently asked questions on child care. At *http://www.fpg.unc.edu/~eco/pages/training_resources.cfm#ChildDevelopment*, you'll find each state's link to early learning and development standards, benchmarks, or guidelines for children from birth to age 5.

National Respite Network and Resource Center
www.archrespite.org

This website provides information about respite care providers in each state and how to access these services.

Legal Issues

Child Care Law Center (CCLC)
www.childcarelaw.org/pubs-audience.shtml#parents

The CCLC, a national nonprofit legal services organization, is the only organization in the United States devoted exclusively to the complex legal issues that affect child care. This section of its website provides parent resources regarding child care for children with disabilities, including information about the Americans with Disabilities Act and child care, resources that address public benefits, civil rights, housing, economic development, regulation and licensing, and land use.

Disability Rights Advocates (DRA)

www.dralegal.org

The DRA is a nonprofit, no-fee law firm that advocates for disability rights through high-impact litigation, as well as research and education.

Other Parenting Resources

Children's Disabilities Information

www.childrensdisabilities.info/autism/index.html

Lists of support groups for parents of children with ASD, as well as many other resources, are available here.

Easter Seals

http://autismblog.easterseals.com

Numerous resources for families of children with ASD—primarily, a blog for parents to communicate their questions and concerns for community input—are available here.

FamilyEducation

www.familyeducation.com/home

This website offers child learning activities, health and nutritional, and general parenting tips from infancy through age 6 for typically developing children and children with special needs.

KidSource Online

www.kidsource.com/NICHCY/toll.free.phone.disa.all.2.html

This section of a website run by the NICHCY (see above) features a selected list of toll-free numbers for national organizations concerned with disability and children's issues, including respite care, education, disability awareness, mental health, and financial planning.

Parent to Parent USA

www.p2pusa.org

Parent to Parent USA is a national nonprofit organization that provides emotional and informational support to parents and other family members of children with special needs. The organization matches each parent looking for information and support with an experienced, trained parent of a child with special needs.

Sibling Support Project

www.siblingsupport.org

The Sibling Support Project is a national program dedicated to the brothers and sisters of people who have developmental disabilities and other special needs. Its website offers information about workshops, conferences, publications, and opportunities for siblings to connect with one another.

Toys, Books, and Activities

BabyCenter
www.babycenter.com/0_games-to-play-with-your-toddler_1485454.bc
www.babycenter.com/preschooler-games-activities
www.babycenter.com/302_activities-play_1517839.bc
This website describes fun, simple games to play with your toddler (top link), preschooler (middle link), or older child (bottom link) to boost development.

Kids Fun and Games
www.kids-fun-and-games.com/index.html
This site lists play ideas for outdoor and indoor games, crafts, dress-up, and birthday parties.

Education.com
www.education.com/topic/books-toddlers
Information about developmentally appropriate books and literacy activities for young children is available here.

Everyday Health
www.everydayhealth.com/autism/toys-and-games.aspx
This section of the Everyday Health site (see above) provides a list of recommended toys for children with ASD, divided by age groups (0–2 years, 2–4 years, and 5+ years), with a brief description of how each toy can be used to teach developmentally appropriate skills.

KidsSource OnLine
www.kidsource.com/NICHCY/literature.html
This section of KidSource OnLine (see above) features the NICHCY bibliography of children's books that are written about or include characters with disabilities. The list is grouped according to disability and is coded for age/grade-level appropriateness.

University of Wisconsin–Madison, Cooperative Children's Book Center (CCBC)
www.education.wisc.edu/ccbc/books/choices.asp
Run by this university's School of Education, the CCBC produces an annual list of highly recommended books published for children (by age group) in that calendar year.

US Recall News
www.usrecallnews.com/section/toy-recalls
Each year's updated Toy Recall List is available here, as well as additional recall lists for other items (such as baby equipment).

Further Reading
Diagnosis and Interventions

Charner, K., Murphy, M., and Clark, C. *The encyclopedia of infant and toddler activities for children birth to 3.* Lewisville, NC: Gryphon House, 2006.

Doidge, N. *The brain that changes itself.* New York: Penguin Books, 2007.

Ingersoll, B. *Teaching social communication to children with autism.* New York: Guilford Press, 2010.

Harris, Sandra L., and Weiss, Mary Jane. *Right from the start: Behavioral intervention for young children with autism: A guide for parents and professionals* (2nd ed.). Bethesda, MD: Woodbine House, 2007.

Robinson, Ricki. *Autism solutions: How to create a healthy and meaningful life for your child.* Buffalo, NY: Harlequin, 2011.

Rogers, Sally J., and Dawson, Geraldine. *Early Start Denver Model for young children with autism.* New York: Guilford Press, 2010.

Stone, Wendy, L., and DeGeronimo, Theresa F. *Does my child have autism?: A parent's guide to early detection and intervention in autism spectrum disorders.* San Francisco: Jossey-Bass, 2006.

Sleep

Durand, V. Mark. *Sleep better.* Baltimore: Brookes, 1998.

Durand, V. Mark. *When children don't sleep well: Interventions for pediatric sleep disorders: Parent workbook.* New York: Oxford University Press, 2008.

Siblings

Bishop, Beverly. *My friend with autism: A coloring book for peers and siblings.* Arlington, TX: Future Horizons, 2011.

Cassette, Mary. *My sister Katie: My 6 year old's view on her sister's autism.* Bloomington, IN: AuthorHouse, 2006.

Healy, Angie. *Sometimes my brother: Helping kids understand autism through a sibling's eyes.* Arlington, TX: Future Horizons, 2005.

Leimbach, Marti. *Daniel isn't talking.* New York: Nan A. Talese/Doubleday, 2006.

Marshak, Laura, and Prezant, Fran P. *Married with special-needs children: A couple's guide to keeping connected.* Bethesda, MD: Woodbine House, 2007.

Meyer, Donald J., ed. *Uncommon fathers: Reflections on raising a child with a disability.* Bethesda, MD: Woodbine House, 1995.

Songs, Finger Plays, and Other Games to Play with Young Children

Cole, Joanna, and Calmenson, Stephanie (Tiegreen, Alan, illustrator). *The eentsy, weentsy spider: Fingerplays and action rhymes.* New York: HarperCollins, 1991.

Delaney, T. *101 games and activities for children with autism, Asperger's, and sensory processing disorders.* New York: McGraw Hill, 2009.

Katz, Alan (Catrow, David, illustrator). *Take me out of the bathtub and other silly dilly songs.* New York: Simon and Schuster, 2001.

Index

About the Authors

Sally J. Rogers, PhD, is Professor of Psychiatry at the MIND Institute at the University of California, Davis. She is a pioneering autism researcher known for her work on early intervention for preschoolers, imitation deficits, family interventions, and autism in infancy. With Geraldine Dawson and colleagues, Dr. Rogers developed the Early Start Denver Model, the treatment approach that is the basis for this book.

Geraldine Dawson, PhD, is Professor of Psychiatry and Director of the Duke Center for Autism Diagnosis and Treatment at Duke University. She served as Founding Director of the renowned University of Washington Autism Center. An internationally recognized autism expert with a focus on early detection and intervention, brain imaging, and genetic studies, Dr. Dawson is a passionate advocate for families.

Laurie A. Vismara, PhD, is a clinical research scientist at the MIND Institute at the University of California, Davis, and a board-certified behavior analyst. Dr. Vismara's interests include developing innovative ways to teach early intervention techniques to professionals and parents.